preventive medicine and public health

The National Medical Series for Independent Study

preventive medicine and public health

EDITOR

Brett J. Cassens, M.D., M.B.A., F.A.C.P.

Clinical Assistant Professor of Medicine
Jefferson Medical College
Thomas Jefferson University
Medical Director, Jeff-Care
Philadelphia, Pennsylvania

A WILEY MEDICAL PUBLICATION
JOHN WILEY & SONS
New York • Chichester • Brisbane • Toronto • Singapore

Harwal Publishing Company, Media, Pennsylvania

Library of Congress Cataloging in Publication Data

Preventive medicine and public health.

(The National medical series for independent study)
(A Wiley medical publication)
Includes index.
1. Medicine, Preventive—Outlines, syllabi, etc.
2. Public health—Outline, syllabi, etc. 3. Medicine, Preventive—Examinations, questions, etc. 4. Public health—Examinations, questions, etc. 5. National Board of Medical Examiners—Examinations—Study guides. I. Cassens, Brett J. II. Series. III. Series: Wiley medical publication. [DNLM: 1. Public Health—examination questions. 2. Public Health—outlines. 3. Preventive Medicine—examination questions. 4. Preventive Medicine—outlines.
WA 18 P944]
RA430.5.P74 1987 614′.076 86-14859
ISBN 0-471-82343-0

10 9 8 7 6 5 4 3 2

Dedication

This book is dedicated to Samuel P. Martin, III, M.D., in appreciation for his many acts of kindness and encouragement, and to Donald H. Stille, whose many years of devotion and patience have made projects like this feasible.

Contents

	Contributors	ix
	Preface	xi
	Acknowledgments	xiii
	Publisher's Note	xv
	Introduction	xvii
	Pretest	1
1	General Principles of Epidemiology	15
2	Experimental Designs and Research Approaches	35
3	Statistics	43
4	Epidemiology and Prevention of Selected Acute Illnesses	79
5	Epidemiology and Prevention of Selected Chronic Illnesses	119
6	Maternal Health Issues	139
7	Health Care of the Young	153
8	Injuries	165
9	Mental Health	179
10	Mental Retardation	191
11	Substance Abuse	201
12	Occupational Medicine	211

13 Environmental Health Issues 235

14 Legal Aspects of Medical Practice and Community Medicine 267

15 Medical Ethics 285

16 Health Care Manpower 295

17 Health Care Services 307

18 Health Care Financing 327

Post-test 337

Index 351

Contributors

Donald J. Balaban, M.D., M.P.H.
Research Associate Professor
of Family Medicine
Director of Research
The Greenfield Research Center
Jefferson Medical College
Thomas Jefferson University
Philadelphia, Pennsylvania

Lawrence D. Budnick, M.D., M.P.H.
Clinical Assistant Professor
Institute of Environmental Medicine
New York University School of Medicine
Regional Epidemiologist
New York State Department of Health
New York, New York

Anthony J. Buividas, M.B.A.
Vice-President, American Health
Management and Consulting Corporation
Wayne, Pennsylvania

Brett J. Cassens, M.D., M.B.A., F.A.C.P.
Clinical Assistant Professor
of Medicine
Jefferson Medical College
Thomas Jefferson University
Medical Director, Jeff-Care
Philadelphia, Pennsylvania

Sally Faith Dorfman, M.D., M.S.H.S.A.
Assistant Professor of Obstetrics and
Gynecology and Epidemiology and
Social Medicine
Director, Family Planning Program
Development and Research
Albert Einstein College of Medicine
New York, New York

Christina L. Herring, M.D.
Clinical Associate Professor of Psychiatry
and Human Behavior
Jefferson Medical College
Thomas Jefferson University
Volunteer Faculty
Thomas Jefferson University Hospital
Philadelphia, Pennsylvania

Stephen Michael Hessl, M.D., M.P.H.
Clinical Assistant Professor of Community
Health and Preventive Medicine
Northwestern University Medical School
Chairman, Division of Occupational
Medicine
Cook County Hospital
Chicago, Illinois

Daniel Oleh Hryhorczuk, M.D., M.P.H.
Assistant Professor of Environmental and Occupational Health Sciences
University of Illinois School of Public Health
Head, Section of Clinical Toxicology
Attending Physician
Division of Occupational Medicine
Cook County Hospital
Chicago, Illinois

Marie C. McCormick, M.D., Sc.D.
Associate Professor of Pediatrics
University of Pennsylvania School of Medicine
Attending Physician
Children's Hospital of Philadelphia
Philadelphia, Pennsylvania

Thomas K. McElhinney, Ph.D.
Adjunct Associate Professor of Humanities and Social Sciences
Hahnemann University
Philadelphia, Pennsylvania

Peter Orris, M.D., M.P.H., F.A.A.O.M.
Clinical Assistant Professor of Preventive Medicine
Northwestern University Medical School
Attending Physician
Divisions of Occupational and General Internal Medicine
Cook County Hospital
Medical Director, Managed Care
Mt. Sinai Hospital
Chicago, Illinois

Mark L. Richards, M.B.A., C.P.A.
Assistant Executive Director, Reimbursement and Planning
Thomas Jefferson University Hospital
Philadelphia, Pennsylvania

Arnold J. Rosoff, J.D.
Associate Professor of Legal Studies and Health Care Systems
The Wharton School
University of Pennsylvania
Associate, Wolf, Block, Schorr, and Solis-Cohen, Attorneys
Philadelphia, Pennsylvania

Samuel L. Rotenberg, Ph.D.
Regional Toxicologist
Hazardous Waste Management Division
United States Environmental Protection Agency, Region III
Philadelphia Pennsylvania

Florence B. Schwartz, M.S.
formerly Research Associate and Consultant
Division of General Pediatrics
University of Pennsylvania School of Medicine
Philadelphia, Pennsylvania

Robert G. Sharrar, M.D., M.Sc.
Director, Division of Disease Control/Health Program Analysis
Department of Public Health
Philadelphia, Pennsylvania

William C. Steinmann, M.D., M.Sc.
Assistant Professor of Medicine
University of Pennsylvania School of Medicine
Chief, Section of General Medicine
Veterans Administration Medical Center
Philadelphia, Pennsylvania

Gail K. Wright, B.A.
Research Assistant
The Greenfield Research Center
Department of Family Medicine
Jefferson Medical College
Thomas Jefferson University
Philadelphia, Pennsylvania

Preface

It is the hope of the authors that this text will give students an appreciation for the fundamental importance of epidemiology and preventive medicine. Epidemiology contributes data to aid in the development of priorities and the measurement of achievements in health care, while preventive medicine offers the hope of intervention before disease strikes. Both of these objectives will continue to grow in importance as the United States seeks to define affordable health care goals for a steadily aging population.

Brett J. Cassens

Acknowledgments

Producing a book, particularly one with the breadth of *Preventive Medicine and Public Health*, requires remarkable patience and cooperation of authors and editors alike. Working with this energetic, bright group of authors has been a memorable and broadening experience. I commend all of them for their commitment to the project.

The brunt of the birthing process was shared with Jane Edwards, busy herself with two deliveries. Her guidance and support were invaluable. Thanks also to Debra Dreger, Keith LaSala, and Jim Harris for their support of this project.

Publisher's Note

The objective of the *National Medical Series* is to present an extraordinarily large amount of information in an easily retrievable form. The outline format was selected for this purpose of reducing to the essentials the medical information needed by today's student and practitioner.

While the concept of an outline format was well received by the authors and publisher, the difficulties inherent in working with this style were not initially apparent. That the series has been published and received enthusiastically is a tribute to the authors who worked long and diligently to produce books that are stylistically consistent and comprehensive in content.

The task of producing the *National Medical Series* required more than the efforts of the authors, however, and the missing elements have been supplied by highly competent and dedicated developmental editors and support staff. Editors, compositors, proofreaders, and layout and design staff have all polished the outline to a fine form. It is with deep appreciation that I thank all who have participated, in particular the staff at Harwal—Debra L. Dreger, Jane Edwards, Gloria Hamilton, Deborah G. Huey, Susan Kelly, Wieslawa B. Langenfeld, Keith LaSala, June Sangiorgio Mash, and Jane Velker.

The Publisher

Introduction

Preventive Medicine and Public Health is one of six clinical science review books in the *National Medical Series for Independent Study*. This series has been designed to provide students and house officers, as well as physicians, with a concise but comprehensive instrument for self-evaluation and review within the clinical sciences. Although *Preventive Medicine and Public Health* would be most useful to students preparing for the National Board of Medical Examiners examinations (Part II, Part III, FLEX, and FMGEMS), it should also be useful to students studying for course examinations. These books are not intended to replace the standard clinical science texts but, rather, to complement them.

The books in this series present the core content of each clinical science, using an outline format and featuring 300 study questions. The questions are distributed throughout the book, at the end of each chapter and in a pretest and post-test. In addition, each question is accompanied by the correct answer, a paragraph-length explanation of the correct answer, and specific reference to the outline points under which the information necessary to answer the question can be found.

We have chosen an outline format to allow maximal ease in retrieving information, assuming that the time available to the reader is limited. Considerable editorial time has been spent to ensure that the information required by all medical school curricula has been included and that the question format parallels that of the National Board examinations. We feel that the combination of the outline and the board-type study questions provides a unique teaching device.

We hope that you will find this series interesting, relevant, and challenging. The authors, as well as the John Wiley and Harwal staffs, welcome your comments and suggestions.

Pretest

QUESTIONS

Directions: Each question below contains five suggested answers. Choose the **one best** response to each question.

1. "Police power," a term of art in constitutional law, describes the inherent authority of

(A) the police to order suspects to undergo medical tests that are believed necessary to obtain evidence related to a crime
(B) the police to order licensed health care professionals to perform tests on individuals suspected of having committed crimes
(C) the state to adopt and enforce measures reasonably necessary for the protection of public health, welfare, safety, and morals
(D) a public health department to enter private homes and places of business to search for public health hazards even in the absence of a court-granted search warrant
(E) a law enforcement agency to use killing or maiming force to apprehend an escaping person who has been adjudicated a felon

2. Which of the following statements best describes the federal government's response in the 1960s to the perceived physician shortage?

(A) The government foresaw a surplus while medical educators thought there was a shortage
(B) The government avoided construction of new schools but heavily financed the expansion of existing schools
(C) Increased federal funding continues to support the effort to eliminate areas with physician shortages
(D) Funds were allocated under the Health Professions Education Assistance Act to construct new health professional schools
(E) None of the above

3. A normal distribution curve is determined by the

(A) mean and sample size
(B) mean and standard deviation
(C) range and sample size
(D) range and standard deviation
(E) mean and range

4. The correct rank order for the five leading causes of death is

(A) injuries, heart disease, cancer, stroke, pneumonia
(B) heart disease, injuries, cancer, stroke, pneumonia
(C) heart disease, cancer, injuries, stroke, pneumonia
(D) heart disease, cancer, stroke, injuries, pneumonia
(E) heart disease, cancer, stroke, pneumonia, injuries

5. Etiologic agents that cause disease can be detected by using the

(A) prevalence rate
(B) case fatality rate
(C) adjusted rate
(D) incidence rate
(E) disease index

6. The figure below depicts the breakdown (by age, race, and sex) of cases of tuberculosis reported in 1982 in the United States.

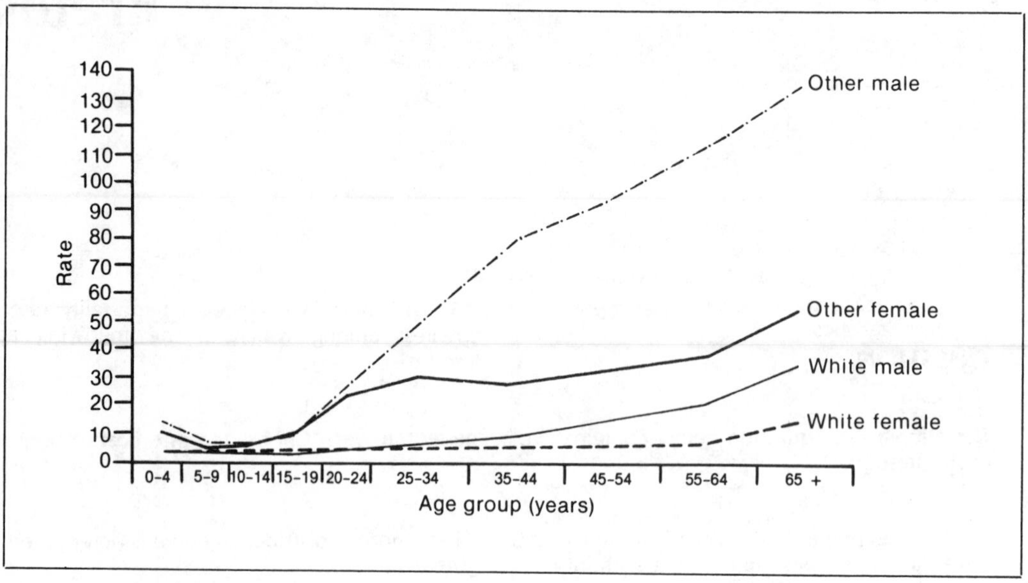

This figure is an example of

(A) a Venn diagram
(B) an epidemic curve
(C) a frequency polygon
(D) a histogram
(E) a cumulative frequency graph

7. Which of the following health practitioners is eligible for a Fifth Pathway?

(A) A third-year resident in surgery
(B) A middle-aged general practitioner seeking licensure in Florida
(C) A Canadian medical school graduate
(D) An American graduating from a foreign medical school
(E) A nurse practitioner

8. The most common sexually transmitted disease in this country is

(A) herpes
(B) gonorrhea
(C) syphilis
(D) genital warts
(E) *Chlamydia*

9. All of the following statements regarding the duty of health care providers to report to the authorities information learned in the course of treating patients are true EXCEPT

(A) the basic, *legal* principle is that patients' confidences must be respected unless there is compelling reason to divulge them
(B) the American Medical Association's code of medical ethics prohibits physicians from divulging patients' confidences
(C) most states require that providers report the treatment of conditions, such as gunshot or knife wounds, that are indicative of a crime or other breach of the peace
(D) some states require mental health professionals to report to the authorities indications that a mentally disturbed individual plans to harm an identifiable individual or group
(E) civil immunity protecting those who divulge patients' confidences is lost if the disclosure was not necessary and was prompted by the provider's desire to cause harm or embarrassment to the subject of the disclosure

10. All of the following statements concerning the labor force in the 1980s are true EXCEPT

(A) the percentage of people engaged in manufacturing is declining
(B) black workers comprise less than 15% of the labor force
(C) the proportion of the labor force engaged in service work has increased over the last several years
(D) occupational illnesses and injuries have begun to decline after a decade of growth
(E) over 100,000 occupational illnesses are reported yearly by the United States Bureau of Labor Statistics

11. Confidence limits are calculated using

(A) the median and the range
(B) the median and its standard error
(C) the mean and the range
(D) the mean and its standard error
(E) none of the above

12. The most common prenatal cause of mental retardation is

(A) accidents of delivery
(B) maternal infections
(C) genetic transmission
(D) maternal ingestion of alcohol or other drugs during pregnancy
(E) nutritional deficiencies

13. Which of the following statements concerning the extent of mental illness in the United States is true?

(A) There are very few readmissions since mental patients often stay in hospitals for long periods of time
(B) About 60 million people have some form of mental disorder that could benefit from professional help
(C) There are more patients in hospitals with mental disorders at any one time than with all other diseases combined
(D) There is a much higher incidence of mental illness in Europe than in the United States because of the way mental illness is designated
(E) There are many more psychiatric inpatients than outpatients, with manic-depressive illness the most common diagnosis

14. In 1984 the percentage of women in the labor force was

(A) 14%
(B) 21%
(C) 28%
(D) 36%
(E) 43%

15. The motor vehicle-related mortality rate is greatest among which of the following age groups?

(A) Less than 15 years
(B) 15–24 years
(C) 25–44 years
(D) 45–64 years
(E) Greater than 65 years

16. All of the following statements concerning the problem of adolescent pregnancy are true EXCEPT

(A) there is a higher incidence of infant mortality among infants born to adolescent mothers
(B) intensive management of adolescent pregnancies has had little impact on reducing the increased risk of low-birth-weight infants
(C) adolescent mothers are unprepared psychologically and educationally for parenthood
(D) adolescent parents are at increased risk for failure to complete their education
(E) adolescent parents usually are faced with numerous economic constraints

17. A key characteristic distinguishing Health Maintenance Organizations (HMOs) from Preferred Provider Arrangements (PPAs) include a

(A) utilization review program
(B) maximum fee schedule for participating physicians
(C) participation agreement for physicians and hospitals
(D) claims review
(E) choice of providers

Directions: Each question below contains four suggested answers of which **one or more** is correct. Choose the answer

A if **1, 2, and 3** are correct
B if **1 and 3** are correct
C if **2 and 4** are correct
D if **4** is correct
E if **1, 2, 3, and 4** are correct

18. Clinical study designs that routinely incorporate the use of a control or comparison group include

(1) clinical trials
(2) case-control studies
(3) cohort studies
(4) case series reports

19. Safe doses for threshold responses of chemicals are determined

(1) by applying uncertainty factors
(2) by the technical ability to control the chemical in a medium
(3) to be protective of the most sensitive human population
(4) from controlled laboratory experiments with human volunteers

20. Correct statements about the Medicare program include which of the following?

(1) The program covers patients 65 years of age and older
(2) The program covers individuals who are disabled or who suffer from end stage renal disease
(3) The payment of inpatient hospital services is based on Diagnosis Related Groups
(4) The Medicare program pays physicians according to a maximum fee schedule for each procedure

21. Examples of nonthreshold effects include which of the following?

(1) Respiratory failure
(2) Cancer formation
(3) Central nervous system depression
(4) Mutagenesis

22. The owner of a local restaurant reported that his short order cook was just diagnosed as having hepatitis A virus (HAV). Recommendations to prevent further spread of HAV should include which of the following?

(1) The short-order cook should not work until he is over his acute illness
(2) Immune serum globulin (IG) should be given to all restaurant employees
(3) IG should be given to all household contacts
(4) IG should be given to all customers who ate in the restaurant during the previous 2 weeks

23. The goal of quality health care is addressed by accreditation, a process which

(1) is carried out by a nongovernmental organization
(2) adheres to guidelines established from within the profession
(3) is a voluntary process
(4) applies to individuals, institutions, or programs

24. Nonparametric tests include the

(1) Wilcoxon two-sample test
(2) Student's t test
(3) Mann-Whitney U test
(4) Poisson test

25. Oral contraceptive use among women over age 35 who smoke is associated with which of the following disease states?

(1) Cerebrovascular disease
(2) Cervical cancer
(3) Coronary heart disease
(4) Breast cancer

26. Exposure to lead may cause which of the following conditions?

(1) Nerve conduction abnormalities
(2) Behavioral changes
(3) Nephropathy
(4) Inflammation of the liver

27. In civil suits, punitive damages are sometimes awarded for which of the following reasons?

(1) To collect additional money to support the court system
(2) To punish the wrongdoer for an act that is particularly culpable
(3) To allow a token recovery in cases where the defendant's wrongdoing has been established but the plaintiff has not been able to prove that he suffered any monetary loss
(4) To deter others from committing the same kind of socially undesirable act as committed by the defendant

28. In one city, 5 white children and 7 black children are bitten by rats. The white children are aged 3, 3, 4, 5, and 6 years; the black children are aged 1, 2, 2, 3, 4, 4, and 5 years. Based on this information, it can be determined that

(1) the median age for the black children is less than that for the white children
(2) the mean age for the black children is more than that for the white children
(3) there are two modal ages for the black children and one for the white children
(4) the range of ages for the black children equals that for the white children

29. Results from clinical trials may be invalidated by

(1) an inadequate number of subjects
(2) biased observations
(3) unmasked observations
(4) an unrepresentative sample

30. Schizophrenia is associated with

(1) urban areas characterized by high mobility and social disorganization
(2) a peak occurrence at 25 to 34 years of age
(3) a higher rate in the lower socioeconomic groups
(4) a better prognosis if the patient is married

31. The sensitivity of a screening test is

(1) the test's ability to identify correctly those persons who truly have the disease
(2) equal to 1 minus the specificity of a test
(3) independent of disease prevalence in the population under study
(4) calculated by dividing the number of persons with the disease who screen positive by the total number of persons who screen positive

32. The risks of fatal motor vehicle-related injuries are increased by

(1) alcohol use
(2) high school driver education
(3) compact cars
(4) night driving

33. A nurse who works on a dialysis unit presents with jaundice. Her HBsAg is positive, and her anti-hepatitis A IgM is negative. Recommendations to prevent further spread should include which of the following?

(1) Administer HBIG to her spouse
(2) Administer HBIG to her children
(3) Advise her not to share her toothbrush or razor
(4) Administer HBV vaccine to her spouse

34. Nurse midwives are registered nurses who

(1) have completed 9 months to a year of additional training in obstetrics
(2) are both licensed by individual states and certified by a national organization
(3) deliver infants of uncomplicated pregnancies with the close cooperation of a physician
(4) can provide virtually all of the basic reproductive services and gynecologic care for women as well as newborn care

35. Routine prenatal well-woman care should include

(1) weight checks
(2) urine testing
(3) blood pressure checks
(4) electronic fetal monitoring

36. A good ethical decision includes

(1) rational consideration of a proposed action
(2) equal attention to alternative choices
(3) consistency with similar cases
(4) an internal logic that is coherent

37. Measures of central tendency include the

(1) median
(2) range
(3) mode
(4) variance

SUMMARY OF DIRECTIONS

A	B	C	D	E
1, 2, 3 only	1, 3 only	2, 4 only	4 only	All are correct

38. Down's syndrome, which occurs when there is extra chromosomal material related to chromosome 21, is characterized by which of the following clinical presentations?

(1) Cardiac abnormalities, especially septal defects
(2) Increased muscle mass and hypertonia
(3) Thick hands with a transverse palmar crease and short inwardly curved little fingers
(4) Slight to moderate mental retardation

39. Postgraduate year-I (PGY-I) programs are

(1) accredited by the Accreditation Council for Graduate Medical Education
(2) continuing to increase in number despite a projected surplus of physicians
(3) the replacement for the former "internship"
(4) designed to rotate the resident briefly through all major departments of the hospital

Directions: The groups of questions below consist of lettered choices followed by several numbered items. For each numbered item select the **one** lettered choice with which it is **most** closely associated. Each lettered choice may be used once, more than once, or not at all.

Questions 40–43

For each statement listed below, select the term that it best describes.

(A) Therapeutic privilege
(B) Emergency consent
(C) Abandonment
(D) Good samaritan
(E) Battery

40. A physician should document carefully when a treatment relationship with a patient has terminated to avoid liability.

41. When a health care provider undertakes, without a person's permission, to render care to that person, tort liability is possible even if no harm was intended and the patient suffered no physical injury as a result of the physician's treatment.

42. Rendering care to a patient without his or her expressed consent may not be considered a tort under certain circumstances.

43. Some jurisdictions will not allow a physician to defend against a charge of unauthorized care if he or she received, or expected to receive, compensation for the services rendered in emergency situations.

Questions 44–48

Match the following statements with the appropriate sexually transmitted disease.

(A) Gonorrhea
(B) Cytomegalovirus
(C) Syphilis
(D) Herpes simplex virus
(E) Pelvic inflammatory disease

44. Ranks as the number one reportable communicable disease in the United States

45. Causes sterility in approximately 150,000 women each year

46. Has been associated with carcinoma of the cervix, vulva, and penis

47. Increases the risk of ectopic pregnancy 10-fold

48. A chronic infection, which can cause blindness, psychosis, or cardiovascular disease

Questions 49–52

For each theory of addiction, select the investigator with whom it is most likely to be associated.

(A) Menninger
(B) Adler
(C) Rado
(D) Khantzian
(E) Vaillant

49. Practitioners should assess the addict's ego functions and then find a substitute for each immature defense.

50. Specific drug effects interact with distinct personality factors and behavior patterns.

51. The self-destructive drive is the prime component which is derived from guilt associated with anger toward parents.

52. The cause of addiction is powerful feelings of inferiority related to a perpetual state of insecurity.

Questions 53–56

For each epidemiologic concept listed below, select the term that most appropriately describes it.

(A) Epidemiologic triangle
(B) Infectious disease spectrum
(C) Herd immunity
(D) Disease surveillance
(E) Disease eradication

53. Group expression of an illness

54. A unique combination of events resulting in disease

55. Periodic outbreaks of disease

56. Determination of the frequency with which disease occurs

Directions: The group of questions below consists of lettered choices followed by several numbered items. For each numbered item, select the one lettered choice with which it is most closely associated. Each lettered choice may be used once, more than once, or not at all. Choose the answer

A if the item is associated with **(A) only**
B if the item is associated with **(B) only**
C if the item is associated with **both (A) and (B)**
D if the item is associated with **neither (A) nor (B)**

Questions 57–60

For each type of cancer listed below, select the risk factor that is most likely to be associated with it.

(A) Family history
(B) High-fat diet
(C) Both
(D) Neither

57. Lung cancer
58. Breast cancer
59. Colorectal cancer
60. Cervical cancer

ANSWERS AND EXPLANATIONS

1. The answer is C. (*Chapter 14 VIII A 1 a, b*) Under our legal system, the state and federal governments, so long as they act within the bounds of their respective constitutions, have an inherent power to take reasonable steps necessary to maintain order and protect the public. This power can be exercised when the state has a legitimate interest in an activity and takes action reasonably related to the protection of that interest. Police power must be balanced against the fundamental rights of the individual.

2. The answer is D. (*Chapter 16 I A 1–2*) Virtually everyone was convinced that a severe physician shortage existed in the 1960s and encouraged federal intervention. The 1963 Health Professions Education Assistance Act funded both construction of new schools and expansion of existing schools. No monies were allocated for the ongoing organization of the schools, however. The number of medical schools increased by 30%, and the total enrollment of medical students rose by 67% under this federal program.

3. The answer is B. (*Chapter 3 III E 1, 3*) The shape of the normal distribution curve is determined by the mean and the standard deviation. In a normal distribution, 68% of the population lies within 1 standard deviation of the mean and 95% within 2 standard deviations. A normal curve cannot be described by the range or the sample size.

4. The answer is D. (*Chapter 8 III B 1 a, b; IV A 1, 2*) Injuries are the fourth leading cause of death, with unintentional injuries accounting for about 91,000 deaths and intentional injuries about 50,000 deaths per year. Diseases of the heart are the leading cause of death (750,000 deaths), followed by malignant neoplasms (430,000 deaths), cerebrovascular diseases (150,000 deaths), and pneumonia (52,000 deaths).

5. The answer is D. (*Chapter 1 IV A 3, B 2 a, b, 3 d, C 2*) An incidence rate is defined as the number of new cases of a specific disease during a specified time period divided by the estimated midinterval population at risk. Because incidence rate is a measure of the rate at which healthy people develop disease during a specified time period, it is a statement of probability, and as such, it can be used to determine factors that cause disease. A prevalence rate contains all current cases (old and new) in the numerator, and is, therefore, determined by both the incidence and duration of disease and cannot be used to determine etiologic factors. Case fatality rate only reveals what happens once the disease occurs. Adjusted rates are fictitious rates and are only used to compare overall rates in different populations. Indexes are used when the true population at risk cannot be determined.

6. The answer is C. (*Chapter 3 II C 6*) A frequency polygon is a representation of the distribution of categories of continuous and ordered data with the frequency plotted against the midpoint of each category and a line drawn through each plotted point. A Venn diagram consists of at least two circles and demonstrates the degrees of overlap and exclusivity. A histogram does not use a continuous line. An epidemic curve is a histogram that depicts the time course of an illness, disease, or abnormality in a defined population within a specified location and time period.

7. The answer is D. [*Chapter 16 II A 2 b (7)*] The Fifth Pathway is a program designed to facilitate the entry of American graduates of foreign medical schools into residency training programs in the United States by providing lectures and clinical rotations not provided by the foreign medical schools. Though a small program—only 374 students entered the Fifth Pathway program in 1984—the need for the Fifth Pathway has been questioned when the United States is confronted with a physician surplus.

8. The answer is E. (*Chapter 4 V A 2 a (1), E 1 a, 2 f*) Although gonorrhea is the most commonly reported disease, *Chlamydia* is believed to be the most common sexually transmitted disease with approximately 3 million cases occurring each year. *Chlamydia* has not been a reportable disease because there is no easy way to confirm the diagnosis. However, it causes a significant proportion of the nongonococcal urethritis and acute epididymitis in men, and mucopurulent cervicitis and pelvic inflammatory disease in women.

9. The answer is B. (*Chapter 14 VIII D 1, 2*) The American Medical Association's (AMA's) code of medical ethics places great importance on the maintenance of patients' confidences; however, the AMA does recognize situations in which revealing information about a patient's condition or treatment may be both ethically and legally required. A patient's confidentiality can be disregarded when there is a higher duty owed to the community or when the law requires the reporting. Disclosures should be made only to the proper authorities, and they should not go beyond what is required by the situation and by the law. Civil immunity is granted to health care providers who disclose patients' confidences in good faith and with reasonable justification; however, disclosures are not protected if they are unnecessary or are motivated by malice or a desire to embarrass the patient.

10. The answer is D. (*Chapter 12 I B, C 1, 2; Table 12-1*) From 1979 to 1984, the percentage of the labor force engaged in manufacturing and agriculture declined, while those engaged in service and trade increased. Approximately 86.7% of the labor force were white and 10.6% were black in 1984. Occupational injuries increased from 4.9 million in 1983 to 5.3 million in 1984, the first yearly increase in this decade. The United States Bureau of Labor Statistics reported 124,800 new cases of occupational illnesses in 1984, which represented an increase of 19,000 cases over 1983.

11. The answer is D. (*Chapter 3 III G 2*) Confidence limits are based on the arithmetic mean and the standard error of the mean. The upper and lower 95% confidence limits are equal to the mean plus and minus, respectively, two times the standard error of the mean. Neither the range nor the median is useful in calculating confidence limits or other probability statements.

12. The answer is C. (*Chapter 10 III B 1 a–c*) Etiologic classifications of mental retardation are based on when the condition is acquired—that is, prenatally, at birth, or postnatally. Genetic diseases, the most common cause of mental retardation, account for about 50% of all cases. Maternal infections and ingestion of alcohol or other drugs during pregnancy can cause mental retardation prenatally, but the percentage of cases is small. Natal causes of mental retardation, including accidents of delivery, account for only 2% of cases of neonatal death and severe neurologic impairment. Nutritional deficiencies are rare in the United States.

13. The answer is C. [*Chapter 9 I B 2 b; II B 2 a; III A 1, 3; V A 3, C 2 b (1)*] About 30 million Americans have some form of mental disorder that could benefit from professional help. In fact, there are more patients in hospitals with mental disorders at any one time than with all other diseases combined, including cancer and heart disease. However, there are more outpatients than inpatients, with the most common diagnosis being depression, not manic-depressive illness. American studies usually report a higher incidence rate of mental illness than European studies because more liberal criteria are used to designate mental illness by American psychiatrists.

14. The answer is E. (*Chapter 12 I A 1*) In 1984, the labor force in the United States numbered 113,544,000 of a total population of 176,383,000 individuals who were 16 years or older. Of these, approximately 56.2% were men and 43% were women. The percentage of women in the labor force has increased by 2.2% since 1980 and 6.2% since 1975.

15. The answer is B. (*Chapter 1 IV B 3 d; Chapter 8 IV B 1 a, b*) Approximately 46,000 people die annually as a result of motor vehicle-related injuries. Of these, individuals 15–24 years of age have the greatest motor vehicle-related injury mortality rates with about 37 deaths per 100,000 population per year. Case fatality rate, however, (i.e., the number of deaths assigned to a specific cause divided by the total number of cases) as a result of motor vehicle-related injuries is greatest among the elderly.

16. The answer is B. (*Chapter 7 III D 2 d, E 1 b*) Although there is a higher incidence of infant mortality among infants of adolescents, the intensive management of adolescent pregnancies has had a significant impact on reducing the increased risk for low-birth-weight infants. By age 19, 55.5% of the adolescent population has had sexual intercourse, which leads the way for the problem of adolescent pregnancy. Adolescent parents usually are unprepared psychologically and educationally for parenthood, and they are at increased risk for failure to complete their education and to secure employment, thereby limiting their future economic well-being.

17. The answer is E. (*Chapter 18 IV A–B*) Health Maintenance Organizations (HMOs) are medical care organizations that accept responsibility for the provision and delivery of a predetermined set of comprehensive health services to insureds who voluntarily choose an HMO for health insurance coverage. HMOs generally restrict coverage to services provided by physicians participating in the plan except for emergencies. Preferred Provider Arrangements (PPAs) are arrangements between a network of health providers—that is, physicians, hospitals, and other health suppliers—and a health benefit purchaser—that is, insurance companies or self-insured employers. In a PPA, the patient may choose a provider outside of the "preferred" network but usually pays a higher deductible or copayment.

18. The answer is A (1, 2, 3). (*Chapter 2 III B, D–F*) Clinical trials, which are most commonly used to compare treatments, routinely use controls who receive placebo or no active drug or alternative treatments for comparison of efficacy. Both case-control and cohort studies, which assess possible risk of association, also use controls for comparison. In case-control studies, nondiseased subjects (controls) serve as comparison for those with disease. In cohort studies, the comparison is between those who were exposed and those who were not exposed to the possible etiologic agents. Case series reports often compare results with the results of other studies; however, these comparisons should never be used for statistical analyses.

19. The answer is B (1, 3). (*Chapter 13 III B 1 a–d, 2 a–e*) Threshold or safe doses are determined for the most sensitive toxic end point and in the most sensitive human population. If the safe dose were not determined for the most sensitive human population, then it could not protect that population from potential toxic effects. Uncertainty factors—the numbers used to estimate threshold doses from available toxicologic data—are used to be sure that the most sensitive toxic end point is considered and that the most sensitive human population is protected. Controlled laboratory experiments with humans rarely provide the basis for the most sensitive toxic end point for a variety of reasons. The most sensitive end points are often chronic effects, and human studies are usually not carried out over extended time periods. The ability to control a chemical is determined by both the available technology and by management decisions. While in the past the chemical industry may have determined safe exposures based on the cost of controls, this criteria is not health based, whereas safe doses are explicitly determined based on health.

20. The answer is A (1, 2, 3). (*Chapter 18 V A, C, D*) The Medicare program was established under Title XVIII of the Social Security Act primarily for patients 65 years of age and older. The program was expanded several years later to include individuals who are disabled or who suffer from chronic renal disease. The current inpatient payment system is based on Diagnosis Related Groups. The claims system is administered on a regional basis by private insurance companies called carriers. Payment for a procedure is made at the low end of the individual physician's median charge or the "prevailing" (75th percentile) charge for each geographic location and specialty. Thus, there is no uniform maximum fee schedule.

21. The answer is C (2, 4). (*Chapter 13 II A 1, 2*) Only toxic effects that are the result of the interaction of a chemical with genetic material are considered nonthreshold effects. All other interactions of a chemical result in threshold toxic effects. Both mutagenesis and carcinogenesis are believed to result from permanent alterations in genetic material. Mutational events may be either in germ cells, in which case they are heritable, or in somatic cells, in which case they only affect the organism in which the event occurs. Although mechanisms of carcinogenesis are complex and are not well understood, some alteration of genetic material is regarded as an early requirement. Each of the other two toxic end points, respiratory failure and central nervous system depression, are toxic effects that may be caused by a variety of chemicals acting systemically but not at the level of DNA.

22. The answer is A (1, 2, 3). [*Chapter 4 VI A 3 b (1)–(2)*] Hepatitis A virus (HAV) is excreted in the stools from about 1 to 2 weeks before the onset of illness until about 1 week after the onset of jaundice. An infected individual should not work in an occupation that prepares or serves food for public consumption during this interval of time. Immune serum globulin (IG) should be administered to all household contacts and restaurant employees. IG does not have to be administered to customers since the cook only handled the food before it was cooked. However, IG may be given to customers if: the employee handled food that was not cooked before it was eaten, the hygienic practices of the food handlers are deficient, and customers can be identified and treated within 2 weeks of exposure.

23. The answer is A (1, 2, 3). (*Chapter 17 VI B 1*) Accreditation is a process carried out by a nongovernmental organization whereby an institution or educational program is recognized as voluntarily meeting a set of quality standards. These standards are established from within the profession to assure adequate programs of education or care. Medical schools, for example, are accredited by the American Association of Medical Colleges. Individuals are certified rather than accredited.

24. The answer is B (1, 3). (*Chapter 3 III K 2*) Nonparametric tests are analytic tests of the null hypothesis for samples and populations, regardless of their size or the underlying distribution. The Wilcoxon two-sample test and the Mann-Whitney U test are nonparametric. Student's t test is based on the t distribution and the Poisson test on the Poisson distribution.

25. The answer is B (1, 3). (*Chapter 5 II C 4; III C 3; IV C 3 a–e, 4 b*) Oral contraceptive use among women over 35 who smoke is associated with an increased incidence of heart disease and an increased risk of stroke. While oral contraceptive use appears to be a risk factor for cervical cancer, the risk appears to be associated with increased sexual activity and subsequent infections rather than increased age and smoking. The development of breast cancer is associated with first pregnancy after age 30, a family history of breast cancer, exposure to ionizing radiation, an early menarche, high socioeconomic status, high fat consumption, and age over 40 years.

26. The answer is A (1, 2, 3). (*Chapter 12 IV A 4 c*) Exposure to lead, which is toxic in adults if it is chronic, can result in nervous system abnormalities, such as motor weakness, nerve conduction abnormalities, and behavioral abnormalities; hematologic abnormalities, such as anemia; nephropathy; and reproductive tract abnormalities, such as fetal toxicity and abnormal sperm. Liver inflammation, or hepatitis, is not associated with lead exposure.

27. The answer is C (2, 4). (*Chapter 14 II G 1 c*) Punitive damages, that is, damages in excess of normal compensation, may be awarded to punish a defendant for an act that is particularly culpable and to deter wrongdoers from acting similarly in the future. When punitive damages are awarded, the defendant must pay the plaintiff (not the state to support the court system), along with any other types of damages awarded. A token recovery in cases where the defendant's wrongdoing has been established but when the plaintiff is unable to prove a monetary loss as a result describes the situation in which *nominal* (not punitive) damages are awarded.

28. The answer is B (1, 3). (*Chapter 3 II A 1–3, B 1*) The median is the value in a series that divides the series into two equal parts. The median age for the black children (3 years) is less than that for the white children (4 years). The mode is the value that occurs most frequently in a series. Among the black children there are two modal ages—2 and 4 years—whereas among the white children the modal age is 3 years. The mean is the sum of all values in a series divided by the number of values. The mean age for the black children (3 years) is less than the mean age for the white children (4.2 years). The range of ages, or the difference between the highest and lowest ages, is higher among the black children (4 years) than it is among the white children (3 years).

29. The answer is A (1, 2, 3). (*Chapter 2 III F 4*) A clinical trial is an experimental design used to assess differences between two or more groups receiving different interventions or treatments. The design is such that at least one control group is included for comparison of the planned interventions. A population with a clinical characteristic requiring intervention must be identified. Subjects must be allocated, preferably randomly, to each of the treatment interventions. Randomization minimizes the potential adverse effect from chance occurrence. Treatments are then administered in an identical or controlled manner to ensure uniformity of nontreatment covariants. Preferably, observations should be made while observers and patients are masked to the type of interventions being made to avoid biased observations. This is called a double-blind study as compared to a single-blind study when only the subject or the observer is masked to the intervention. An insufficient number of subjects may lead to failure to detect true differences that may exist (beta error). It should also be noted that statistically significant results can occur due to chance even in the most rigorous study design, such as a well-designed clinical trial where treatments are randomized and subjects and observers are masked. This occurrence of detecting a significant difference, which does not exist but is due to chance, is called an alpha error and is usually coupled with a probability (P) of less than 0.05 by most investigators.

30. The answer is E (all). [*Chapter 9 II B 1 a–d, 2 b (3)*] Admission rates for schizophrenia for both sexes involve people 20 to 40 years of age, with a peak occurrence at 25 to 34 years of age. The differential in rates of schizophrenia among various population groups was most striking among different socioeconomic groups. For example, Faris and Dunham found that areas in Chicago with high rates of schizophrenia were characterized by high mobility and social disorganization. The high rate of schizophrenia among the lower socioeconomic groups is supported by hospitalization statistics. Married schizophrenics seem to have a better prognosis than unmarried schizophrenics.

31. The answer is B (1, 3). (*Chapter 3 IV C 1*) Screening test parameters are measures of the clinical usefulness of a test when compared with a definitive diagnostic test. Sensitivity is a test's ability to identify correctly those persons who truly have the disease and is calculated by dividing the number of persons with the disease who screen positive by the total number of persons with the disease. The sensitivity of a test is independent of the prevalence of disease in the population being screened. The positive predictive value is a test's ability to identify those persons who truly have the disease from among all those persons whose screening tests are positive.

32. The answer is E (all). (*Chapter 8 II B 3 d, E 2 b; VI B 4*) The risks of motor vehicle-related injuries are increased by all of the factors listed in the question. Not only are small automobiles associated with an increased risk of fatal injuries, but about half of all drivers who die in motor vehicle crashes have blood alcohol concentrations above the legal limit. Although driver education programs are aimed at influencing and improving driving behavior, populations with these programs have relatively more motor vehicle-related injuries among young drivers than populations without these programs. This is no doubt a result of licensure at young ages and an increase in the proportion of young people who drive. Night driving (from 10:00 p.m. to 3:59 a.m.) is associated with over one-third of all fatalities although less than one-fifth of crashes occur during that time.

33. The answer is B (1, 3). [*Chapter 4 VI B 2 a (3), 3 a, f (3), (4)*] Hepatitis B virus (HBV) is transmitted by sexual activity and by contaminated blood; therefore, immune globulin (HBIG) should be administered to the spouse of the dialysis nurse because it gives immediate protection against HBV. HBV vaccine should only be given to all family members if the patient becomes a chronic carrier of the HBsAg. A chronic carrier of the HBsAg is defined as an individual with a positive blood test on two determinations separated by a 6-month period.

34. The answer is E (all). (*Chapter 16 V B 1–3*) Registered nurses from any of the three educational programs—diploma, associate degree, and bachelor degree programs—can enter a midwife program of 9 to 12 months. They can provide a broad range of services to women and newborn children. States license all nurses, and some states have separate nurse midwife laws. The American College of Nurse Midwifery certifies midwives and accredits midwifery programs. Some states require certification for practice.

35. The answer is A (1, 2, 3). (*Chapter 6 IV B*) Routine prenatal well-woman care should include a Pap smear; a breast examination; advice on nutrition, exercise, and hygiene; and screening for sexually transmitted diseases. Weight, urine, and blood pressure should be checked routinely at every visit. Electronic fetal monitoring is an option that has specific indications during pregnancy and labor. Electronic fetal monitoring is not always an essential component of prenatal care.

36. The answer is E (all). (*Chapter 15 IV A 1, C 1–5, D 1 a, b*) A good ethical decision presents all of the options. All complete arguments not only present their own case but also demonstrate an understanding of opposing positions and objections. A good decision is also marked by consistency and an internal logic.

37. The answer is B (1, 3). (*Chapter 3 II A*) Measures of central tendency include the median, mode, and mean, which are summary measures for a sample or population that describe the middle values or the values occurring most often. Measures of dispersion include the range, variance, standard deviation, and coefficient of variation, which are summary measures for a sample or population that describe the scatter of the series.

38. The answer is B (1, 3). (*Chapter 10 IV A 3 a–e*) Down's syndrome, which occurs when there is extra chromosomal material related to chromosome 21—that is, there is either an extra chromosome 21 or a translocation where the long arm of chromosome 21 becomes attached to another chromosome. Clinical features include moderate to severe mental retardation and hypotonia, cardiac anomalies, especially septal defects, thick hands with a transverse palmar crease and short inwardly curved little fingers, oblique palpebral fissures, abundant neck skin, a small flattened skull, high cheek bones, and a fissured, thickened tongue.

39. The answer is A (1, 2, 3). (*Chapter 16 II A 3*) Internships are now integrated into the course of the entire residency and are now known simply as the first postgraduate year (PGY-I). Residency training programs must be accredited by the Accreditation Council on Graduate Medical Education, comprised of representatives of several major medical and hospital organizations. Residency positions continue to increase but also are more narrowly focused. Residents most commonly rotate only within their department of specialty and the emergency department. In 1982, the American Medical Association (AMA) adopted recommendations calling for a return to the concept of a PGY-I rotating through all major departments. The proposal met with little enthusiasm.

40–43. The answers are: 40-C, 41-E, 42-B, 43-D. (*Chapter 14 III C 1 a, b; V F 4; VI A 2; VII A 1 b, 3 a, b*) A physician cannot unilaterally terminate a treatment relationship with a patient. He or she must have the patient's consent to the termination or must give the patient sufficient notice of termination to allow the patient to secure care elsewhere. A successful suit on grounds of abandonment is unlikely if the patient lives in an area where care from alternative sources is readily available.

The doctrine of battery is the root premise of our entire law on consent and informed consent. Our legal system places great weight upon the individual right of bodily inviolability. Battery is regarded as a deliberate tort, even in cases where the individual doing the touching has acted in good faith and with good intentions. However, a technical violation is not likely to lead to an award of significant damages.

The doctrine of emergency consent requires that before care is rendered, steps reasonable under the circumstances are taken to locate the patient's next of kin to get authorization for treatment. In the absence of this consent, the physician is entitled to assume, unless there is a reliable indication to the contrary, that the patient would have authorized the treatment if he or she had been able to state a preference. Still, the care rendered must not extend beyond that necessary to preserve life and prevent serious harm to the patient's health.

A physician who expects compensation for emergency services rendered is not acting as a "good samaritan." This may be consistent with the general concept of a "good samaritan" as one who is motivated by altruism; however, it is not consistent with the practical intent of the "good samaritan" statutes, which is to encourage physicians to render care under the difficult circumstances of emergencies.

44–48. The answers are: 44-A, 45-E, 46-D, 47-E, 48-C. (*Chapter 4 V A 4 b, c, d, B 1 f*) Sexually transmitted diseases are the most common communicable diseases in this country, and gonorrhea is the most commonly reported disease. The long-term morbidity of these diseases is significant. Pelvic inflammatory disease (PID), which can be caused by a number of organisms, can cause infertility in 4% of women after a single episode and 60% after the third episode. Furthermore, 6% of pregnancies occurring in women with a previous history of PID are ectopic. Long-term sequelae of herpes simplex virus (HSV) infection cause various types of cancers, and chronic syphilis infection can lead to blindness, psychosis, and cardiovascular disease.

49–52. The answers are: 49-E, 50-D, 51-A, 52-B. (*Chapter 11 IV A 2–4, 6, 8*) Vaillant urged practitioners to assess carefully the addict's ego functions and then work to find a substitute for each immature defense. He felt attempts should also be made to control self-destructive behavior and provide a context for involvement and acceptance.

Khantzian focused on how specific drug effects interact with distinct personality factors and behavior patterns. He suggested that individuals select one drug over another in an attempt to cope with specific problems, which would be unbearable without the particular drug effect.

Menninger held that a self-destructive drive is the primary component of drug addiction. Addiction is considered the means by which individuals with a powerful, but unconscious, urge to destroy themselves could destroy themselves. This urge, Menninger thought, originated from the guilt associated with a child's anger toward his or her parents for frustrating early needs for oral gratification.

Adler attributed the cause of addiction to powerful feelings of inferiority related to a perpetual state of insecurity and a desire to escape responsibility.

53–56. The answers are: 53-B, 54-A, 55-C, 56-D. (*Chapter 1 III A–E*) The infectious disease spectrum describes a group expression of illness in response to exposure to a particular biologic agent. Group expression ranges from no clinical evidence of disease to death from the disease.

Epidemiologic triangle describes the unique combination of events that results in disease. A harmful *agent* must come in contact with a *susceptible host* in the *proper environment*. The disease process can be prevented by eliminating the agent likely to cause disease, by immunizing susceptible hosts, or by modifying the physical environment.

Periodic outbreaks of disease occur when the proportion of susceptible individuals is high; these outbreaks subside as the proportion of immune individuals increases (herd immunity). Herd immunity explains why epidemics occur in a cyclic or periodic fashion. Outbreaks occur when the population contains a lot of susceptible individuals and disappear when most of the population is immune from either natural exposure or immunizations.

Disease surveillance refers to the process of determining the frequency with which certain diseases occur in the community. A good surveillance program consists of the collection, consolidation, analysis, and dissemination of relevant data.

57–60. The answers are: 57-A, 58-C, 59-C, 60-D. (*Chapter 5 IV C 1 a–e, 2 a–e, 3 a–e, 4 a–g*) Most studies consistently demonstrate that cigarette smoking is a major risk factor in the development of lung cancer. This risk increases with an early age at the onset of smoking and as the number of cigarettes smoked increases. In addition to the risks inherent with exposure to industrial carcinogens, air pollution, and radiation, there is also a tendency for lung cancer to aggregate in families, primarily adenocarcinoma and alveolar cell carcinoma, the cell types less closely related to smoking. The risk imparted by familial predisposition resembles that of cigarette smoking, and the combined effect seems to be synergistic.

Risk factors for the development of breast cancer include a first pregnancy after age 30, exposure to radiation, a high-fat diet, a family history of breast cancer, an early menarche, age over 40 years, and high socioeconomic status. Increased intake of fat and animal protein increases the risk of developing breast cancer by promoting growth and sexual development and a consequent early age at menarche; by increasing adiposity, leading to a greater conversion of androstenedione to estrone; by increasing prolactin release from the pituitary; or by increasing bile salt production in the gut, leading to altered bacterial flora and the production of carcinogenic substances. The risk of breast cancer to women whose mother *or* sisters had breast cancer is twofold, and the risk to those whose mother *and* sisters had breast cancer is threefold.

Fiber deficiency and a high-fat diet appear to be related to colorectal cancer. In addition, there appears to be a familial predisposition. Other risk factors include heavy alcohol (particularly beer) consumption, high socioeconomic status, and being white.

Sexual promiscuity, leading to infections and other sexually transmitted diseases, oral contraceptive use (perhaps leading to promiscuity), early age at first coitus, and smoking are the most important risk factors for developing cervical cancer.

1
General Principles of Epidemiology

Robert G. Sharrar

I. EPIDEMIOLOGY

A. Definitions

1. Derived from three Greek roots (*epi* meaning upon, *demos* meaning people, and *logia* meaning study), the term epidemiology was originally applied to the study of outbreaks of acute infectious diseases and was defined as the science of epidemics.
2. Epidemiology now refers to the study of the distribution and determinants of diseases or conditions in a defined population. Epidemiology is based on two fundamental assumptions:
   - **a.** Diseases do not occur by chance.
   - **b.** Diseases are not randomly distributed in the population; thus, their distribution indicates something about how and why that disease process occurred.
3. Maxcy defined epidemiology as "the field of science dealing with the relationship of the various factors which determine the frequencies and distributions of an infectious process, a disease, or a physiologic state in a human community." Three aspects of this definition need emphasis. Epidemiology is a:
   - **a.** Science concerned with the observation, identification, description, experimental investigation, and theoretical explanation of natural phenomenon.
   - **b.** Study of cause and effect—that is, the relationships among variables that determine an outcome.
   - **c.** Study of events in a defined population.
4. Frost states that epidemiology "at any given time is something more than the total of its established facts. It includes their orderly arrangements into chains of inference which extend more or less beyond the bounds of direct observation." This definition emphasizes the fact that epidemiology is primarily a method of reasoning—that is, a way of looking at a complex population with many variables and making sense out of the events that occur within the population. It is applied common sense.

B. Epidemiologist. Since epidemiology is a multidisciplinary subject, epidemiologists have diverse backgrounds, including human and animal medicine, microbiology, statistics, computer programming, administration, toxicology, and entomology.

1. The goals of the epidemiologist are:
   - **a.** To identify factors that cause disease or disease transmission.
   - **b.** To prevent the spread of communicable and noncommunicable diseases and conditions.
2. An epidemiologist is trained to identify and prevent diseases in a given population, while a clinician is trained to identify and treat disease in an individual.
3. An epidemiologist studies diseases in a population with many variables over which he has no control, while a basic scientist studies diseases in a laboratory modifying one variable at a time.

C. Types of epidemiologic studies

1. **Descriptive studies** describe the distribution of cases by the variables of person, place, and time in order to study and explain acute outbreaks of disease, to follow secular trends of disease occurrence over time, and to develop hypotheses about disease transmission (see section V).
2. **Analytic studies**—such as the retrospective or case control and the prospective or cohort—

identify causal relationships or factors associated with disease. Analytic studies do not prove cause and effect, but they are used to generate hypotheses that can be tested (see Chapter 2).

3. **Experimental studies**—such as vaccine field trials and clinical studies that evaluate therapy—are carefully designed to prove an association between a factor and disease outcome (see Chapter 2).

D. **Uses of epidemiology.** Study of the distribution and determinants of disease in a defined population helps to:

1. Identify factors that cause disease.
2. Identify factors or conditions that can be used or modified to prevent the occurrence or spread of disease.
3. Explain how and why diseases and epidemics occur.
4. Evaluate the effectiveness of vaccines and different forms of therapy.
5. Establish a clinical diagnosis of disease.
6. Identify the health needs of the community.
7. Evaluate the effectiveness of health programs.
8. Predict the future health needs of a population.

II. INFECTIOUS DISEASE PROCESS.

For an infectious disease to occur, the following six conditions or events must take place.

A. **Etiologic agents.** There must be an etiologic agent that produces disease, such as:

1. **Protozoa**—single-cell parasites of the animal kingdom (e.g., malaria and amebae).
2. **Metazoa**—multicellular parasites of the animal kingdom (e.g., tapeworms and blood flukes).
3. **Fungi**—unicellular structures belonging to the plant kingdom that can exist in either the yeast phase, characterized by cells that reproduce asexually by budding, or the mycelial phase, characterized by long branching filaments. Most fungi are beneficial to man. Some of the diseases that are caused by fungi include ringworm and histoplasmosis.
4. **Bacteria**—single-cell structures that reproduce sexually or asexually, grow on cell-free media, and can exist in an inanimate environment. Some bacteria enter a dormant state and form spores where they are protected from the environment and where they remain viable for years.
   a. Normal bacteria found on the skin and in the mouth, gastrointestinal tract, and vagina are necessary for life.
   b. Bacteria can cause disease in humans by:
      (1) **Invading and multiplying in a portion of the body that is normally sterile**, such as the lungs, urine, and bloodstream.
      (2) **Producing a toxin or poison** that can exert its influence at a body site distant from where bacterial replication is taking place; for example, tetanus is caused by a certain type of wound infection, but it presents clinically as a central nervous system disorder.
      (3) **Initiating a hypersensitivity response.** An individual with a group A beta hemolytic streptococcal infection may develop rheumatic fever or acute glomerulonephritis. In the process of eliminating the infection, an antibody is produced that also attacks the heart valves or the glomeruli of the kidney. Thus, the heart valve and glomeruli are damaged by antibodies (not the *Streptococcus* organism) that combine with these tissues to form immune complexes.
   c. Bacteria, for the most part, infect the extracellular body space and have different metabolic pathways than humans. Consequently, antimicrobial agents have been developed that selectively kill bacteria without harming the host.
5. **Rickettsiae**—microorganisms that are between bacteria and viruses in terms of size and characteristics. They are similar to bacteria because they respond to some antimicrobial agents and to viruses because they are obligate intracellular parasites.
   a. In man, rickettsial organisms must live intracellularly where they borrow certain enzymes and coenzymes, which they cannot make, from the cell. Usually, they infect the endothelial cells lining the walls of blood vessels.
   b. Most rickettsial species exist in nature in ticks and mites; humans are not necessary for survival of the species. Rocky Mountain spotted fever is a rickettsial infection.
6. **Viruses**—obligate intracellular parasites—which are among the smallest of the biologic agents known to infect man. They consist of encapsulated genetic material (DNA or RNA).

a. To infect humans, a virus must first attach to a cell, then squirt its genetic material inside the cell. The genetic material migrates to the nucleus where it combines with the genetic material of the host cell and takes control. Normal cell functions cease, and the cell begins to exist for the sole purpose of making more viral particles. When sufficient viral particles are made, the cell breaks open releasing the viral particles, which infect new cells.

b. Viral infections are difficult to treat because:

(1) Antiviral agents that selectively kill viruses without harming the host cell have been difficult to develop.

(2) They destroy cells, which may result in permanent damage. For example, polioviruses and arboviruses destroy certain nerve cells that do not regenerate. However, the lining of the trachea, which can be destroyed by influenza viruses, and the hepatocytes, which can be destroyed by hepatitis viruses, do regenerate.

B. Reservoirs. There must be a reservoir where the biologic agent can propagate (i.e., live, multiply, and die in the natural state). The three reservoirs are:

1. Humans. Certain biologic agents can multiply only in humans, causing either an acute clinical or subclinical problem. **Clinical cases** are not normally a public health problem since these individuals withdraw from society and seek medical attention. However, **subclinical cases** are problematic as these individuals may transmit the agent to others without knowing they are infected. These asymptomatic individuals are called **carriers.** There are three carrier states.

a. **Incubatory carrier.** Patients incubating a communicable disease may transmit the infection shortly before they become symptomatic (e.g., chickenpox and hepatitis A).

b. **Convalescent carriers.** Patients who have recovered from an acute illness may continue to shed the organism, particularly enteric infections caused by *Salmonella* or *Shigella*.

c. **Chronic carriers.** Patients may develop chronic infections and transmit the infection for long periods of time, usually over 1 year. *Salmonella typhi* and hepatitis B can cause lifelong infections.

2. Animals. Diseases that can be transmitted under natural conditions from vertebrate animals to humans are called zoonoses (e.g., rabies, tularemia, and leptospirosis).

3. Environment. Certain biologic agents, such as *Cryptococcus neoformans*, live free in the environment.

C. Portals of entry and exit. There must be a portal of exit from a reservoir and a portal of entry into a susceptible host in order for a disease to be caused elsewhere.

1. Portal of exit. There are five portals of exit from a human or animal reservoir.

a. **Respiratory tract.** Organisms in the respiratory tract, such as influenza and tuberculosis, can be spread by expectoration.

b. **Genitourinary tract.** Organisms can exit the body via urine and secretions of the genital tract; for example, leptospirosis is found in the urine of infected animals, and sexually transmitted diseases are transmitted via the genital tract.

c. **Alimentary tract.** Organisms can exit the body via saliva, such as rabies, or the lower gastrointestinal route, such as hepatitis A and the enteric diseases.

d. **Skin.** Organisms in superficial lesions, such as impetigo, syphilis, and chicken pox, can be easily dislodged. Other organisms, such as malaria and hepatitis B, exit the body via the percutaneous route through breaks in the skin, insect bites, and needles.

e. **In utero transmission.** During pregnancy, organisms, such as rubella, cytomegalovirus, or syphilis, can be transmitted from the mother across the placenta to the developing fetus, resulting in a wide range of fetal abnormalities.

2. Portal of entry. There must be a portal of entry into a susceptible host. In general the portal of entry is similar to the portal of exit; for example, if an individual releases an agent by coughing, the susceptible host will inhale it, and if an organism leaves one genitourinary tract, it will enter another genitourinary tract.

D. Mode of transmission. An organism must be transmitted, either directly or indirectly, from one place to another.

1. Direct transmission occurs when the reservoir and the susceptible host are in close proximity.

a. **Person-to-person spread** occurs from skin-to-skin contact as with sexually transmitted diseases (e.g., syphilis, herpes, and hepatitis B) or direct contact with a free-living organism in the environment (e.g., sporotrichosis).

b. **Droplet spread** occurs when infectious aerosols produced by coughing, talking, and sneezing transmit infection to susceptible hosts. However, transmission only occurs within

3 to 6 feet because droplets that fall to the ground are not able to enter the host [e.g., mumps and rhinovirus (common cold)].

2. **Indirect transmission** occurs when the reservoir and the susceptible host are separated. This separation can be as small as a few feet or as large as thousands of miles.
   a. **Vector spread** involves mosquitoes, fleas, and ticks. Infectious agents may be transmitted through purely mechanical means, such as on the feet or wings of the insect, or it may actually grow and multiply in the vector. For example, the mosquito is not only a means of spreading malaria but also is an important part of the life cycle of the malaria parasite.
   b. **Vehicle spread** involves the transportation of an infectious agent on inanimate objects (fomites), such as toys, school supplies, bedding, or biologic equipment, or in contaminated food, water, milk, or biologic supplies. An epidemiologic investigation of 29 cases of *Salmonella new brunswick*, a rare serotype, involving 17 states, suggested that a commercial product, instant nonfat dry milk, was the vehicle of infection.
   c. **Airborne spread** involves droplet nuclei 1–5 μ in size, which are produced by talking, singing, coughing, or sneezing and float on air currents for varying periods of time. Droplet nuclei may also be created by a variety of atomizing devices, such as a dentist's drill, or laboratory procedures, such as centrifugation. Particles this small can reach the lungs, settle by gravity, and produce disease (e.g., influenza and tuberculosis). The airborne route is obviously the most difficult to block.

E. **Susceptible host.** There must be a susceptible host. Microbiologic agents surround us and are inside us. People stay healthy because of their own host defense mechanisms.

1. **General factors of resistance** include the following:
   a. **Intact skin** prevents most organisms from entering the body.
   b. **Cough reflex** eliminates organisms from the lungs.
   c. **Gastric juices** digest food as well as the organisms we swallow.
   d. **Diarrhea** eliminates harmful agents from the gastrointestinal tract.
   e. **Normal bacterial flora** prevents pathogenic organisms from growing.

2. **Specific factors of resistance** include the following:
   a. **Leukocytes**, with the assistance of serum factors, ingest and destroy bacteria (phagocytosis).
   b. **Serum factors and fibroblasts** encapsulate or wall off invading organisms.
   c. **The immune system** consists of cell-mediated immunity and circulating antibodies.
      (1) **Cell-mediated immunity** is responsible for delayed hypersensitivity and the regulation of antibody production; for example, patients with aquired immune deficiency syndrome (AIDS) have abnormalities in the T-cell lymphocytes and, consequently, are infected by common organisms, which surround us and which do not cause disease in normal people.
      (2) **Circulating antibodies** are proteins that inactivate specific antigens or organisms and prevent replication in the body. Antibodies are disease-specific (e.g., the measles antibody only protects against measles).
         (a) **Active immunity** occurs when the host develops long-lasting antibodies to fight infection. Antibody production results from either natural disease or vaccines. It normally takes several weeks of exposure or immunization before protective antibodies are produced.
         (b) **Passive immunity** occurs when antibodies are given to the host. Although of short duration, passive immunization provides immediate protection. Passive antibodies protect the newborn infant during the first several months of life and can also be used to prevent certain diseases, such as hepatitis A and measles, if immune serum globulin is given shortly after exposure.

III. EPIDEMIOLOGIC CONCEPTS

A. **The epidemiologic triangle** states that in order for a disease process to occur, there must be a unique combination of events—that is, a harmful agent that comes into contact with a susceptible host in the proper environment. The occurrence of a disease can be blocked by intersecting the triangle at any of its three sides.

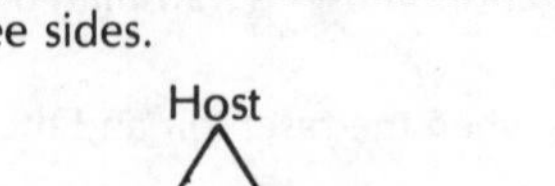

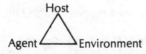

A disease or outcome is never caused by one event but rather a chain of events that form a web (epidemiologic web), which, because of its complexity, can never be fully understood.

1. **The agents of disease** can be biologic (e.g., microorganisms), chemical (e.g., toxins or poisons), nutritional (e.g., excess food, lack of food, or vitamin deficiency), physical forces (e.g., automobiles), or energy (e.g., ionizing radiation).
   a. While an agent may be necessary for a disease, it may not be a sufficient cause for disease.
      (1) Inoculum size or dose is important.
      (2) Particular serotypes or strains of a species may be more likely to cause disease than other strains of the same organism.
      (3) The agent must be able to enter the host.
   b. A disease may be prevented by eliminating the agent; for example, the strategy of the World Health Organization to eradicate smallpox worldwide was to eliminate the smallpox virus, which no longer exists in the natural state.

2. **Host factors** that determine the occurrence of a disease include biologic traits with which a host is born and social traits, which a host develops or acquires.
   a. **Biologic traits** include genetic characteristics, race, ethnic origin, sex, and age. Age is one of the most important epidemiologic factors because:
      (1) Young children are more likely to have subclinical infection.
      (2) Adults are immune to certain diseases because of prior exposure.
      (3) Children and adults are exposed to different agents of disease.
   b. **Social traits** are acquired as the host goes through life. Marital status, life-style, diet, residence, and travel are a few factors that determine disease outcome. Modification of dietary habits and uses of tobacco and alcohol or changes in employment or area of residence can prevent disease. Vaccines can make a host resistant to certain diseases; for example, individuals immunized against measles by a vaccine will not contract the disease even if they come into contact with the measles virus circulating in the community.

3. **Environmental factors** that determine the occurrence of disease may be physical, biologic, or social.
   a. **Physical factors** include climate (e.g., temperature and moisture), setting (e.g., urban versus rural), gravity, and pollution (e.g., water and air). Diseases can be prevented by modifying the physical environment; for example, the simple processes of filtering and chlorinating the water supply and separating the water and sewage systems has virtually eliminated typhoid fever in most urban areas in the United States.
   b. **Biologic factors** include environmental factors that are necessary to maintain the agent or allow for its transmission; for example, malaria does not occur in Katmandu, Nepal because the mosquitoes that transmit malaria cannot fly at high altitudes.
   c. **Social factors** include the political, social, and economic bases of society and its institutions; for example, certain diseases and conditions, such as tuberculosis, are more common in the lower socioeconomic strata where crowding may play a role.

B. **The infectious disease spectrum** describes a group expression of illness in response to exposure to a particular biologic agent. In some diseases (e.g., polio), the clinical cases represent only the "tip of the iceberg," while in others (e.g., measles), subclinical cases are thought to be rare.

1. If a group of susceptible people are exposed to a biologic agent, the following outcomes will occur. A certain proportion will:
   a. Have no clinical or laboratory evidence of infection.
   b. Have no clinical evidence of infection but may have laboratory evidence of infection. These individuals will continue normal daily activities but are capable of spreading the disease.
   c. Develop mild to severe clinical illness. These individuals will interrupt normal daily activities, seek medical help, modify their behavior, and are therefore, less likely to spread their illness.
   d. Die from the disease.

2. Although one agent can have many clinical presentations, many different agents can produce the same clinical disease. For example, the clinical manifestations of pneumonia are fever, cough, and an abnormal chest x-ray; however, these symptoms and findings can be caused by chemicals, parasites, fungi, bacteria, rickettsiae, or viruses.

C. **Herd immunity** describes the spread of a communicable disease within a group based on the proportions of susceptible and immune individuals in the group. Epidemics or outbreaks of disease occur when the proportion of susceptible individuals is high and disappear as the proportion of immune individuals increases.

1. The proportion of immune individuals within a group that is necessary to prevent an outbreak of disease varies according to the disease and its mode of transmission. In general, diseases

spread by the airborne route require a higher proportion of immune individuals to prevent an outbreak than diseases spread by direct contact.

2. Vaccine preventable diseases (e.g., measles) may occur because of improper immunization (e.g., immunization at the wrong age), poor storage of vaccine, or unidentifiable host factors. Thus, because of these vaccine failures and because measles is an airborne transmitted disease, outbreaks have occurred in populations that were 90% immunized.

3. Because of herd immunity, a disease can be eradicated without achieving 100% immunization levels. For example, smallpox was eradicated by immunizing around a case to prevent further spread and not by achieving 100% immunization levels (see section III E).

D. **Disease surveillance** refers to the process of determining the frequency with which certain diseases occur in the community by collection, consolidation, analysis, and dissemination of relevant data. The legal bases for disease surveillance are regulations adapted by State Boards of Health, which derive their authority to issue regulations from Acts of the State Legislatures.

1. **Objectives** of disease surveillance are to:
   a. Know what diseases are occurring so effective control can be initiated.
   b. Evaluate the effectiveness of the control programs.
   c. Increase our knowledge of disease processes either because gaps exist in the available knowledge of many acute and chronic diseases or because shifts from the customary pattern of a particular disease have occurred.

2. **Sources** of disease surveillance data include:
   a. Individual case reports.
   b. Laboratory reports.
   c. Emergency room visits.
   d. Hospital discharge summaries.
   e. Case investigations revealing additional cases.
   f. Death certificates.
   g. Surveys.

E. **Disease eradication** requires the total annihilation of the agent so that the epidemiologic triangle (see section III A) will never occur again. Smallpox was eradicated because of unique epidemiologic features of this disease.

1. The agent of smallpox was a virus that only lived in man and that always caused clinical disease. There were no chronic carriers of this virus.

2. A susceptible host could be made immune to this disease by immunization with an effective vaccine.

3. Disease surveillance identified all known cases, and mass immunization campaigns eliminated the susceptible hosts so that the virus had no reservoir in which to reside. The smallpox virus then became extinct and can no longer cause disease. Therefore, smallpox vaccinations are no longer required.

4. Because of herd immunity, eradication was achieved without 100% immunization levels.

IV. TOOLS OF THE TRADE.

To determine factors that cause disease, epidemiologists must be able to describe and compare the occurrence of disease within a population. The characteristics of the populations affected most by disease are used to determine the factors that cause the disease.

A. Quantitative measurements

1. **Ratio** is the expression of the relationship between two items. These items may be either related to or independent of each other. Mathematically, a ratio is expressed as X:Y, where X is the count of one item and Y is a count of another. Both counts are taken during the same time interval. For example,

   in a classroom of 15 boys and 5 girls, the male to female ratio is 15:5 or 3:1.

2. **Proportion** is the expression of the relationship of one part to the whole. The numerator is always included in the denominator, and since the base always equals 100, a proportion is expressed as a percent. Mathematically, a proportion is expressed as

$$\frac{X}{Y} \bullet K.$$

The values of X and Y are determined during the same time interval. For example,

in a classroom of 15 boys and 5 girls, the
proportion of females students is 25%.

3. Rate is the expression of the probability of occurrence of a particular event in a defined population during a specified period of time. Mathematically, a rate is expressed as

$$\frac{X}{Y} \bullet K,$$

where X = the number of events or cases, Y = the total population at risk, and K is a round number or base chosen to express the rate as a number greater than one. The values of X and Y are determined during the same time interval. Examples are given in section IV B.

4. Index is used when the true denominator or population at risk cannot be determined. A related denominator is used as a measure of the population at risk. An index is then a pseudo-rate. An example is given in section IV B 3 c.

B. Specific measurements

1. Natality rates measure the rate of birth.

a. Crude birth rate is the number of live births reported during a given time interval divided by the estimated midinterval population. It is expressed per 1000 population. (Note that the total population is used in the denominator even though many individuals are not at risk of becoming pregnant.) The crude birth rate in the United States in 1980 was 15.9 live births per 1000 population.

b. Fertility rate is the number of live births reported during a given time interval divided by the estimated number of women in the 15–44-year-old age group at midinterval. It is expressed per 1000 population. The fertility rate in the United States in 1980 was 68.4 live births per 1000 women aged 15–44.

2. Morbidity rates measure the rate of illness.

a. Incidence rate is the number of new cases of a specific disease reported during a given time interval divided by the estimated midinterval population at risk. A high incidence rate means a high occurrence of disease; a low incidence rate means a low occurrence of disease.

(1) Because incidence rate is a measure of the rate at which healthy people develop disease during a specified time period, it is a statement of probability.

(2) Since incidence rates are affected by any factor that affects the development of a disease, they can be used to detect etiologic factors.

b. Prevalence rate is the number of current cases (old and new) of a specified disease during a specified time period divided by the estimated midinterval population at risk. **Point prevalence** refers to a specific point in time, and **period prevalence** refers to a given time interval.

(1) Since prevalence rate contains all known cases in the numerator, it is used primarily to measure the amount of illness in a community and thus can be used to determine the health care needs of that community.

(2) Prevalence rates are influenced by both the incidence of disease and by the duration of illness.

c. Attack rate is the number of new cases of a specified disease reported during a specific time interval divided by the total population at risk during the same time interval. It is normally expressed as percent. It is an incidence rate that is calculated in an epidemic situation using a particular population observed for a limited period of time.

d. Secondary attack rate is the number of new cases in a group minus the initial case or cases during a specified time period divided by the number of susceptible individuals in the group minus the initial case or cases. Note that the initial case or cases that introduced the disease into the group are removed from both the numerator and denominator. The secondary attack rate measures spread within an epidemiologic unit.

3. Mortality rates measure the rate of death.

P19 Morton

a. Crude death rate is the total number of deaths reported during a given interval divided by the estimated midinterval population. It is expressed per 1000 population. (Note that the total population is used even though the risk of death is different for different age groups.) The crude death rate in the United States in 1980 was 8.8 deaths per 1000 population.

b. Cause-specific death rate is the number of deaths assigned to a specified cause during a given time interval divided by the estimated midinterval population. It is expressed per 100,000 population. The cause-specific death rate for diseases of the heart in the United States in 1980 was 336.0 deaths per 100,000 population.

c. Maternal mortality rate is defined as the number of deaths related to pregnancy during a given time interval divided by the number of live births reported during the same time interval. Although the true population at risk should be the number of pregnant women, this is an impossible figure to determine. The number of live births is chosen because it reflects the number of pregnant women; thus, this is a **pseudorate or index**. The maternal mortality rate in the United States in 1980 was 9.2 deaths per 100,000 live births.

d. Case fatality rate is the number of deaths assigned to a specified disease divided by the number of cases of the disease. It is frequently expressed as a percent. It predicts the risk of dying if the disease is contracted.

e. Proportionate mortality ratio (PMR) is the number of deaths from a given cause in a specified time period divided by the total deaths in the same time period. It is usually expressed as a percent. The PMR:

(1) Is not a rate and does not measure the probability of dying from a particular cause.
(2) Is primarily used to determine the relative importance of a specific cause of death in relation to all causes of death within a population.
(3) Was reported in 1980 for the top three leading causes of death in the United States as follows:
(a) Heart disease: 38.2%
(b) Cancer: 20.9%
(c) Stroke: 8.6%

C. Types of rates. The type of rate calculated depends on the available data and the purpose of the calculation.

1. Crude rates, such as the crude birth and death rates discussed above are summary rates for an entire population.

a. They are simple to calculate because only the number of events and the total population are necessary.

b. They cannot be used to compare events in different populations because the rate is dependent on the age-sex composition of the total population; for example, a high death rate and a low birth rate would be expected in a community with many senior citizens as compared to a community with many young people.

2. Adjusted rates are summary rates for the total population, but they are fictitious rates. Statistical techniques are used to calculate summary rates for populations differing in some important characteristics, the most important of which is age. Thus, adjusted rates equalize the differences in the population at risk so that the rates are comparable. However, adjusted rates are difficult to calculate because the demographic composition of the population must be known.

a. Age-adjusted rates are most frequently used to compare mortality in different populations.

b. The two methods used to compute age-adjusted rates are the direct and indirect.

(1) The direct method calculates the rate that would have been observed if the populations being compared had the same age distribution. To perform this calculation:
(a) The age-specific rates in the populations being compared must be known.
(b) A standard population from elsewhere must be borrowed (this standard population can be a composite of all populations being compared, the United States population, or a hypothetical population).
(c) Multiply the known age-specific rates times the chosen standard population in that age group to determine the number of events that would have occurred (the total number of events divided by the standard population chosen is the adjusted rate).

(2) The indirect method calculates the number of events that would have been observed if the two populations being compared had the same age-specific rates. The indirect method is used when the age-specific rates are unknown, as in developing countries, or unstable because of small numbers in the population being studied. To perform this calculation:
(a) The age composition of the populations being compared and the total number of observed events in each population must be known.
(b) Age-specific rates from a larger population with more stable rates must be borrowed.
(c) Multiply the known population in a specified age group times the borrowed age-specific rate to determine the expected number of events that would have occurred in that age group (the total expected number of events would be the sum of the expected events in each age group).
(d) Calculate the standardized ratio (SR), which is defined as the total observed events in a population divided by the total expected events in that population times 100 [if the SR is over 100, it means that more events are occurring in the population than expected; if the SR is less than 100, it means that fewer events are occurring than

expected; when mortality or morbidity is being compared, the SR is called the standardized mortality or morbidity ratio (SMR)].

3. **Specific rates** are calculated for various segments of the population. These rates are:
   - **a.** Difficult to calculate because more information about the demographic composition of the population must be known than with other rates (i.e., the number of observed events and the number of individuals at risk in each segment of the population).
   - **b.** Specific for a particular population segment and therefore can be used to compare events in different populations.

D. Examples of rates. Table 1-1 compares the observed death rates in community A and community B.

1. Note that the crude death rate is 10/1000 in both communities. Thus, it might be concluded that the risk of death is equal in both communities. However, crude rates cannot be used to compare rates in different populations.

2. Adjusted rates can be calculated with these data.
   - **a. Direct method.** Borrow a standard population which can be the composite of the two separate populations (Table 1-2).
     - **(1)** The direct age-adjusted death rate of A is:

$$\frac{423.6}{50{,}000} \times 1000 = 8.5/1000.$$

     - **(2)** The direct age-adjusted death rate of B is:

$$\frac{591.2}{50{,}000} \times 1000 = 11.8/1000.$$

     - **(3)** Since the direct age-adjusted death rate in community B is higher than in community A, it can be concluded that the risk of death is higher in community B.
   - **b. Indirect method.** Borrow standard age-specific rates from a larger population (Table 1-3).
     - **(1)** The standardized mortality ratio (SMR) of community A is:

$$\text{SMR} = \frac{\text{Observed deaths (Table 1-1)}}{\text{Expected deaths (Table 1-3)}} \times 100 = \frac{250}{288.2} \times 100 = 86.7.$$

     - **(2)** The SMR of community B is:

$$\text{SMR} = \frac{250}{204.4} \times 100 = 122.3.$$

     - **(3)** Since the SMR in community B is higher than in community A, it can be concluded that the risk of death is higher in community B.

3. In Table 1-1, the age-specific death rates in the 0–20-, 21–49-, and 50–69-year-old age groups are higher in community B than in community A. These are directly comparable without any need for adjusting.

V. EPIDEMIOLOGIC VARIABLES.

The characteristics and circumstances of a given population that comprises a community are various, and environmental factors are in constant flux. These epidemiologic variables are grouped into the three main categories of time, person, and place. The analysis of the distribution of cases by these variables (descriptive epidemiology) is frequently used to determine how and why diseases occur. Specifically, the epidemiologist looks for a clustering of cases in a segment of the population during a short period of time in a definite geographic space.

Table 1-1. Crude Death Rate

	Community A			Community B		
Age Group	**No. Deaths**	**No. in Age Group**	**Age-Specific Death Rate***	**No. Deaths**	**No. in Age Group**	**Age-Specific Death Rate***
0–20	10	4,000	2.5	40	8,000	5.0
21–49	40	9,000	4.4	60	10,000	6.0
50–69	100	10,000	10.0	100	6,000	16.7
70+	100	2,000	50.0	50	1,000	50.0
Total	250	25,000	10.0	250	25,000	10.0

*Per 1000

Table 1-2. Adjusted Death Rate Using Direct Method

	Community A			Community B		
Age Group	Age-Specific Death Rate*	Standard Population	Expected No. Deaths	Age-Specific Death Rate*	Standard Population	Expected No. Deaths
0–20	2.5	12,000	30.0	5.0	12,000	60.0
21–49	4.4	19,000	83.6	6.0	19,000	114.0
50–69	10.0	16,000	160.0	16.7	16,000	267.2
70+	50.0	3,000	150.0	50.0	3,000	150.0
Total		50,000	423.6		50,000	591.2

*Per 1000

Table 1-3. Adjusted Death Rate Using Indirect Method

	Community A			Community B		
Age Group	**No. in Age Group**	**Borrowed Age-Specific Rate***	**Expected No.**	**No. in Age Group**	**Borrowed Age-Specific Rate***	**Expected No.**
0–20	4,000	3.3	13.2	8,000	3.3	26.4
21–49	9,000	5.0	45	10,000	5.0	50.0
50–69	10,000	13.0	130	6,000	13.0	78.0
70+	2,000	50.0	100	1,000	50.0	50.0
Total	25,000		288.2	25,000		204.4

*Per 1000

A. **Time** refers to the date and, in some instances, the hour of the onset of illness. The occurrence of a disease can be observed over a long period of time (years) to determine secular trends, over a moderate period of time (months) to determine seasonal variation, or over a short period of time (days or weeks) in an epidemic situation.

1. **Secular trends** reflect changes in the periodicity and the natural history of a disease over many years.
   a. Many diseases have a **periodicity** that can be used to predict their future behavior. This periodicity is believed to be related to the proportion of susceptible and immune individuals in the population. For example, because of slight changes (antigenic drift) on the surface of the influenza virus, increased influenza activity is seen every few years. Major changes (antigenic shift) on the surface of the influenza virus occur at longer intervals and are capable of causing worldwide epidemics (pandemics), which happened in 1947, 1957, and 1968.
   b. Changes also occur in the **natural history** of a disease. Figure 1-1 shows the reported cases of viral hepatitis by 4-week periods in the United States from July 1952 to July 1972. (Note that the separate reporting of infectious hepatitis and serum hepatitis did not occur until 1966.) This graph shows that the 7-year periodicity between 1954 and 1961 was not reported in 1968. Note also that the baseline has shifted upwards and that the seasonal pattern (winter peaks and summer troughs) of the 1950s and 1960s has flattened. These data suggest that there has been a change in the natural history of hepatitis.

2. **Seasonal variations** that occur with some diseases may provide information about the reservoir or the mode of transmission. Human susceptibility does not vary significantly throughout the year. Influenza, which is a fall-winter disease in the temperate zone, also occurs in the tropics.
   a. **Legionnaires' disease** is more common in the summer months because it is caused by contaminated air-cooling systems. However, since cases occur throughout the year, there must be other sources of infection.
   b. **Arthropod-borne viral encephalitis**, which is transmitted by the bite of infective mos-

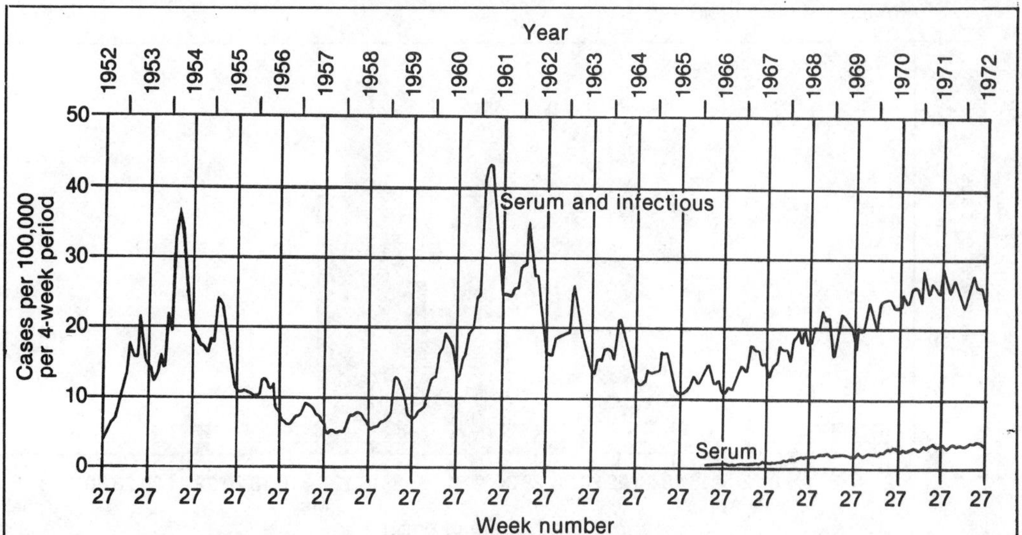

Figure 1-1. Reported cases of viral hepatitis by 4-week periods in the United States since July 1952. (Reprinted from Centers for Disease Control, *Hepatitis Surveillance Report*, No. 35, July 1972, p. 5.)

quitoes, occurs in temperate regions in the late summer and early fall. Environmental factors such as temperature and rainfall influence the size of the vector population.

c. Tularemia is a zoonotic disease (see section II B 2) that is more common in the summer months in the western states and in the winter months in the eastern states. In western states, tularemia is primarily transmitted by the bite of a tick; in eastern states, it is primarily contracted by skinning rabbits and muskrats during the hunting season, by eating insufficiently cooked food, or drinking contaminated water.

3. Epidemic curves are used to describe the distribution of cases during short periods of time and is helpful in determining the source of infection and the possible mode of transmission. In foodborne outbreaks, the calculation of the incubation period (i.e., the time interval from exposure to onset of clinical disease) can be used to determine the etiologic agent.

a. Type I epidemic curves are characterized by a rapid rise and fall of cases so that all cases fall within the range of one incubation period. They are caused by a common source of exposure at one point in time. If the incubation period of the disease is known and if all of the cases occur within one incubation period, the days can be counted backwards and the source of infection determined. Figure 1-2 shows the epidemic curve describing an outbreak of infectious hepatitis in Ogemaw County, Michigan.

(1) The curve suggests a common source outbreak since all of the cases fall within a 30-day period, which is consistent with the known incubation period for hepatitis A [i.e., 15–50 days (average 25–30)].

(2) The cases were epidemiologically linked to the index case (onset April 6) who prepared glazed doughnuts and applied icing to pastry.

b. Type II, or propagated, epidemic curves are characterized by cases occurring over more than one incubation period of the disease. The shape of the curve suggests either person-to-person transmission or a continuing common source outbreak. Figure 1-3 shows the epidemic curve describing an outbreak of viral hepatitis transmitted from person to person.

B. Person refers to characteristics that describe the host (see section III A 2). While no two people are exactly alike, many people share certain characteristics, which place them in a certain segment of the population. For example, people in a segment of the population because of a particular characteristic (age) may be placed in a different segment of the population with a different characteristic (sex). The occurrence of a disease in certain segments of the population can reveal information about host immunity, host exposure, or source of infection.

1. In the era before measles vaccine, 90% of reported cases occurred in children younger than 10 years of age, and 95% occurred by 15 years of age. Adults did not get measles because they were immune from childhood exposure.

2. In the adult population, certain diseases are more common in one sex than the other primarily because exposure to biologic agents that cause disease is different. Women are more likely to get *Salmonella* and *Shigella* infections because of their exposure to children. In the 1960s and 1970s, malaria was more common in men, many of whom acquired the disease during military service in Southeast Asia.

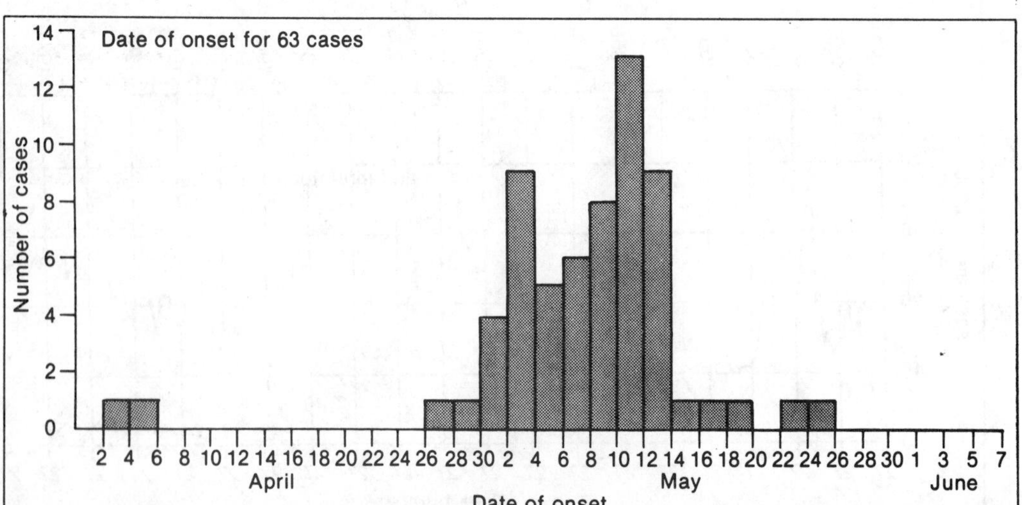

Figure 1-2. Reported cases of infectious hepatitis in Ogemaw County, Michigan, from April to May 1968. (Reprinted from National Communicable Disease Center, *Hepatitis Surveillance Report*, No. 29, September 1968, p. 13.)

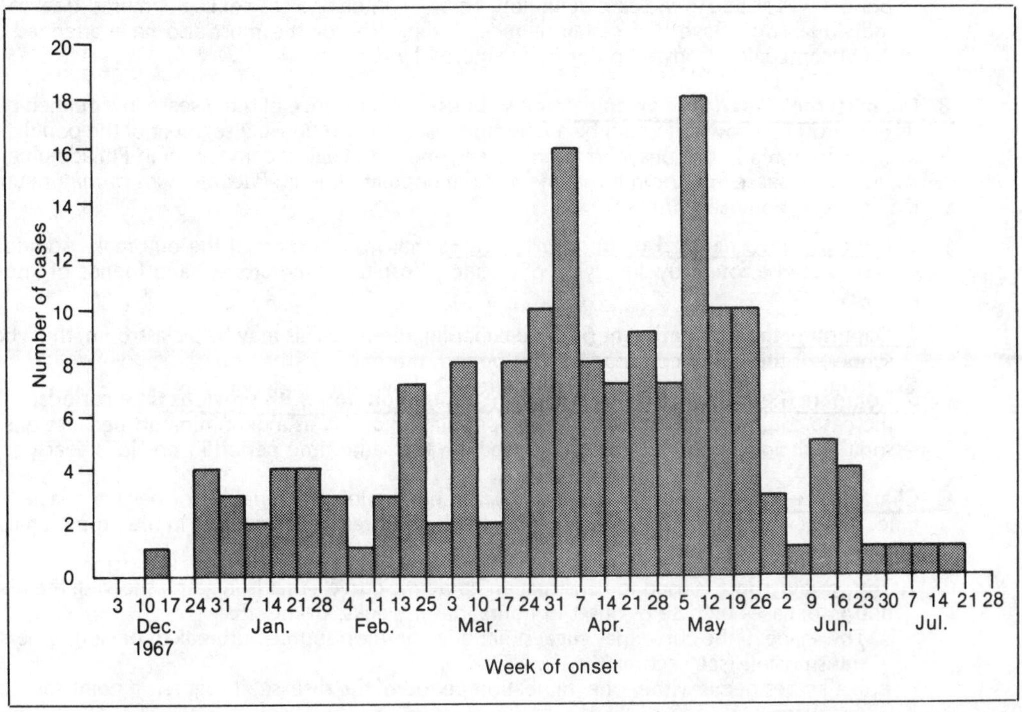

Figure 1-3. Reported cases of viral hepatitis by week of onset in Santa Lucía, Uruguay, from December 1967 to July 15, 1968. (Reprinted from National Communicable Disease Center, *Hepatitis Surveillance Report*, No. 29, September 1968, p. 24.)

3. During the 1960s and 1970s, the pattern of hepatitis changed. Before 1965, it was primarily hepatitis A that was more common in rural areas in individuals aged 5–14 years. Since then, hepatitis has shown a higher urban than rural incidence and a shift to males aged 15–29 years. Since many of these men admitted to parenteral drug abuse, this shift is probably due to hepatitis B.

4. In a foodborne outbreak, a particular food can be incriminated by showing that people who ate a particular item (exposed) were more likely to get sick than the group who did not (not exposed). (See the table that accompanies study questions 5 and 6.)

C. Place refers to a specific geographic point or area and to the features, factors, or conditions that exist in or describe the environment in which the disease occurred. It is the spot where the agent of disease and the susceptible host come together (see section III A 3). It can be as specific as a place of residence or as broad as an urban area. Place is primarily used to determine the source of infection, but it may be used to determine the mode of transmission.

VI. INVESTIGATION OF AN EPIDEMIC. Epidemics, like diseases, do not occur by chance; they require a unique combination of events, including a harmful agent coming into contact with a group of susceptible hosts in the proper environment. The purpose of an investigation of an epidemic is to describe the outbreak and to explain how and why the outbreak took place. There are seven basic steps in conducting an investigation.

A. Verify the diagnosis of the disease under investigation.

1. **Laboratory tests** may be used; however, make certain that the results are reliable.

2. **Clinical criteria** may be used when laboratory results are not available or are unreliable.
   a. Subclinical or mild illnesses will be missed.
   b. Similar, but unrelated illnesses, will be included in the case count.

3. **Epidemiologic criteria** may be added to the clinical and laboratory diagnosis to restrict further the cases under investigation. For example, during the 1976 investigation of Legionnaires' disease in Philadelphia, no laboratory test was available to confirm a diagnosis. Consequently, a clinical diagnosis of a febrile respiratory illness was created. Since the clinical definition was so broad as to include a large number of unrelated cases, an epidemiologic com-

ponent was added to the case definition. To be counted as a case of Legionnaires' disease, an individual must have had certain clinical findings; he or she must also have attended the American Legion Convention or have entered Hotel A.

B. Establish the existence of an epidemic. An unusual occurrence of the disease in a defined population must be shown. It could be a common disease in an unusual segment of the population (e.g., pneumonia in persons who attended an American Legion convention in Philadelphia) or an unusual disease in a common segment of the population (e.g., *Pneumocystis carinii* pneumonia in young homosexual men).

1. **Look for unrecognized or unreported cases** that may be part of the outbreak. Additional cases may be found by surveying physicians, hospitals, laboratories, and friends of known cases.

2. **Determine the population at risk** of developing disease. This may be a classroom, the whole school, or the entire community.

3. **Compare the incidence of disease in the population now with previous time periods**, using the case count as a numerator and the population at risk as a denominator. Because of seasonal variations, compare the incidence with the same time period in previous years.

C. Characterize the distribution of cases by the epidemiologic variables of person, place, and time. The key to understanding how and why the outbreak occurred lies in the proper analysis of the distribution of cases.

1. **The variable time** is used to construct an epidemic curve—that is, a graph showing the distribution of cases by date of onset in hours, days, weeks, or months.
   - **a.** The shape of the curve may suggest either a common source outbreak or person-to-person transmission (see section V A 3).
   - **b.** If all cases occur within one incubation period of the disease, it suggests a point source of exposure.
   - **c.** If the cases occur over several incubation periods, it suggests either person-to-person transmission or a continuing common source of exposure.
   - **d.** If the incubation period of the disease is known, the curve could tell the probable time and possible source of infection.
   - **e.** If the time of exposure can be determined, the incubation period of the disease can be determined.
   - **f.** If the time of exposure is known, the incubation period can be used to establish a diagnosis in foodborne outbreaks. Chemical food poisoning due to ingestion of cadmium or copper have incubation periods that can be measured in minutes. Staphylococcal food poisoning has an onset in 2–6 hours, *Bacillus cereus* and *Clostridium perfringens* in 12–18 hours, and *Salmonella* and *Shigella* in 24–72 hours.

2. **The variable place** can be used to detect a source of infection by looking for possible clustering. Cases can be plotted by place of residence, place of work, position in a classroom, or any other geographic coordinates. Since clustering may only reflect population density, maps should be drawn comparing rates in different areas.

3. **The variable person** can be used to examine a population from different angles (segments) to determine the characteristics of the segment contracting the disease compared to the characteristics of the segment without the disease.

D. Develop an hypothesis that can adequately explain the distribution of cases observed. In developing an hypothesis, the odd case is extremely helpful. The exceptions frequently provide important information. The hypothesis should explain:

1. The source of infection.

2. The mode of transmission.

3. Every case (remember that epidemic disease frequently occurs on top of endemic disease, and some cases may be part of the normal background pattern).

E. Test the hypothesis

1. **Demonstrate differences in attack rates** in people exposed and not exposed to the source of infection. You must be able to show that the ill group was more often exposed to the risk factor than the well group (controls).
2. **Apply statistical tests** to data to determine if variations are random or if they are statistically

significant (see Chapter 3). A statistically significant result may not be epidemiologically significant.

3. **Collect clinical and environmental specimens** for processing in a laboratory.

4. **Ignore the laboratory data** if they do not support the epidemiologic data.

F. **Formulate a conclusion** based upon all pertinent evidence and the results of the hypothesis testing. A final report describing all aspects of the investigation should be prepared.

G. **Institute control measures.** Control measures should be instituted as early as possible in the outbreak investigation. Control measures are directed at one of the six conditions or events in the infectious disease process. The control measure selected depends upon the disease under consideration.

BIBLIOGRAPHY

Lilienfeld AM, Lilienfeld DE: *Foundations of Epidemiology*, 2nd ed. New York, Oxford University Press, 1980

Mausner JS, Bahn AK: *Epidemiology: An Introductory Text*. Philadelphia, WB Saunders, 1974

Principles of Epidemiology. A Three-Day Training Course. Prepared by the Training Program, Health Agencies Branch, Epidemiology and Demonstrations Activity, Centers for Disease Control, Atlanta, Ga. 1974

STUDY QUESTIONS

Directions: Each question below contains five suggested answers. Choose the **one best** response to each question.

1. The most important tool for the epidemiologist is a

(A) stethoscope
(B) calculator
(C) swab
(D) syringe
(E) vaccine

2. The most important biologic trait that determines what disease an individual will contract is

(A) sex
(B) genetic predisposition
(C) ethnic origin
(D) age
(E) race

3. The most difficult mode of transmission to prevent is

(A) person-to-person spread
(B) droplet spread
(C) vector spread
(D) vehicle spread
(E) airborne spread

4. The first step in conducting an epidemic investigation is to

(A) determine the case count
(B) calculate the incubation period
(C) determine the population at risk
(D) verify the diagnosis
(E) collect appropriate samples

Questions 5 and 6

Approximately 100 people attended a buffet dinner at which they were served fried chicken, sliced ham, Swedish meatballs, green beans, potato salad, and apple pie. Thirty guests developed vomiting and diarrhea within 6 hours of the dinner. An epidemiologic investigation, interviewing 60 guests (25 ill and 35 not ill), revealed the following data:

	Consumed Food			Did Not Consume Food		
Food Served	**Ill**	**Not Ill**	**Attack Rate**	**Ill**	**Not Ill**	**Attack Rate**
Chicken	20	28	42%	5	7	42%
Ham	12	17	41%	13	18	42%
Meatballs	23	24	49%	2	11	15%
Green beans	15	24	38%	10	11	48%
Potato salad	18	26	41%	7	9	44%
Apple pie	22	34	39%	3	1	75%

5. The incriminated food item is most likely to be

(A) chicken
(B) ham
(C) meatballs
(D) potato salad
(E) apple pie

6. The most likely etiologic agent is

(A) *Salmonella*
(B) *Staphylococcus*
(C) *Clostridium perfringens*
(D) *Bacillus cereus*
(E) *Shigella*

Directions: Each question below contains four suggested answers of which **one or more** is correct. Choose the answer

A if **1, 2, and 3** are correct
B if **1 and 3** are correct
C if **2 and 4** are correct
D if **4** is correct
E if **1, 2, 3, and 4** are correct

7. Adjusted rates have which of the following characteristics?

(1) They are easy to calculate
(2) They can be used for international comparisons
(3) They are frequently used in epidemic investigations of acute disease
(4) They are fictitious rates

8. The prevalence rate of a disease has which of the following characteristics?

(1) It measures all of the current cases in the community
(2) It is dependent upon the duration of illness
(3) It is dependent upon the incidence of disease
(4) It can be used to determine the health care needs of a community

9. Epidemiologic principles are used to

(1) evaluate drug therapy
(2) plan future health needs of the community
(3) help to establish a diagnosis
(4) determine a patient's prognosis

Directions: The group of questions below consists of lettered choices followed by several numbered items. For each numbered item select the **one** lettered choice with which it is **most** closely associated. Each lettered choice may be used once, more than once, or not at all.

Questions 10–14

For each disease listed below, select the step in the infectious disease process that should be blocked to prevent transmission.

(A) Agent
(B) Reservoir
(C) Mode of transmission
(D) Portal of entry
(E) Susceptible host

10. Meningococcal meningitis

11. Polio

12. Sexually transmitted diseases

13. Tuberculosis

14. *Salmonella* infection

Directions: The group of questions below consists of lettered choices followed by several numbered items. For each numbered item, select the one lettered choice with which it is most closely associated. Each lettered choice may be used once, more than once, or not at all. Choose the answer

A if the item is associated with **(A) only**
B if the item is associated with **(B) only**
C if the item is associated with **both (A) and (B)**
D if the item is associated with **neither (A) nor (B)**

Questions 15–18

For each situation listed below, select the study design that would be most useful to solve the problem.

(A) Descriptive studies
(B) Analytical studies
(C) Both
(D) Neither

15. A drug company wants to evaluate a new vaccine before it can be marketed.

16. Public health officials want to control a measles outbreak in a local school.

17. Investigation of a newly identified disease, such as legionnaires' disease or acquired immune deficiency syndrome, has just been initiated.

18. A clinician wishes to determine the cause of an unusual cancer.

ANSWERS AND EXPLANATIONS

1. The answer is B. (*I B 1 a, b; IV A–C*) The epidemiologist is interested in identifying factors that cause disease or disease transmission and in preventing the spread of disease within a given population. To do this an epidemiologist must be able to describe and compare the occurrence of disease in different segments of the population. A calculator is needed to calculate the rates for comparison.

2. The answer is D. (*III A 2*) Host factors that determine the occurrence of a disease include biologic traits (i.e., genetic characteristics, race, ethnic origin, sex, and age) with which a host is born and social traits (i.e., life-style, diet, employment, residence, and marital status), which a host acquires or develops. Age is the most important biologic factor because it is directly related to the ability of the body to respond to disease, acquired immunity, and exposure. For example, susceptible children are more likely to have subclinical disease than susceptible adults, and adults who have acquired immunity over time because of prior exposure are more likely to have no disease. In addition, adults in the workplace are exposed to different agents than children in school.

3. The answer is E. (*II D 1–2*) An organism must be transmitted, either directly or indirectly, from one place to another. Direct transmission includes person-to-person spread by skin contact and droplet spread produced by coughing, sneezing, talking, or singing within close proximity of a susceptible host. Indirect transmission occurs when the reservoir and the susceptible host are separated; this type of transmission involves vector spread, vehicle spread, and airborne spread. Diseases disseminated by the airborne route are the most difficult to prevent and, thus, are able to infect large numbers of individuals in a relatively short period of time. For example, a new strain of influenza virus can spread throughout the world in a relatively short period of time.

4. The answer is D. (*VI A 1–3, B*) The first step in conducting an epidemic investigation is to verify the diagnosis of the disease under investigation. The establishment of a clinical, laboratory, or epidemiologic case definition is necessary to determine an accurate case count so that the existence of an epidemic can be established. Once the existence of an epidemic has been established, the full investigation can then begin.

5 and 6. The answers are: 5-C, 6-B. (*II D 2 b; VI C 1 f, E 1–4*) In conducting an investigation of a foodborne outbreak, the investigator must be able to demonstrate that the ill group was more often exposed to the incriminated food item than the well group. The specific attack rate must be significantly higher in the group that ate the food as compared to the group that did not eat the food. If there is no significant difference in attack rates, the food item is not responsible for the outbreak. The data given in the question show that the Swedish meatballs were responsible. Note that two ill persons did not eat Swedish meatballs. These cases could have occurred by cross-contamination of serving spoons or as a result of an unrelated diarrhea-causing agent.

The short incubation period for staphylococcal food poisoning is a result of the fact that it is caused by a heat-stable enterotoxin, which is produced in the food. The other bacterial causes of food poisoning require some multiplication in the gastrointestinal tract to produce symptoms; they, therefore, have a longer incubation period.

7. The answer is C (2, 4). [*IV C 2 b (1)–(2)*] Adjusted rates are summary rates for the total population, but they are fictitious—that is, in a sense, adjusted rates, by using a standard population or standard age-specific rates, equalize the differences in the population at risk so that the rates are comparable. Adjusted rates are difficult to calculate because the demographic composition of the population must be known. They are frequently used to compare birth and death rates in different populations and for international comparisons because they take into consideration the age composition of the different populations; however, they are seldom used for epidemic investigations of acute diseases.

8. The answer is E (all). [*IV B 2 b (1), (2)*] The prevalence rate is the number of current cases (old and new) of a specified disease during a specified time period divided by the estimated midinterval population at risk. Since the prevalence rate includes *all* cases in the community, it is determined by both the incidence and the duration of the disease process. It can also be used to determine the health care needs of the community since it measures the total illness within the community.

9. The answer is A (1, 2, 3). (*I A 2, D 1–8*) Epidemiology is the study of the distribution and determinants of diseases or conditions in a defined population and as such cannot determine the prognosis of a disease process in a particular patient. Since the social and occupational characteristics of an individual determines to what diseases he or she will be exposed, these factors can be used to establish a diagnosis. Clinical trials use epidemiologic principles to evaluate the effectiveness of new drugs. Because epidemiology can be used to predict future occurrence of disease, it can also predict future health care needs of a community.

10–14. The answers are: 10-A, 11-E, 12-D, 13-B, 14-C. (*II A–E*) Chemoprophylaxis with either rifampin or sulfonamide is used to eliminate pharyngeal carriage of *Neisseria meningitidis* from household contacts of a known case of meningococcal meningitis to prevent secondary spread. The hope is that the family will be recolonized by a less pathogenic strain of the meningococcus, which would stimulate a natural immunity.

Polio vaccine is used to immunize a susceptible host against the wild poliovirus. Once immunity has been established in the host, exposure to the wild virus will not cause disease.

Most sexually transmitted diseases can be prevented by using a condom, which blocks the portal of entry into a susceptible host. Note that the condom does not block the agent's portal of exit from its reservoir.

New cases of tuberculosis can be prevented by eliminating the reservoir of infections. The reservoir of infection consists of individuals who have been infected with the tubercle bacillus, including patients with sputum-positive pulmonary tuberculosis who can infect other people and individuals with only a positive tuberculin skin test in whom a dormant infection can be reactivated, causing disease. Chemotherapy can prevent spread from a patient with pulmonary tuberculosis, and chemoprophylaxis with isoniazid can prevent reactivation.

Salmonella infections are spread by poor personal hygiene or by a common vehicle such as contaminated food. *Salmonella* infections are controlled by emphasizing good hand-washing techniques and by not allowing infected individuals to work in an occupation that prepares or serves food for public consumption. The spread of all enteric diseases is prevented by having a safe water supply and an adequate sewage system.

15-18. The answers are: 15-D, 16-A, 17-C, 18-B. (*I C 1–3*) The effectiveness of a new vaccine can only be determined by carefully designed experimental studies, which show protection in the immunized group as compared to the nonimmunized group.

Descriptive studies, which describe the distribution of disease by the epidemiologic variables of person, place, and time, are used to determine who is getting the disease and why the outbreak occurred. Public health officials can then use this information to apply proper control measures to prevent further spread.

The investigation of a new disease process always begins with descriptive studies to determine which segments of the population are contracting the disease. After these segments are identified, case control studies (analytical studies) are designed to identify risk factors that cause disease or to explain why certain individuals within these population segments develop disease.

Unusual diseases or rare diseases are usually studied with analytical studies of the case control variety. Because of the small number of cases that occur, a case control study has to be used to identify causal relationships or factors associated with disease. Hypotheses that are generated by this technique can be tested with additional studies.

2
Experimental Designs and Research Approaches

William C. Steinmann

I. INFORMATION ROUTINELY SOUGHT BY CLINICAL STUDIES

A. To assess the health status or clinical characteristics of a well-defined population or group of subjects, the kind of information that should be sought includes:

1. The annual rate for suicide in teenagers.
2. The immunization status of children in the community.
3. The incidence of rabies in the state.

B. To probe the natural history of disease, the kind of information that should be sought includes:

1. The clinical course of retinopathy in diabetics over a 10-year follow-up period.
2. The prognosis of patients with solitary calcified pulmonary nodule.

C. To examine clinical decision-making processes, the kind of information that should be sought includes:

1. The best sequence of tests for screening and diagnosis of a patient with a solitary pulmonary nodule.
2. The best screening test for glaucoma in the general population by general practitioners.
3. The likelihood that patients with bright red blood per rectum have colorectal cancer.

D. To determine and assess treatment outcomes, the kind of information that should be sought includes:

1. The tumor response of laryngeal cancer in patients who receive radiation treatment.
2. Medical treatment versus coronary artery bypass surgery for angina pectoris.

E. To identify and assess risk factors, the kind of information that should be sought includes:

1. The incidence of lung cancer in smokers compared to nonsmokers.
2. The likelihood that offspring of patients with rheumatoid arthritis will develop this disease.
3. The likelihood that patients with colonic polyps will develop colorectal cancer.

II. PRINCIPLES OF CLINICAL STUDY DESIGN

A. Study characteristics, which are determined by the clinical information sought, include:

1. The specific type of study design that will be employed.
2. The way in which the study will be conducted, including:
   a. The criteria that are used for subject selection and treatment.
   b. The way in which data are collected.
   c. The way in which data are analyzed.

B. Strengths and limitations of a clinical study are defined by the study methodology, which in turn affects the validity and generalizability of the results and possible conclusions.

1. Each study design has well-defined and well-recognized strengths or weaknesses.

2. The methods employed within any study design for the selection and treatment of subjects, data collection, and analysis can vary greatly, thereby strengthening or weakening the study design.

C. **Major methodologic considerations** are important in the conduct of a clinical study, particularly issues of subject selection, data collection, and statistical analysis.

1. **Subject selection.** It is important to consider:
   a. Whether or not the clinical subjects represent the target population, such as the general population.
   b. How the subjects were selected; for example, if they were selected at random, it is important to determine whether all of the eligible subjects had an equal chance to be included in the study, who was excluded, and how may those who were excluded differ from those who participated. If they were not selected at random, were the selection criteria objective enough to eliminate systematic error.
   c. Whether or not there was a group (controls) with which to compare results.

2. **Data collection**
   a. **Prospective data collection** involves the collection of data after the study objectives are defined and the study design has been completed.
   b. **Retrospective data collection** involves the collection of data prior to the definition of the study objectives and the design of the study; for example, the data can be abstracted from chart reviews to assess clinical outcomes.
   c. Data can be collected **directly** by examination of patients or **indirectly** by review and abstraction from hospital case records.
   d. Treatments can be standardized to eliminate the possible influence of systematic error (**bias**).
   e. Observations of outcomes or results can be standardized to prevent bias.
   f. Treatments or other interventions can be allocated randomly—that is, patients have an equal chance of falling into any of the treatment groups.
   g. Observers and subjects can be masked or blinded to ensure that observations are made and treatments are administered in an unbiased manner.
   h. There may or may not be a control group with which to compare results.

3. **Statistical analysis.** It is important to determine if:
   a. The number of subjects is sufficient to generate enough statistical power to determine a true difference that may have existed between the comparison groups and thus avoid a **beta error**, which is the failure to detect a true difference when it exists because the sample size is inadequate.
   b. The appropriate statistical tests or methods are employed based on characteristics of the data collected, including whether or not the distribution of the variables are:
      (1) Normal or Gaussian.
      (2) Continuous or discrete.
   c. The likelihood that differences found between two or more groups were due to chance and an **alpha error** occurred, which means a difference was detected even though no real difference existed.

D. **Additional influences** that deserve consideration in assessing study methodologies include:

1. The resources that were available for the study.
2. The ethical constraints that were imposed by the study design.
3. The population that could reasonably have been expected to participate in the study.
4. The costs and risks that had to be considered in the design of the study.
5. All studies have limitations, and the key is whether:
   a. These affect the validity of the study design.
   b. The results despite limitations are generalizable to a comparison population such as individual practices.

E. **Terminology or principles** used in assessing clinical data from clinical studies follow.

1. **Efficacy** describes the true treatment intervention effect under ideal conditions.
2. **Effectiveness** describes the true treatment or intervention effect under clinical conditions or in "routine" practice.
3. **Reliability** describes the reproducibility of test results.
4. **Validity** describes the accuracy and reliability of a test (i.e. the extent to which the test measures what it is supposed to measure).

5. **Causality** denotes direct effect. It requires that criteria, such as biologic plausibility, reproducibility, consistency, and temporal association, be met. Rarely can cause and effect be defined by a single clinical study.
6. **Bias** is a systematic error that is unintentionally made.
7. **Sensitivity** of a test describes the population of true abnormals or test-positives correctly identified.
8. **Specificity** of a test describes the population of true normals or the test-negatives correctly identified.

III. SPECIFIC CLINICAL STUDY DESIGNS

A. Case report

1. **Description.** A case report is a brief, objective report of a clinical characteristic or outcome from a single clinical subject or event.
2. **Study questions.** A case report can address almost any clinical question or issue, including screening test results or treatment outcomes or natural history findings. It is commonly used to report unusual or unexpected events, such as adverse drug reactions.
3. **Methodology**
   - **a.** A single noteworthy event must first be identified.
   - **b.** Data collection is generally retrospective with a review and a descriptive summary of subjects or events.
   - **c.** No statistical analysis or comparison group is included in the design.
   - **d.** Although few conclusions can be drawn based on evidence from a single event or observation, they:
     - **(1)** Are valuable for first report of unexpected findings.
     - **(2)** Can generate hypotheses for testing.
     - **(3)** Can define issues for further study.
4. **Strengths and limitations.** A case report is often the first evidence of an unexpected or unusual event, but rarely are the results generalizable.
5. **Examples**
   - **a.** A report of advanced proliferative diabetic retinopathy in a patient with no other clinical evidence of diabetes is an appropriate subject for a case report.
   - **b.** The initial report of phocomelia in a newborn of a woman on thalidomide is an important example of how a single case report can trigger further important investigations.

B. Case series report

1. **Description.** A case series report is an objective report of a clinical characteristic or outcome from a group of clinical subjects.
2. **Study questions.** A case series report can address almost any clinical problem, including screening test results or treatment outcomes and natural history findings. However, it is most commonly used to describe clinical characteristics, such as signs and symptoms of disease or disease outcomes—for example, the natural history of a series of patients with specific disease.
3. **Methodology**
   - **a.** Subjects must be identified with regard to the clinical events or characteristics in question.
   - **b.** Data collection may be retrospective or prospective, but a comparison or control group is usually not included.
   - **c.** Descriptive statistics are calculated to define the proportion of subjects with the characteristics under study. Results are often incorrectly compared with the results from other populations or studies of similar subjects.
   - **d.** Conclusions generally are limited because there is no comparison group within the study.
4. **Strengths and limitations**
   - **a.** Because the selection of study subjects is often unrepresentative or otherwise biased, the generalizability of the results is often limited. The denominator—that is, the population from which the subjects were drawn—rarely is defined, nor is the selection criteria for subjects, which further limits generalizability.
   - **b.** The lack of a control or comparison group also limits the generalizability of results.
   - **c.** Conclusions are often incorrectly considered to be generalizable and valid based on the large number of study subjects.

d. Study results are strengthened when a consecutive series of subjects, that is, all eligible subjects, are included over a specified period of time.

5. Examples

a. Intraocular pressure control in 100 consecutive patients with primary open-angle glaucoma who were treated with laser trabeculoplasty and followed for 1 year is an appropriate subject for a case series report.

b. Identification of several children born to mothers who had taken thalidomide, which gave evidence of possible association of this drug with birth defects, exemplifies a case series report.

C. Incidence and prevalence studies

1. Description. Incidence and prevalence studies are actually a type of case series report but differ in that the entire study population is well-defined and then uniformly surveyed regarding the parameters in question.

2. Study questions. Usually incidence and prevalence studies concern the occurrence of disease, but they also address the rate of other events, such as the adverse side effects of drugs or even death.

a. Incidence is the occurrence of an event or characteristic over a period of time—for example, the rate of staphylococcal food poisoning following lunch in a particular restaurant. Incidence is used to:

(1) Describe the rate of disease occurrence over time.

(2) Assess survival—that is, the incidence of death over time or at a specific time after follow-up—for example, the 5-year survival rate for breast cancer.

(3) Compare risk of disease between two or more populations.

b. Prevalence is the presence of an event or characteristic at a single point in time—for example, the rate of previously undiagnosed glaucoma in a population of elderly individuals screened for ophthalmic disorders. Prevalence is used to:

(1) Describe the burden of disease, especially undiagnosed disease.

(2) Define the rate of clinical characteristics in subjects with a specified disease—for example, weight loss in patients presenting with terminal disorders.

3. Methodology

a. A target population to be followed over a period of time for an incidence study or to be surveyed at a single point in time for a prevalence study must be identified.

b. Events or characteristics must be measured and recorded by periodic reassessment over time for the incidence study and at a particular time for the prevalence study.

c. A rate, the occurrence of the measured target event over the entire population, must be calculated.

d. No statistical analytic component is included although rates within populations or subpopulations can be compared.

4. Strengths and limitations. True rates are determined, which can serve as comparison measures between populations. However, they may provide poor estimates of infrequent or rare events. They may be adversely affected by sampling, which may be unrepresentative. They usually require description of population characteristics, such as age, race, and sex, to be meaningful.

5. Examples

a. Incidence. The rate of colon carcinoma developing in an elderly population over 1 year is an appropriate subject for an incidence study.

b. Prevalence. The rate of unrecognized heart murmur in children presenting for their first preschool physical is an appropriate subject for a prevalence study.

D. Case-control study

1. Description. A case-control study is an observational or descriptive analytic study in which diseased and nondiseased or affected or nonaffected subjects are identified after the fact and then compared regarding specific characteristics to determine possible association or risk for the disease in question.

2. Study questions. Most often a case-control study is used to address issues of the risk of association for disease—that is, the differences between diseased and nondiseased populations in the characteristic under investigation—for example, a comparison of the rate of cigarette smoking between those individuals who have lung cancer and those who are cancer free. They are also used in clinical decision analysis to assess the differences between diseased and nondiseased populations in test positivity—for example, the likelihood that patients with urinary tract infections have greater than 10 white cells in unspun urine samples before treatment compared to those without infection.

3. Methodology

a. Diseased and nondiseased populations must be identified, usually retrospectively.

b. The prevalence of characteristics under investigation and other characteristics that possibly may be related to the presence of disease and characteristic under study must be assessed.

c. Statistical comparison can be made between study groups of the characteristics under investigation to assess the likelihood that differences in these characteristics between diseased and nondiseased groups are real and not due to chance (alpha error).

d. Conclusions are useful for the generation of hypotheses and for initial evidence of putative risk associations. Results cannot be used for define causality.

4. Strengths and limitations

a. A case-control study is relatively easy and inexpensive to conduct since prospective or long-term follow-up is not required.

b. There is a potential for bias in the selection of subjects since a case-control study is not population based.

c. Bias in data collection may also occur since the presence or absence of disease is usually known to the subject and may be known to the study observer (unmasked). Bias may also influence the recall of previous exposure by the subject if possible associations are known to him or her, such as the association between cigarette smoking and lung cancer.

d. The incidence rate of disease in a population cannot be determined nor compared between populations to assess possible risk (relative risk). However, the **odds ratio**, which provides an estimate of the relative risk of characteristics between diseased and nondiseased populations can be calculated.

5. Examples

a. A comparison of prior estrogen use in uterine cancer cases compared to age-matched controls without cancer to assess possible risk for exposure to estrogens is an appropriate subject for a case-control study.

b. The case-control study comparing thalidomide ingestion in mothers of children with phocomelia with ingestion in mothers with normal children clearly demonstrates that thalidomide ingestions were more common in mothers with affected children than in mothers with children who did not have phocomelia.

E. Cohort study

1. Description. A cohort study is an observational or descriptive analytic study in which exposed and nonexposed populations are identified and followed prospectively over time to determine the rate of a specific clinical disease or event.

2. Study questions. Most often a cohort study is used to address issues of risk for the development of disease between populations exposed and not exposed to a factor under study—for example, a population of smokers and nonsmokers are followed over time to provide comparison rates between smokers and nonsmokers for lung cancer or heart disease. A cohort study also can be used in clinical decision analysis to assess the predictive value of test positivity or negativity—for example, to determine the proportion of patients with positive sedimentation rates at screening who have a diagnosis of cancer on a subsequent definitive workup.

3. Methodology

a. A population of exposed and nonexposed (or test positive and negative) individuals must be identified and followed prospectively.

b. Exposure to the risk factors under study and other potentially associated variables must be quantitated initially and over time.

c. The incidence of the target event, such as cancer, over time must be measured.

d. The incidence rate of an event for both exposed and nonexposed populations must be calculated. This calculation can then be compared to determine the relative risk and incidence in exposed and nonexposed individuals. Statistical comparison of the rates of disease occurrence or outcome parameter between the exposed and nonexposed groups allows one to assess the likelihood that the observed differences are real and not due to chance (alpha error). In addition, the attributable risk can be determined which is simply the difference in the incidence of the event or disease between exposed and nonexposed populations. While relative risk is commonly used to assess possible etiology, attributable risk is used to measure the burden of disease in a population.

4. **Strengths and limitations.** Although costly and time-consuming due to a large number of subjects often needed and the prolonged duration of time required for follow-up of the disease occurrence, a cohort study allows for determination of a population-based rate of the event under question and the relative risk. Potential bias in recall and observations is lessened since exposure can be determined prior to the onset of disease or event. As with a case-control study, causality cannot be determined by results from this type of study since other important criteria must be met.

5. **Examples**
   a. Follow-up in a population of adults exposed and not exposed as children to radiation of the neck to assess risk from thyroid cancer is an appropriate subject for a cohort study.
   b. The cohort study of physicians comparing the incidence of lung cancer between individuals who smoked and those who did not was a landmark study in defining the association of cigarette smoking and lung cancer.

F. Clinical trial

1. **Description.** A clinical trial is an experimental design used to assess differences between two or more groups receiving different interventions or treatments.

2. **Study questions.** A clinical trial is usually employed to compare outcomes between different treatments, such as antibiotic treatments for a specific disease or chemotherapy for a specific cancer. It can also be used in clinical decision analysis to compare outcomes, such as when comparing the differences in mortality from cancer among populations receiving different screening interventions.

3. **Methodology**
   a. A population with a clinical characteristic requiring intervention must be identified.
   b. Subjects must be allocated, preferably randomly, to each of the treatment interventions. Treatments are administered in an identical or controlled manner to ensure uniformity of nontreatment covariants, which may affect outcomes.
   c. Treatment outcomes and other results, such as side effects, costs, or benefits, must be measured. Preferably observations should be made while observers and patients are masked to the type of interventions (double masked or blind).
   d. Rates of measured outcomes between the different treatment groups can be statistically compared.
   e. The strongest evidence of differences in clinical outcome due to treatment effect are provided by the conclusion.

4. **Strengths and limitations.** A clinical trial allows for control of other clinical variables, which can also affect outcomes under investigation. Randomization minimizes the potential adverse effect from systematic error (bias). However, unmasking either the observer or subject often leads to biased observations and may invalidate the results. An insufficient number of subjects may lead to failure to detect true differences that may exist (beta error).

5. **Examples**
   a. Comparison of chemotherapy versus chemotherapy plus radiation for laryngeal carcinoma is an appropriate topic for a clinical trial.
   b. The recent randomized, controlled clinical trial for breast cancer showed that radical mastectomy was in some cases no more effective than lumpectomy.

STUDY QUESTIONS

Directions: Each question below contains five suggested answers. Choose the **one best** response to each question.

1. Bias is unlikely to invalidate cohort studies used to assess risk of exposure because

(A) data collection is retrospective
(B) data collection is prospective
(C) large numbers of subjects are usually included
(D) exposure is usually determined prior to disease occurrence
(E) actual relative risk can be determined

2. The validity of results from clinical trials can be compromised by all of the following EXCEPT the

(A) observer unmasked to treatment
(B) patient unmasked to treatment
(C) nonrandom allocation of treatments
(D) small number of subjects
(E) lack of control group

Directions: The group of questions below consists of lettered choices followed by several numbered items. For each numbered item select the **one** lettered choice with which it is **most** closely associated. Each lettered choice may be used once, more than once, or not at all.

Questions 3–7

For each case history that follows, select the study design that it most appropriately illustrates.

(A) Case series report
(B) Case-control study
(C) Clinical trial
(D) Cohort study
(E) Case report

3. A total of 300 newly diagnosed patients with laryngeal cancer are allocated to treatment with either surgical excision alone or surgical exision plus radiation treatment.

4. A 39-year-old man who presents with a mild sore throat, fever, malaise, and headache is treated with penicillin for presumed streptococcal infection. He returns after a week with hypotension, fever, rash, and abdominal pain. He responds favorably to chloramphenicol, after a diagnosis of Rocky Mountain spotted fever is made.

5. A total of 3500 patients with thyroid cancer are identified and surveyed by patient interviews regarding past exposure to radiation.

6. A total of 10,000 Vietnam veterans, half of whom are known by combat records to have been in areas where Agent Orange was used and half of whom are known to have been in areas where no Agent Orange was use, are asked to give a history of cancer since discharge.

7. Patients admitted for carcinoma of the stomach are age and sex matched with fellow patients without a diagnosis of cancer and surveyed as to smoking history to assess the possible association of smoking and gastric cancer.

ANSWERS AND EXPLANATIONS

1. The answer is D. (*III E 4*) Bias is unlikely to invalidate cohort studies used to assess relative risk of exposure since exposure is usually determined prospectively and prior to the onset of disease. Hence, subjects are unaware of their disease status as are those who are recording the exposure. Although a large number of subjects may be needed, this would not invalidate the results if the investigators ensured that the sample size is adequate to provide the statistical power to determine a true difference in exposure if it usually existed and thus avoid a beta error problem. Although prospective data collection will help prevent bias in observations, knowledge of possible associations, if present, could invalidate cohort design.

2. The answer is E. (*III F 1–4*) A clinical trial is an experimental design used to assess differences between two or more groups receiving different interventions or treatments. The design is such that at least one control group is included for comparison of the planned interventions. A population with a clinical characteristic requiring intervention must be identified. Subjects must be allocated, preferably randomly, to each of the treatment interventions. Randomization minimizes the potential adverse effect from systematic error (bias). Treatments are then administered in an identical or controlled manner to ensure uniformity of nontreatment covariants. Preferably observations should be made while observers and patients are masked to the type of interventions being made to avoid biased observations. This is called a double-blind study as compared to a single-blind study when only the subject or the observer are masked to the intervention. An insufficient number of subjects may lead to failure to detect true differences that may exist (beta error). It should also be noted that statistically significant results can occur *due* to chance even in the most rigorous study design as in a well-designed clinical trial where treatments are randomized and subjects and observers are masked. This occurrence of detecting a significant difference, which does not exist but is due to chance, is called an alpha error and is usually expressed as a probability (P) with less than 0.05 considered by most investigators as significant.

3–7. The answers are: 3-C, 4-E, 5-A, 6-D, 7-B. (*III A 1–2, B 1–2, D 1–2, E 1–2, F 1–2*) The laryngeal cancer patients are part of a clinical trial since subjects receive one treatment or the other with the intent to compare outcomes between the two treatment groups. This study is strengthened if patients are randomly allocated to the treatment groups to minimize possible selection bias. Obviously, it would be difficult to mask patients and observers to treatment regimens to prevent biased observations. Case reports or case series reports do not include comparison groups, and cohort and case-control studies, which use controls, are used to assess risk association.

The 39-year-old man represents a case report, which is a description of a single interesting case. It is an important report that serves to alert other physicians of the possibility of misdiagnosing a potentially fatal disease if untreated. No control or comparison subjects are included.

The thyroid cancer patients represent a case series report because there is no active group for comparison of exposure with those who have the disease. The report processes information on a unique population as to their experience with previous exposure. In a case-control study, the assessment of risk would also be retrospective. In addition, a population of those without disease would be included from whom a history of past exposure would be obtained for comparison with estimates of relative risk.

The Vietnam veterans represent a cohort study, which relies on classification of subjects as to exposure to Agent Orange and then looks forward in time to assess the incidence of cancer. Sometimes this kind of study where historic data are used to define previous exposure is called an historic cohort design. True incidence rates can be determined for this disease in this population in contrast to case-control studies. In case-control studies, those with disease would first be identified, then past exposure would be assessed for possible risk associations. Unlike case series reports, controls are available for comparison.

The patients admitted for stomach carcinoma represent a case-control study since it defines both diseased and nondiseased populations for comparisons of previous exposure to cigarette smoking. Incidence rates of cancer among exposed or nonexposed individuals obviously could be determined. There is great potential for possible bias in recall of exposure by individuals with cancer given the current knowledge of association of lung cancer and cigarette smoking. Case series reports do not include control groups for comparison nor can they be used for possible assessment of risk association.

3
Statistics

Lawrence D. Budnick

I. INTRODUCTION

A. Statistics

1. **Definition.** Statistics is a scientific field that deals with the collection, classification, description, analysis, interpretation, and presentation of data.
   a. **Descriptive statistics** (see section II) and **analytic statistics** (see section III) refer to the summary measures of data.
   b. **Vital statistics** is the ongoing collection by government agencies of data relating to vital events, including births, deaths, marriages, divorces, and health and disease-related conditions deemed reportable by local health authorities.

2. **Uses.** For the practicing physician, statistics has at least three important functions.
   a. Statistics is a scientific method used in the interpretation of data obtained by other methods.
   b. Statistics provides a powerful reinforcement for other determinants of scientific causality.
   c. Statistical reasoning, albeit unintentional or subconscious, is involved in all scientific clinical judgments.

3. **History.** The following are some of the more noteworthy individuals responsible for the early developments in the field of statistics.
   a. **John Graunt** (1620–1674) studied the Bills of Mortality, which were compiled from English parish registers, and published the first analytic studies of vital statistics in which mortality differences between the sexes and between urban and rural dwellers were noted.
   b. **Pierre-Charles-Alexandre Louis** (1787–1872) studied diseases, including typhoid fever and tuberculosis, and therapeutic procedures, such as bloodletting, and used quantitative results and analytic reasoning ("the numerical method") to discuss his clinical findings. Louis was the premier teacher of medical statistics of his time.
   c. **Lemuel Shattuck** (1793–1859) was instrumental in establishing an effective vital statistics system in the United States. Shattuck's report to the Sanitary Commission of Massachusetts in 1850 laid out the fundamentals for organized public health activities. He founded the American Statistical Association.
   d. **William Farr** (1807–1883) became the first Registrar-General in the General Register Office of England in 1839. Farr's *Annual Reports* used vital statistics and epidemiology to point out the social consequences of diseases. He introduced many of the basic concepts of epidemiology and originated a uniform coding system for diseases that has evolved into the *International Classification of Diseases*.
   e. **John Snow** (1813–1858) analytically studied cholera outbreaks in London and demonstrated the relationship between cholera and water contaminated by sewage. Snow wrote what is considered the first practical book on epidemiology, entitled, *On the Mode of Communication of Cholera*.

B. Data

1. **Definition.** Data are the basic building blocks of statistics and refer to the individual values presented, measured, or observed.

2. **Characteristics**
   a. **Data can be derived from a total population or a sample.**
      (1) A **population** is the universe of units or values being studied. It can consist of individuals, objects, events, observations, or any other grouping.

(2) A **sample** is a selected part of a population. The following are some of the more common types of samples.

(a) In a **simple random sample**, each member of the population has an equal possibility of being chosen for the sample, with chance alone responsible for the selection of any member. The sample can be chosen by using a table of random numbers. Each individual in the population is numbered, and a list of random numbers is drawn from the table, with the sample size needed determining how many numbers to draw. This list of numbers represents the individuals chosen for the simple random sample.

(b) In a **systematically selected sample**, a random starting point at the beginning of an ordered population is chosen, and then the remainder of the sample is chosen according to a predetermined selection schedule.

(c) In a **stratified selected sample**, the population is divided into sampling units that contain individuals, and a random sample of individuals proportionate to the size of the sampling unit is chosen from each sampling unit.

(d) In a **cluster selected sample**, the population is divided into sampling units or groups, and a random sample of groups is chosen. A complete count of the individuals in the chosen groups is undertaken. The sample is made up of **groups**, not individuals.

(e) In a **nonrandomly selected sample**, members of the population are chosen for the sample based on known factors.

b. Data can be ungrouped or grouped.

(1) **Ungrouped data** are presented or observed individually. An example of ungrouped data is the following list of weights (in pounds) for 6 men: 140, 150, 150, 150, 160, and 160.

(2) **Grouped data** are presented in groups consisting of identical data by frequency. An example of grouped data is the following list of weights for the 6 men noted above: 140 lb (1 man), 150 lb (3 men), and 160 lb (2 men).

c. Data can be quantitative or qualitative.

(1) **Quantitative data** are numerical or based on numbers. An example of quantitative data is the measuring of height in inches.

(2) **Qualitative data** are non-numerical or based on a categorical scale. An example of qualitative data is the measuring of height in terms of short, medium, and tall.

d. Data can be discrete or continuous.

(1) **Discrete data** are data for which distinct categories and a limited number of possible values exist. An example of discrete data is the number of children in a family, that is, 2 or 3 children, but not 2.5 children. All qualitative data are discrete.

(2) **Continuous data** are data for which there is an unlimited number of possible values. An example of continuous data is an individual's weight, which may actually be 159.232874. . . lb but is reported as 159 lb.

e. The **quality of measured data** is defined in terms of **the data's accuracy, validity, precision, and reliability**.

(1) **Accuracy** refers to the extent that the measurement measures the true value of what is under study.

(2) **Validity** refers to the extent that the measurement measures what it is supposed to measure.

(3) **Precision** refers to the extent that the measurement is consistent and reproducible.

(4) **Reliability** refers to the extent that the measurement is stable, dependable, and sound.

C. Distributions

1. Definition. A distribution is the complete summary of frequencies or proportions of a characteristic for a series of data from a sample or population.

2. Types of distributions

a. Binomial distribution is a distribution of possible outcomes from a series of data characterized by two mutually exclusive categories (see section III D 2).

b. Uniform distribution, also called **rectangular distribution**, is a distribution in which all events occur with an equal frequency.

c. Skewed distribution is a distribution that is asymmetric.

(1) A skewed distribution with a tail among the lower values being characterized is skewed to the left or **negatively skewed**.

(2) A skewed distribution with a tail among the higher values being characterized is skewed to the right or **positively skewed**.

d. Normal distribution, also called **Gaussian distribution**, is a continuous, symmetrical, bell-shaped distribution and can be defined by a number of measures (see section III E).

e. **Log-normal distribution** is a skewed distribution when graphed using an arithmetic scale but is a normal distribution when graphed using a logarithmic scale.
f. **Poisson distribution** is used to describe the occurrence of rare events in a large population.

II. DESCRIPTIVE STATISTICS

A. **Measures of central tendency** are characteristics that describe the middle or most commonly occurring values in a series; they are used as summary measures for the series. The series can consist of a sample of observations or a total population, and the values can be grouped or ungrouped. In this discussion, ungrouped data are presented and analyzed.

1. **Arithmetic mean**
   a. **Definition.** The arithmetic mean, which also is called simply the **mean**, is the sum of all values in a series divided by the actual number of values in the series.
   b. **Applications and characteristics**
      (1) The arithmetic mean is useful when performing analytic manipulations.
      (2) The arithmetic mean is sensitive to an extreme value in the series.
   c. **Calculation.** The arithmetic mean is determined as:

$$\bar{x} = \frac{\Sigma x_i}{n},$$

where $\bar{x}$ = the arithmetic mean; Σ = "the sum of"; x_i = each of the values in the series; and n = the number of values in the series. In describing a total population, the mean is symbolized by $\bar{\mu}$ and the number of the population by N.

   d. **Example.** The ages (in years) of 7 children seen in an emergency room after a house fire are: 1, 1, 1, 2, 4, 6, and 6. Since the sum of the ages (Σx_i) is 21 years and the number of children (n) is 7, the arithmetic mean ($\bar{x}$) of the ages is 21 years divided by 7, or 3 years.

2. **Median**
   a. **Definition**
      (1) The median is the value that divides the series into two equal groups so that half of the values are greater than and half are less than the median.
      (2) The median is the middle of the **quartiles**, which are the values that divide the series into quarters, and of the **percentiles**, which are the values that divide the series into defined percentages.
   b. **Applications and characteristics**
      (1) The median is not sensitive to one or more extreme values in a series; therefore, in a series with an extreme value, the median is a more representative measure of central tendency than the arithmetic mean.
      (2) The median is not as useful in analytic calculations as the arithmetic mean.
   c. **Calculation**
      (1) **In a series with an odd number of values**, the values in the series are arranged from lowest to highest, and the value that divides the series in half is the median.
      (2) **In a series with an even number of values**, the two values that divide the series in half are determined, and the arithmetic mean of these two values is the median.
      (3) **An alternative method** for calculating the median is to determine the 50% value on a **cumulative frequency curve** (see section II C 7).
   d. **Example.** Among the 7 children discussed above, 3 are younger than and 3 are older than 2 years. The median age of the children, therefore, is 2 years.

3. **Mode**
   a. **Definition.** The mode is the most commonly occurring value in a series of values. A series may have no mode (i.e., no value occurs more than once) or it may have several modes (i.e., several values equally occur at a higher frequency than the other values in the series).
   b. **Applications and characteristics**
      (1) The mode is useful in practical epidemiologic work, such as for determining the peak of disease occurrence in the investigation of a disease outbreak.
      (2) The mode is the most difficult measure of central tendency to manipulate mathematically; no analytic concepts are based on the mode.
   c. **Calculation.** The mode is calculated by determining which value or values occur most in a series.
   d. **Example.** Among the 7 children discussed above, the most common age is 1 year. Therefore, the mode of the ages is 1 year.

4. Geometric mean

a. Definition

(1) The geometric mean is the **nth root** of the product of the values in a series of **n values.**

(2) The geometric mean is most easily determined by calculating first the logarithms of the values, then the arithmetic mean of the logarithms, and finally the antilogarithm of the calculated arithmetic mean. Any logarithm base can be used.

b. Applications and characteristics

(1) The geometric mean is more useful and representative than the arithmetic mean when describing a series of reciprocal or fractional values, such as for a series of serum antibody titers or a series with a skewed distribution.

(2) The geometric mean can be used only for positive values.

(3) It is more difficult to calculate than the arithmetic mean.

c. Calculation. The geometric mean is determined as:

$$GM = \sqrt[n]{(x_1)(x_2)\ldots(x_n)} \text{ or} \qquad (A)$$

$$GM = \text{antilog } 1/n\,[\Sigma(\log x_i)], \qquad (B)$$

where GM = the geometric mean. The geometric mean is easier to calculate using equation B.

d. Example. Five individuals are tested for serum antibody to influenza A/Lilliput and are found to have reciprocal serum titers of 10, 100, 100, 10,000, and 1,000,000 (i.e., the serum titers are 1:10, 1:100, 1:100, 1:10,000, and 1:1,000,000, respectively).

(1) Using a base of 10, the **logarithms of the reciprocal titers** are: 1, 2, 2, 4, and 6, respectively. (Note that with $10^1 = 10$, $10^2 = 100$, $10^3 = 1000$, etc., the logarithms to the base of 10 are 1, 2, 3, etc., respectively.)

(2) Because the sum of the logarithms is 15 and there are 5 values, the arithmetic mean of the logarithms is calculated as 15 divided by 5, or 3.

(3) Finally, the **geometric mean** is calculated as the antilogarithm of 3 (to the base of 10) or 1000 (recall that $10^3 = 1000$). Therefore, the geometric mean reciprocal serum titer for the 5 individuals tested is 1000. (Incidentally, the geometric mean serum titer is 1:1000.)

B. Measures of dispersion are characteristics that are used to describe the variation and scatter of a series of values. The series can consist of a sample of observations or a total population, and the values can be grouped or ungrouped.

1. Range

a. Definition. The range is the difference between the highest and lowest values in a series.

b. Applications and characteristics

(1) The range is used to measure data spread.

(2) The range provides no information concerning the scatter within the series.

c. Calculation. The range is calculated by subtracting the lowest value in the series from the highest value.

d. Example. Five individuals arrested for driving automobiles under the influence of alcohol are aged 17, 18, 18, 21, and 26 years. The range of ages is 26 years minus 17 years, or 9 years.

2. Variance

a. Definition. The variance is the sum of the squared deviations from the mean divided by the number of values in the series minus 1.

b. Applications and characteristics

(1) The principal use of the variance is in calculating the standard deviation.

(2) By itself, the variance is mathematically unwieldy.

c. Calculation. The variance is determined as:

$$V = \frac{\Sigma(\bar{x} - x_i)^2}{n-1} \text{ or} \qquad (C)$$

$$V = \frac{\Sigma x_i^2}{n-1} - \frac{(\Sigma x_i)^2}{n(n-1)}, \qquad (D)$$

where V = the variance (s^2 is another symbol for the variance); Σx_i^2 = the sum of the squares of all x_i; $(\Sigma x_i)^2$ = the square of the sum of all x_i. Usually, the variance is easier to calculate using equation D. In describing a total population, the variance is symbolized by σ^2.

d. Example. The age variance for the 5 drunk drivers, whose mean age is 20 years, can be calculated in two ways using the data in Table 3-1.

Table 3-1. Calculating the Age Variance for Five Individuals

Case No.	Age (years)	Mean Age (years)	Deviation from the Mean	Deviation from the Mean Squared	Age Squared
1	17	20	− 3	9	289
2	18	20	− 2	4	324
3	18	20	− 2	4	324
4	21	20	+ 1	1	441
5	26	20	+ 6	36	676
Total	100	. . .	0	54	2054

(1) The variance can be calculated by using equation C.

(a) The sum of the squares of the deviations, which is 54, is divided by the number of values minus 1, which in this example is 5 minus 1, or 4.

(b) The variance, therefore, equals 13.5. In this example, the unit of the variance is $years^2$.

(2) Alternatively, the variance can be calculated by using equation D.

(a) The squares of the ages of the 5 individuals are summed (Σx_i^2) and then divided by the number of values minus 1, which in this example is 2054 divided by 4, or 513.5.

(b) The squared sum of all the ages is then calculated, which is 100^2 or 10,000.

(c) The squared sum is divided by both the number of values and the number of values minus 1, which in this example is 10,000 divided by 20, or 500.

(d) The variance is calculated by subtracting 500 from 513.5, which equals 13.5—the same as calculated using the first formula.

3. Standard deviation

a. Definition. The standard deviation is the positive square root of the variance.

b. Applications and characteristics. The standard deviation is the most useful measure of dispersion. In certain circumstances, quantitative probability statements that characterize a series, a sample of observations, or a total population can be derived from the standard deviation of the series, sample, or population (see sections III B 2, E).

c. Calculation. The standard deviation is determined as:

$$SD = +\sqrt{V},$$

where SD = the standard deviation (s is another symbol for the standard deviation). In describing a population, the standard deviation is symbolized by σ.

d. Example. The variance of the ages of the 5 drunk drivers is 13.5 $years^2$. The standard deviation of the ages, which is the square root of the variance, is 3.7 years.

4. Coefficient of variation

a. Definition. The coefficient of variation is the ratio of the standard deviation of a series to the arithmetic mean of the series. The coefficient of variation is unitless and is expressed as a percentage.

b. Applications and characteristics

(1) The coefficient of variation is used to compare the relative variation or spread of the distributions of different series, samples, or populations or of the distributions of different characteristics of a single series.

(2) The coefficient of variation can be used only for characteristics that are based on a scale with a true zero value.

c. Calculation. The coefficient of variation is calculated as:

$$CV\ (\%) = \frac{SD}{\bar{x}} \times 100,$$

where CV = the coefficient of variation.

d. Example

(1) In a typical medical school, the mean weight of 100 fourth-year medical students is 140 lb, with a standard deviation of 28 lb. The coefficient of variation for weight is 28 lb divided by 140 lb, or 20%.

(2) The mean height for these students is 66 in, with a standard deviation of 6 in. The coefficient of variation for height is 6 in divided by 66 in, or 9%.

(3) Based on the coefficients of variation, therefore, the relative spread of weight among the students is greater than that of height.

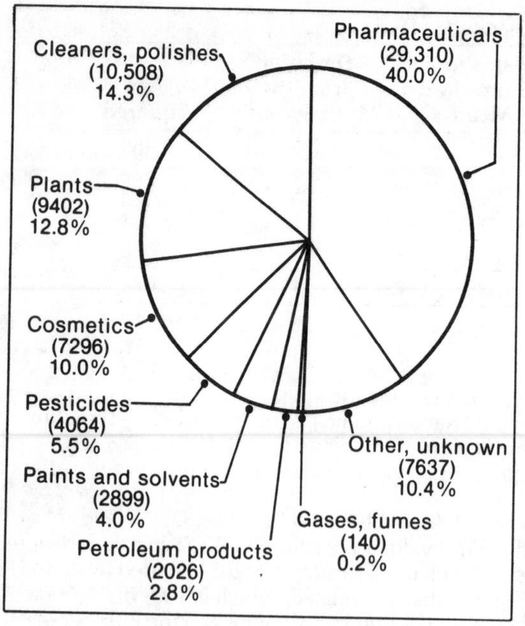

Figure 3-1. Pie chart shows the distribution of exposures to chemical products for children under 5 years of age in the United States in 1981, as reported by poison control centers to the Food and Drug Administration.

C. Graphic or pictorial presentations of data are useful in simplifying the presentation and enhancing the comprehension of data. All graphs, figures, and other pictures should have clearly stated and informative titles, and all axes and keys should be clearly labeled, including the appropriate units of measurement. Visual aids can take many forms; some basic methods of presenting data are described below.

1. Pie chart

a. Description. A pie chart is a pictorial representation of the proportional divisions of a sample or population, with the divisions often represented as parts of a whole circle.

b. Example. Figure 3-1 is a pie chart that depicts the findings of a surveillance system for exposures to chemical products for children. Note that pharmaceuticals accounted for 40.0% of the exposures and comprise the largest part of the "pie."

2. Venn diagram

a. Description. A Venn diagram shows the degrees of overlap and exclusivity for two or more characteristics or factors within a sample or population—in which case each characteristic is represented by a whole circle—or for a characteristic or factor among two or more samples or populations—in which case each sample or population is represented by a whole circle. The sizes of the circles need not be equal but may represent the relative size for each factor or population.

b. Example. Figure 3-2 depicts the reporting sources of deaths due to drowning in a bathtub. Note that the majority of deaths were reported through both surveillance systems.

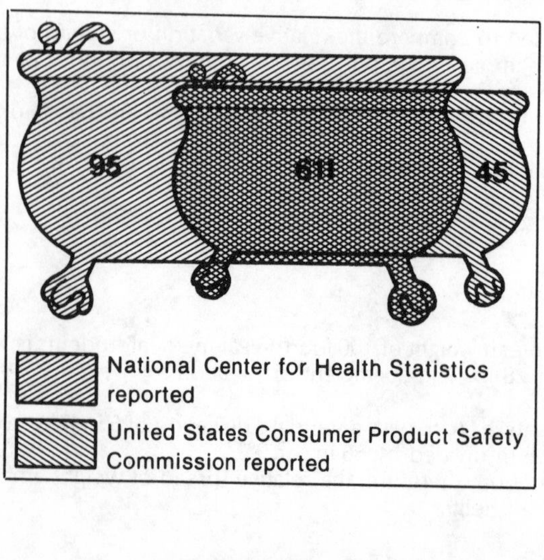

Figure 3-2. Venn diagram shows the number of bathtub-related drownings in the United States in 1979 through 1981, by reporting source.

3. Bar diagram

a. **Definition.** A bar diagram is a tool for comparing categories of mutually exclusive discrete data [see section I B 2 d (1)]. The different categories usually are indicated on the x-axis (abscissa). The frequency of data in each category is indicated on the y-axis (ordinate), and the categories are compared by the heights of the bars. Because the data categories are discrete, the bars can be arranged in any order on the x-axis with spaces between them.

b. **Example.** Figure 3-3 shows the incidence of tuberculosis in the United States in 1979. Note that the tuberculosis rate among nonwhite males exceeds that among white males by more than 40 cases per 100,000 population.

4. Histogram

a. **Description.** A histogram is a special form of bar diagram that represents categories of continuous and ordered data [see section I B 2 d (2)]. The bars are adjacent to each other on the x-axis, and there is no intervening space. The frequency of data in each category is depicted on the y-axis, and the width of the bar represents the interval of each category.

b. **Example.** Figure 3-4 depicts the frequency distribution of nosocomial infection rates among hospitals in a surveillance system in 1979. Note that the lowest nosocomial infection rates occurred more often in the community hospitals.

5. Epidemic curve

a. **Description.** An epidemic curve is a histogram that depicts the time course of an illness, disease, abnormality, or condition in a defined population and in a specified location and time period. The time-intervals are indicated on the x-axis, and the number of cases during each time interval are indicated on the y-axis. An epidemic curve can assist an investigator in determining such outbreak characteristics as the peak of disease occurrence (mode), a possible incubation or latency period, and the type of disease propagation (see Chapter 1, section V A 3).

b. **Example.** Figure 3-5 depicts the number of nursing home residents and employees with an influenza-like illness during one outbreak. Note that the onset of illness for the residents and employees was somewhat parallel and that the unimodal peak among the residents on December 21 is similar to that seen in a **common-source outbreak**.

6. Frequency polygon

a. **Description.** A frequency polygon is a representation of the distribution of categories of continuous and ordered data and, in this respect, is similar to a histogram. The x-axis depicts the categories of data and the y-axis the frequency of data in each category. In a frequency polygon, however, the frequency is plotted against the midpoint of each category, and a line is drawn through each of these plotted points. The frequency polygon can be more useful than the histogram because several frequency distributions can be plotted easily on one graph.

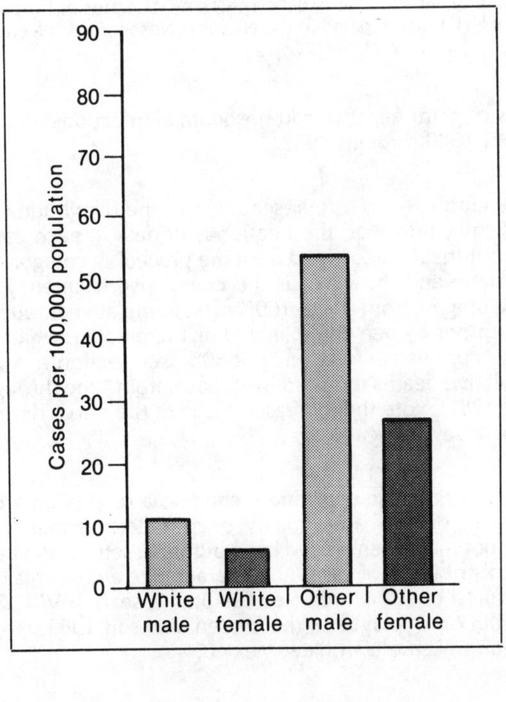

Figure 3-3. Bar chart shows the tuberculosis incidence by race and sex in the United States in 1979.

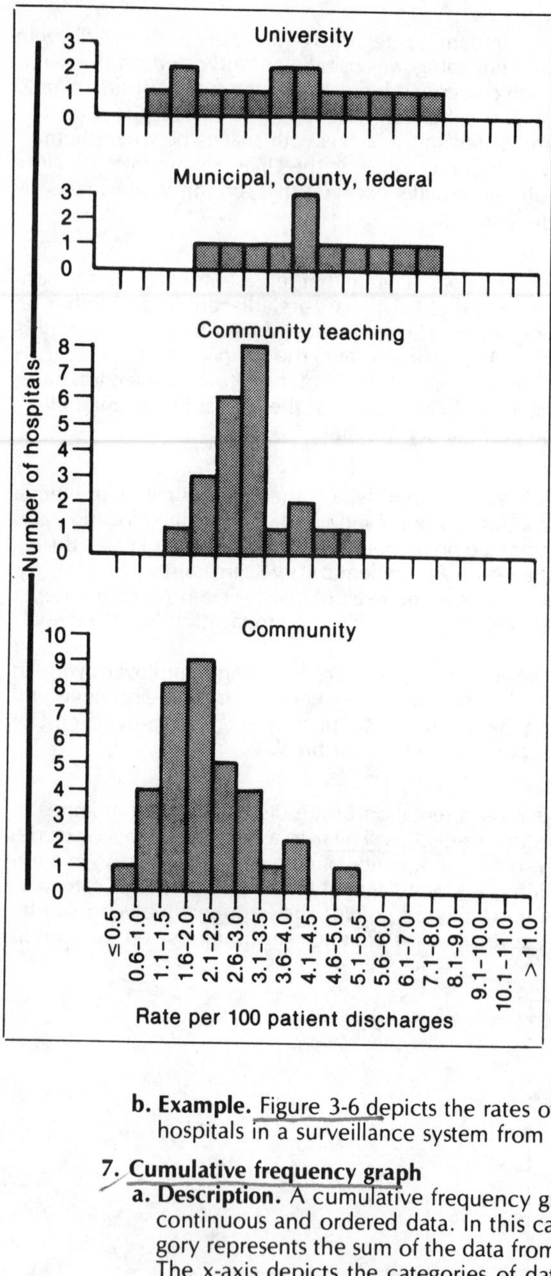

Figure 3-4. Histogram shows the frequency distribution of nosocomial infection rates by category of hospitals that participated in the National Nosocomial Infections Study in 1979.

b. Example. Figure 3-6 depicts the rates of gram-negative rod nosocomial infections among hospitals in a surveillance system from 1980 through 1982.

7. Cumulative frequency graph

a. Description. A cumulative frequency graph also is a representation of the distribution of continuous and ordered data. In this case, however, the frequency of data in each category represents the sum of the data from that category and from the preceding categories. The x-axis depicts the categories of data, and the y-axis is the cumulative frequency of data, sometimes given as a percentage ranging from 0% to 100%. The cumulative frequency graph is useful in calculating distributions by percentile, including the median, which is the category of data that occurs at the cumulative frequency of 50% (see section II A 2).

b. Example. Figure 3-7 depicts the cumulative deaths reported in St. Louis from June through August for the years 1979, 1980, and 1981. Note the increased slope of the curve during mid-July 1980, which occurred during a severe heat wave.

8. Spot map

a. Description. A spot map, also called a **geographic coordinate chart**, is a map of an area with the location of each case of an illness, disease, abnormality, or condition identified by a spot or other symbol on the map. A spot map often is used in an outbreak setting and can help an investigator to determine the distribution of cases and characterize an outbreak if the population at risk is evenly distributed over the area (see Chapter 1, section VI C 2).

b. Example. Figure 3-8 depicts the distribution of plague in the United States in 1983. Note that the greatest concentration of human plague is in New Mexico.

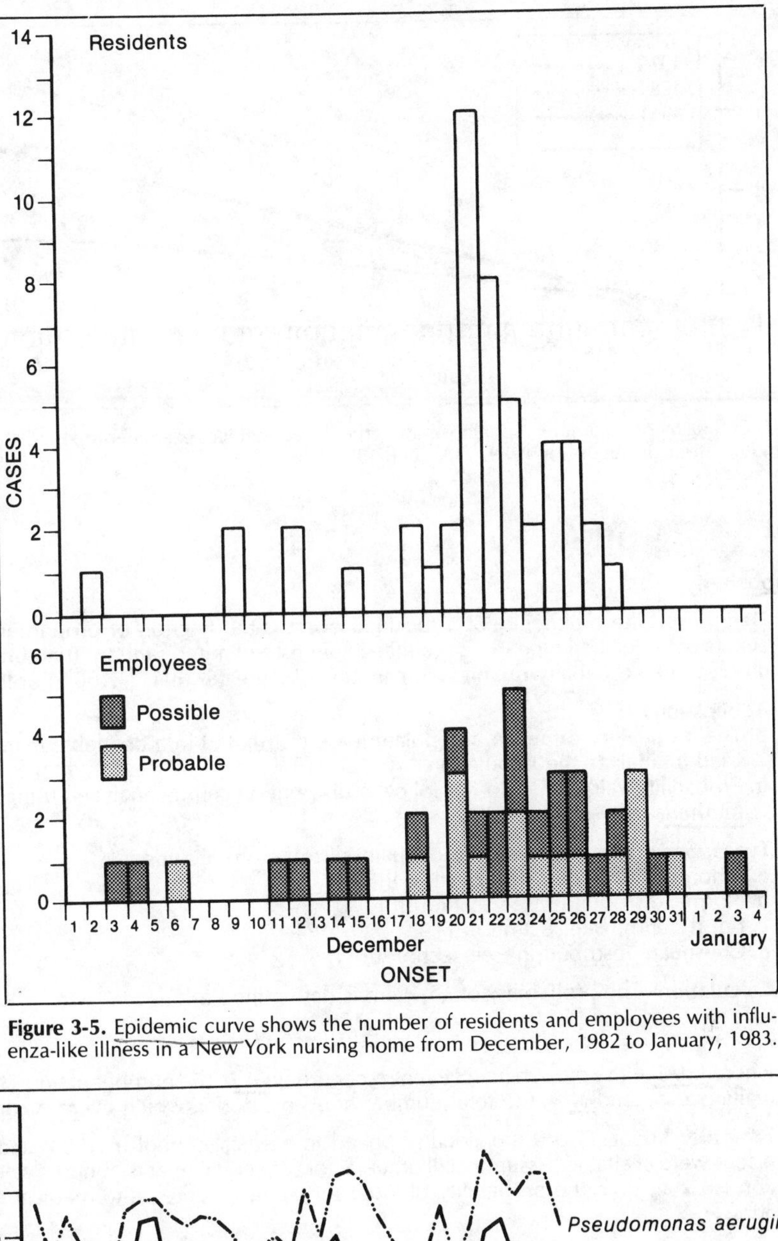

Figure 3-5. Epidemic curve shows the number of residents and employees with influenza-like illness in a New York nursing home from December, 1982 to January, 1983.

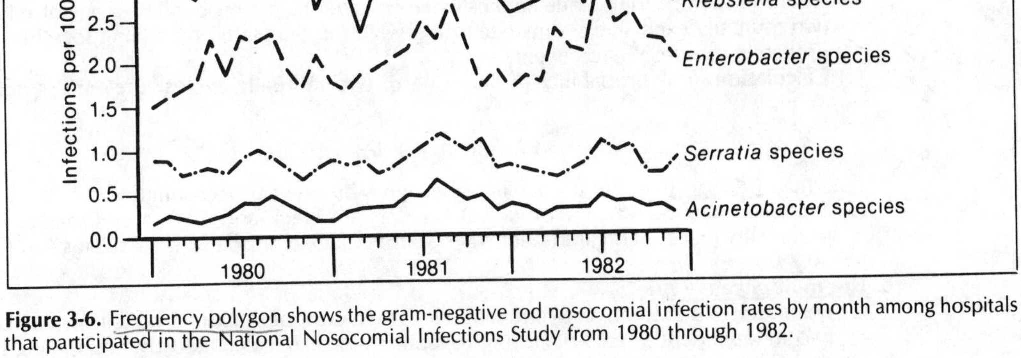

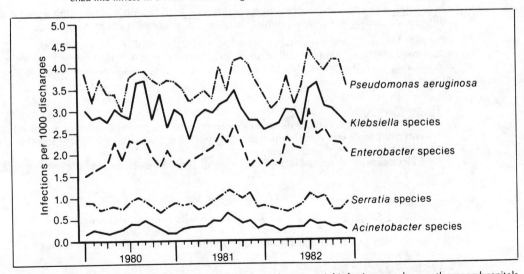

Figure 3-6. Frequency polygon shows the gram-negative rod nosocomial infection rates by month among hospitals that participated in the National Nosocomial Infections Study from 1980 through 1982.

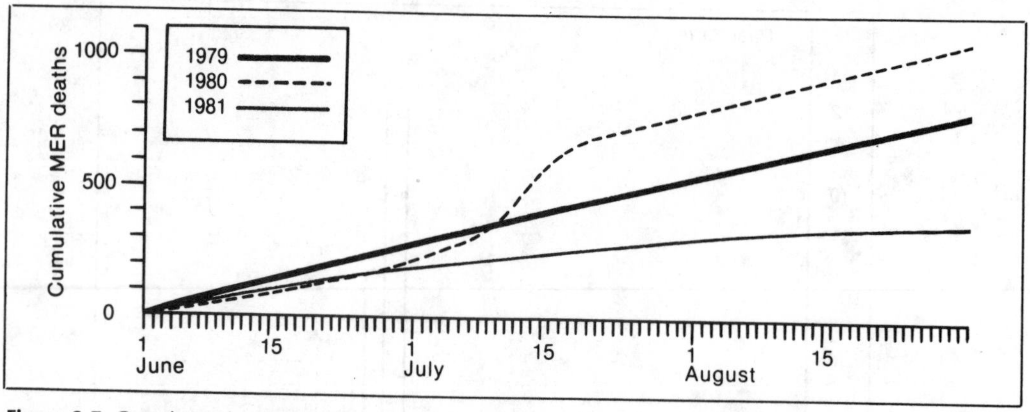

Figure 3-7. Cumulative frequency graph shows the cumulative medical examiner-reported (MER) deaths in St. Louis from June through August for 1979, 1980, and 1981.

III. ANALYTIC STATISTICS

A. Probability

1. **Definition.** The probability of a specified event is the fraction or proportion of all possible events of a specified type in a sequence of almost unlimited random trials under similar conditions. The probability of an event can never be greater than 1 (100%) or less than 0 (0%).
2. **Applications**
   a. The probability values in a population are distributed in a definable manner that can be used to analyze the population.
   b. Probability values that do not follow a distribution can be analyzed using **nonparametric methods** (see section III K).
3. **Types.** Some commonly used probability distributions include:
   a. Binomial distribution (see section III D)
   b. Normal distribution (see section III E)
   c. t distribution (see section III F)
   d. Chi-square distribution (see section III H)
4. **Calculation.** The probability of an event is determined as:

$$Pr(A) = A/N,$$

where Pr(A) = the probability of event A occurring; A = the number of times that event A actually occurs; and N = the total number of events during which event A can occur.

5. **Example.** About 35,200 individuals applied to medical school in 1983, and about 17,200 places were available. Assuming all other factors are equal, that is, random selection (see section I B 2 a), then the probability of a person being accepted into medical school is about 50%.
6. **Rules**
   a. **The additive rule**
      (1) **Definition.** The additive rule applies when considering the probability of one of at least two mutually exclusive events occurring, which is calculated by adding together the probability value of each event.
      (2) **Calculation.** The probability of only one of two mutually exclusive events is determined as:

$$Pr(A \text{ or } B) = Pr(A) + Pr(B),$$

      where Pr(A or B) = the probability of event A or event B occurring.
      (3) **Example.** About 5.4% of all medical students are black and 4.8% are Hispanic. The probability that a medical student will be either black or Hispanic is 5.4% plus 4.8%, or 10.2%.
   b. **The multiplicative rule**
      (1) **Definition.** The multiplicative rule applies when considering the probability of at least two independent events occurring together, which is calculated by multiplying the probability values for the events.

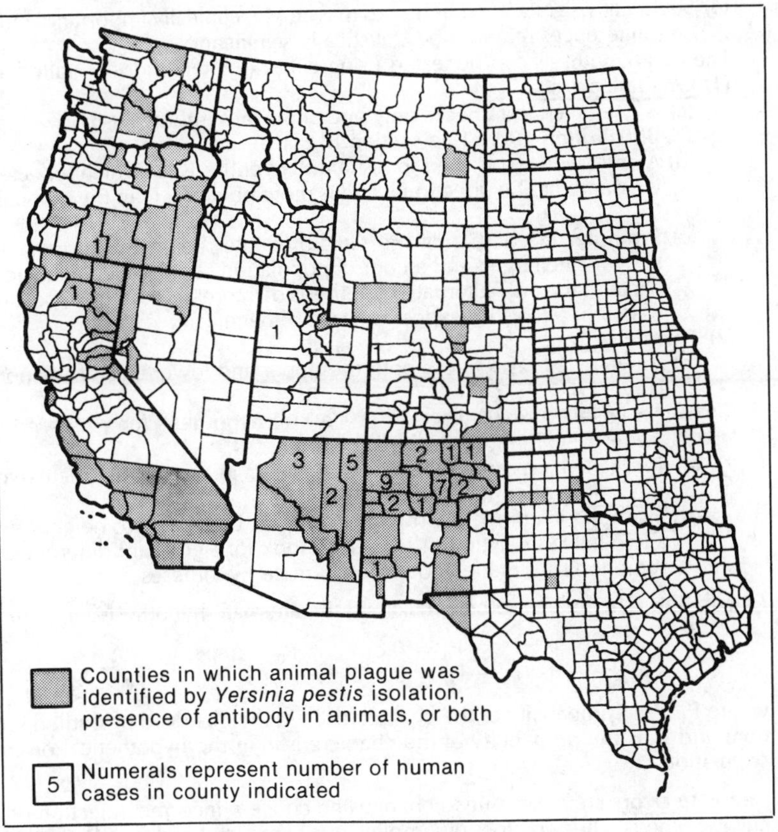

Figure 3-8. Spot map shows the geographic distribution of human and animal plague by county in the United States west of the Mississippi River in 1983.

(2) Calculation. The probability of two independent events occurring together is determined as:

$$Pr(A \text{ and } B) = Pr(A) \times Pr(B),$$

where Pr(A and B) = the probability of both event A and event B occurring.

(3) Example. About 5.4% of all medical students are black and 30.7% of all students are women. Assuming race and sex are independent selection factors, the percentage of students who are black women should be about 5.4% multiplied by 30.7%, or 1.7%.

B. The null hypothesis

1. Definition. The null hypothesis, symbolized as H_0, is the hypothesis that the samples or populations being compared in an experiment, study, or test are similar. Any difference discerned is ascribed to chance and not to any other factor.

2. Applications and characteristics

a. The null hypothesis is initially accepted and considered true for all analytic comparisons.

b. It is used to define **significant difference**. Significant difference, also called **statistical significance**, is the conclusion that a difference between the samples, populations, or both is due to factors other than chance. In other words, a significant difference occurs if the null hypothesis is disproved.

(1) When the null hypothesis is rejected, at least one alternate hypothesis is accepted, that is, factors other than chance account for the difference.

(2) When no significant difference can be shown between two populations, they may still be different; that is, accepting the null hypothesis does not necessarily mean the populations are identical.

(3) The **level of confidence** for rejecting the null hypothesis is arbitrary. One conventional cutoff for defining a significant difference is 5%, that is, if the probability that the difference is due to chance is 5% or less, then the null hypothesis is rejected, and an alternate hypothesis is accepted. This level of confidence refers to the **type I error** (see section III B 4 a).

(4) Statistically significant differences may not be clinically important, and clinically important differences may not be statistically significant.

c. The null hypothesis can be tested using either one-tailed or two-tailed analytic tests.

(1) One-tailed tests

(a) A one-tailed test checks only one of the tails (the upper or lower tail) of the **normal distribution curve** (see section III E 1 b).

(b) A one-tailed test is used to test a null hypothesis for which the alternate hypothesis is assumed to be directional and is more powerful than the two-tailed test for doing so.

(c) Example. In comparing the rates of cancer between a population exposed to a known carcinogen and a control population, a one-tailed analytic test can be used because the only alternate hypothesis of interest is that the exposure was harmful. It is assumed that the exposure was not beneficial.

(2) Two-tailed tests

(a) A two-tailed test checks both the upper and lower tails of the normal distribution curve.

(b) A two-tailed test is used to test a null hypothesis for which no assumptions are made concerning the alternate hypotheses.

(c) Two-tailed tests are especially useful when generating alternate hypotheses and are used more often than one-tailed tests.

(d) Example. In comparing the rates of death between two neighboring communities, a two-tailed analytic test is used to look for significant differences because no assumptions are made about the alternate hypotheses.

3. Calculation. The null hypothesis (H_0) and the alternate hypothesis (H_A) are determined as:

$$H_0: P_1 - P_0 = 0 \text{ or } P_1 = P_0$$
$$H_A: P_1 - P_0 \neq 0 \text{ or } P_1 \neq P_0,$$

where P_1 is the probability of the characteristic in the observed or studied sample or population; and P_0 is the probability of the characteristic in the hypothetical or control sample or population.

4. Sampling errors are errors due to chance and concern incorrect rejection or acceptance of a null hypothesis. The two types of sampling error are **type I** and **type II**. **Systematic errors**, also called **biases**, are discussed in Chapter 2.

a. Type I error

(1) Definition. A type I error, also called an **error of the first kind** or **an α error**, is the rejection of a null hypothesis that is actually true (Table 3-2). If the null hypothesis is false in a study, there can be no type I error.

(2) Applications

(a) Statistical testing is based predominantly on the α error. Many studies testing a null hypothesis arbitrarily use an α error of 0.05 (5%) as the cutoff for rejecting the null hypothesis. In studies that test multiple hypotheses, more stringent (i.e., lower) values for the α error need to be considered; in studies designed to generate hypotheses, other values of the α error may need to be considered.

(b) Sample size determinations depend on the type I error and the type II error (see section III B 4 b) as well as other parameters, such as the prevalence of the problem under study, the standard deviation, the amount of difference to be detected, and the relative number of experimental-to-control subjects.

(3) Example

(a) In a study of hemoglobin levels of students in different high schools, the α error is defined as 5%. The mean hemoglobin level in one school is 14 g/dl and in another 13 g/dl. The probability that this is due to chance is determined to be 15%, which is greater than the acceptable α error. The difference is not considered significant, and the null hypothesis is not rejected.

(b) However, if the study were repeated 100 times, the mean hemoglobin levels may appear significantly different statistically for five (5% of 100) of the trials, although there actually is no true difference between the populations. For these five trials, the null hypothesis has been incorrectly rejected, and a type I error has been made.

Table 3-2. Sampling Errors

	Decision	
Null Hypothesis	**Accept**	**Reject**
True	Correct conclusion	Type I or α error
False	Type II or β error	Correct conclusion

b. Type II error

(1) Definition. A type II error, also called an **error of the second kind** or **a β error**, is the acceptance of a null hypothesis as true when it actually is false (see Table 3-2). If the null hypothesis is true in a study, there can be no type II error. The type II error is inversely related to the type I error.

(2) Application. The type II error is used to determine the **power of a study**, which equals 1 minus β. The power of a study is the probability that the study would reject a null hypothesis as false when it actually is false, that is, that the study would detect a difference of specified size that actually exists. In determining the power for a study, the β error generally is at least double the α error. A power of 80% often is considered acceptable.

(3) Example. In the study of high school students, the β error is defined as 20%. Therefore, the power of the study is 80%. If there is a difference between the hemoglobin levels of the students, the probability of the study detecting the difference is 80% and of not detecting the difference is 20%.

C. Contingency table and degrees of freedom

1. Contingency table

a. Definition

(1) A contingency table depicts the cross-classification of data according to two characteristics, each of which can be divided into two or more discrete and mutually exclusive categories.

(a) A contingency table in which there are more than two categories for either or both characteristics is called an **r × c table**, where r = the number of horizontal rows and c = the number of vertical columns.

(b) A contingency table in which the characteristics are divided into only two categories is called a **2 × 2** or **fourfold table.**

b. Application. The contingency table is a simple method for displaying data and is useful when performing chi-square and other tests (see section III H, I).

c. Structure. The structure of a contingency table is depicted in Table 3-3, in which the value in each cell is represented by a, b, c, or d; the marginal values, which are subtotals, are represented by a + b, a + c, b + c, and c + d; and the grand total, which equals a + b + c + d, is represented by N.

d. Example. Table 3-4C is an example of a fourfold contingency table, in which the sex and eye color of 50 schoolchildren are tabulated.

2. Degrees of freedom

a. Definition

(1) The degrees of freedom is the number of variables in a series or distribution that can be freely assigned values when the sum of the values is fixed.

(2) In a contingency table, the degrees of freedom is the number of cells available in the table that can be freely assigned values, assuming set and established marginal values. Once these cells have been assigned values, the values of all the remaining cells in the table are automatically determined.

b. Application. In a number of probability distributions, such as the **t distribution** (see section III F) and the **chi-square distribution** (see section III H), the probability values vary with the number of degrees of freedom of the sample.

c. Calculation

(1) When the distribution has either a single row or a single column, the number of degrees of freedom is determined as:

$$df = c - 1, \text{ if } r = 1 \text{ or}$$
$$df = r - 1, \text{ if } c = 1,$$

where df = the degrees of freedom.

Table 3-3. The Structure of a Contingency Table

	Characteristic A		
Characteristic B	**Category A-1**	**Category A-2**	**Total**
Category B-1	a	b	a + b
Category B-2	c	d	c + d
Total	a + c	b + d	N

Table 3-4. The Distribution of Eye Color by Sex for 50 Schoolchildren

	Sex		
Eye Color	**Male**	**Female**	**Total**
A. Marginal Values and Total Are Known			
Blue	a	b	15
Brown	c	d	35
Total	20	30	50
B. Value in One Cell Is Known			
Blue	5	b	15
Brown	c	d	35
Total	20	30	50
C. Values in All Cells Are Known			
Blue	5	10	15
Brown	15	20	35
Total	20	30	50

(2) When the table has at least two rows and two columns, the number of degrees of freedom is determined as:

$$df = (r - 1)(c - 1).$$

d. Example. In a fourfold table in which the sex and eye color of 50 schoolchildren are tabulated, the marginal values are 20, 30, 15, and 35, and the total is 50 (see Table 3-4*A*).

(1) It is determined that 5 boys have blue eyes, and all the children have either blue or brown eyes (see Table 3-4*B*). Therefore, the number of boys with brown eyes must be 15, the number of girls with blue eyes must be 10, and the number of girls with brown eyes must be 20 (see Table 3-4*C*). Because it is necessary to determine the value in only one cell to determine the value of all the cells, this table has 1 degree of freedom.

(2) Alternatively, the number of degrees of freedom could be determined from the equation. Since there are two rows and two columns, the number of degrees of freedom is calculated as:

$$(2 - 1)(2 - 1), \text{ which equals } 1.$$

D. Binomial distribution

1. Definition. A binomial distribution of data is the distribution that results when there are only two mutually exclusive, and therefore discrete, outcomes in a series of independent trials of an event.

2. Application. A binomial distribution is used when a problem relates to the probability of two mutually exclusive outcomes in a known number of trials. The probability of each of the two outcomes is the same in each of the trials, but the result of each trial is independent from the results of the other trials. Standard deviations can be derived from the binomial distribution and confidence limits can be established (see section III G 2).

3. Calculation. The probability in a binomial distribution is determined as:

$$f(x) = \frac{n!}{x!\,(n - x)!}\,p^x q^{n-x},$$

where f(x) = the probability of obtaining x values in n trials; p = the probability of one of two possible outcomes (e.g., a success) in a single trial; q = the probability of the other possible outcome (e.g., a failure) in a single trial; n = the size of each independent trial; x = the number of successes in one trial of size n; n − x = the number of failures in the same trial; and ! = the factorial sign. (The factorial sign, which is also read as "prime," indicates the product of the preceding whole number and all smaller whole numbers to 1. Both 1! and 0! are defined as being equal to 1.)

4. Example. When a couple is expecting a baby, the probability of having a girl is about 50%

(p = 0.50), and the probability of having a boy is about 50% (q = 0.50). If a couple has 7 children (n = 7), the probability that they will have 2 girls (x = 2) and 5 boys (n − x = 5) is calculated as:

$$\begin{aligned} f(2) &= \{7!/[(2!)(5!)]\}\,(0.50^2)(0.50^5) \\ &= \{5040/[(2)(120)]\}\,(0.25)(0.03) \\ &= (21)(0.25)(0.03) \\ &= 0.16, \text{ or } 16\%. \end{aligned}$$

A useful shortcut when calculating with factorials is to cancel like terms before multiplying out the factorial expression. In the calculation above, 7!/[(2!)(5!)] can be simplified because 7!, or (7)(6)(5)(4)(3)(2)(1), is equal to (7)(6)(5!). The 5! term, therefore, can be canceled from both the numerator and denominator, which reduces 7!/[(2!)(5!)] to (7)(6)/2.

E. Normal distribution

1. Definition

a. The normal distribution, also called the **Gaussian distribution**, is a theoretical, continuous, symmetrical, unimodal distribution of infinite range.

b. The normal distribution curve is bell-shaped, with lower and upper tails, and is determined by the mean and the standard deviation of the population.

c. The mean, median, and mode of a normally distributed population are equal.

2. Applications

a. The normal distribution can be used to characterize many populations and samples, especially large ones.

b. The normal distribution and normal approximations are the bases of a number of analytic tests, such as chi-square tests (see section III H).

3. The **critical ratio** or **z score** is the number of standard deviations that a value in a normally distributed population lies away from the mean.

a. Increasing the critical ratio corresponds to decreasing the probability for accepting the null hypothesis.

b. The proportion of the population (or the probability of finding a member of the population) within each critical ratio, within ± each critical ratio, and outside ± each critical ratio are listed in Table 3-5.

c. In a normally distributed population, about 68% of the population lies within 1 critical ratio (i.e., within the mean ± 1 standard deviation), about 95.5% lies within 2 critical ratios of the mean, and about 99.7% lies within 3 critical ratios of the mean (Fig. 3-9).

d. In large samples, the critical ratio is used to calculate confidence intervals around the sample mean.

4. Calculation. The critical ratio is determined as:

$$z = \frac{x - \bar{\mu}}{\sigma},$$

where z = the critical ratio; x = the value being tested; $\bar{\mu}$ = the population mean; and σ = the population standard deviation.

5. Example. One thousand randomly selected men have a mean weight of 160 lb, with a standard deviation of 10 lb. The population is normally distributed with respect to weight.

a. About 680 (68%) of the men have weights of 160 ± 1(10) lb (mean ± 1 standard

Table 3-5. Table of Critical Ratio (abbreviated)

Critical Ratio	Probability of Lying: Within the Critical Ratio	Within ± the Critical Ratio	Outside ± the Critical Ratio
1.0	0.341	0.683	0.317
1.645	0.450	0.900	0.100
1.96	0.475	0.950	0.050
2.0	0.477	0.954	0.046
2.576	0.495	0.990	0.010
3.0	0.499	0.997	0.003

Reprinted from Centers for Disease Control: *Analytic Statistics: Statistical Methods—Testing for Significance*. Washington, DC, US Department of Health and Human Services, Public Health Service, May, 1981.

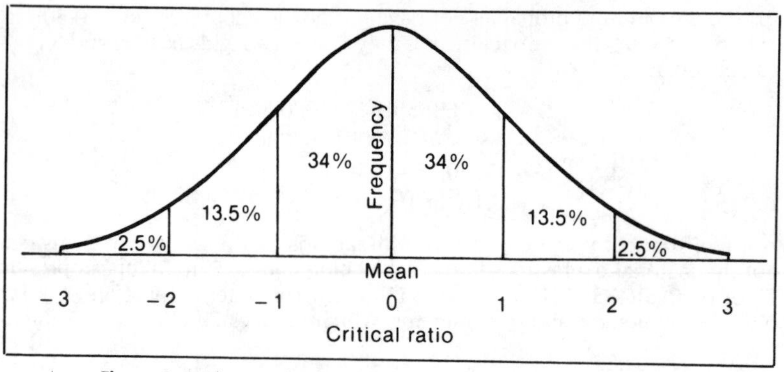

Figure 3-9. The standardized normal distribution by critical ratio.

deviation), that is, weights ranging from 150 to 170 lb; about 950 (95%) have weights of 160 ± 2(10) lb (mean ± 2 standard deviations) or weights ranging from 140 to 180 lb; and about 997 (99.7%) have weights of 160 ± 3(10) lb (mean ± 3 standard deviations) or weights ranging from 130 to 190 lb.

b. Similarly, about 340 (34%) of the men weigh between 160 and 170 lb (mean to mean + 1 standard deviation); about 135 (13.5%) of the men weigh between 140 and 150 lb (mean − 2 standard deviations to mean − 1 standard deviation); and about 2–3 (2.5%) of the men weigh greater than 180 lb (mean + 2 standard deviations).

F. Student's t tests, based on the **t distribution**, which reflects greater variation due to chance than the normal distribution, are used to analyze small samples. The t distribution is a continuous, symmetrical, unimodal distribution of infinite range, which is bell-shaped, similar to the shape of the normal distribution, but more spread out. As the sample size increases, the t distribution closely resembles the normal distribution. At infinite degrees of freedom, the t and normal distributions are identical, and the t values equal the critical ratio values.

1. Student's t test for a single small sample

a. Definition. Student's t test for a single small sample compares a single sample with a population.

b. Applications and characteristics

(1) Student's t tests are used to evaluate the null hypothesis for continuous variables for sample sizes less than 30.

(2) Student's t tests are used in analyses for which a sample standard deviation is substituted as an estimate for an unknown population standard deviation.

(3) Either the proportions or the actual counts of the variables can be employed in Student's t tests.

(4) Probability values are derived from the t value and the number of degrees of freedom by using the t table. (Table 3-6 is an abbreviated t table.) For each degree of freedom, a row of increasing t values corresponds to a row of decreasing probabilities for accepting the null hypothesis.

(5) The probability statements derived from Student's t tests are dependent on the sample size in two ways.

(a) The sample size is related to the value of the t. As the sample size decreases, the t value decreases and the probability that the difference noted is ascribed to chance increases, that is, there is an increased probability for accepting the null hypothesis.

(b) The sample size is directly related to the number of degrees of freedom. As the number of degrees of freedom decreases, for a constant t value, the probability that the difference noted is ascribed to chance increases.

(c) Even though the t distribution is more appropriate than the normal distribution for analyzing small samples, statistically significant differences observed in small samples may be overestimates of true differences.

(6) In small samples, especially those sized less than 30, the t distribution is used to calculate confidence intervals around the sample mean (see section III G 2).

c. Calculation. The t value for comparing a sample mean with a population mean is determined as:

$$t(df) = \frac{\bar{x} - \bar{\mu}}{SD/\sqrt{n}},$$

Table 3-6. t Table (abbreviated)

Degrees of Freedom	Probability 0.10	0.05	0.01
1	6.31	12.71	63.66
2	2.92	4.30	9.93
8	1.86	2.31	3.36
9	1.83	2.26	3.25
10	1.81	2.23	3.17
∞	1.64	1.96	2.58

Reprinted from Centers for Disease Control: *Analytic Statistics: Statistical Methods—Testing for Significance*. Washington DC, US Department of Health and Human Services, Public Health Service, May, 1981.

where t(df) = the t value at the degrees of freedom; df = the number of degrees of freedom, which equals n − 1; $\bar{x}$ = the sample mean; $\bar{\mu}$ = the population mean; SD = the sample standard deviation; and n = the number in the sample. The denominator of the equation is the standard error of the sample mean.

d. **Example.** The mean serum sodium concentration for 9 patients is 150 mg/dl, with a standard deviation of 6 mg/dl. The mean serum sodium concentration for all individuals in the community is 140 mg/dl.

(1) The t value—calculated from the equation with $\bar{x}$ = 150, $\bar{\mu}$ = 140, SD = 6, and n = 9—is equal to 5.

(2) The probability is determined from the t table (see Table 3-6). For (9 − 1) or 8 degrees of freedom and a t value of 5, the probability is less than 0.01 that the observed difference between the sample and population means is due to chance.

(3) If an arbitrary cutoff of 0.05 is accepted for statistical significance, then the difference between the sample mean and the population mean is significantly greater than the difference expected due to chance alone. The null hypothesis is rejected.

2. Student's t test for independent samples

a. Definition. Student's t test for independent samples compares the means of two small samples.

b. Applications and characteristics. The uses and restrictions of Student's t test for independent samples are similar to those for other Student's t tests, except that both sample sizes are less than 30. Student's t test is inappropriate to use if more than two means are compared, unless adjustments for multiple comparisons are made.

c. Calculation. The t value for comparing the means from two independent samples is determined as:

$$t(df) = \frac{|\bar{x} - \bar{y}|}{SD_p \sqrt{\frac{1}{n_x} + \frac{1}{n_y}}}$$

with:

$$SD_p = \sqrt{\frac{\Sigma(\bar{x} - x_i)^2 + \Sigma(\bar{y} - y_i)^2}{(n_x - 1) + (n_y - 1)}},$$

where t(df) = the t value at the degrees of freedom; df = the number of degrees of freedom, which equals $n_x + n_y - 2$; $\bar{x}$ = the mean from sample x; $\bar{y}$ = the mean from sample y; n_x = the number in sample x; n_y = the number in sample y; SD_p = the pooled standard deviation from both samples x and y; and | | = "absolute value of" or the difference between the values expressed with a positive sign. The denominator of Student's t test is the standard error of the difference between the means.

d. **Example.** Serum sodium concentration is measured in two groups of patients. The serum sodium levels (in mg/dl) in one group of 6 patients are 142, 147, 148, 149, 153, and 155, with a mean of 149 mg/dl; and the serum sodium levels in another group of 5 patients are 138, 139, 142, 143, and 144, with a mean of 141 mg/dl. To determine the probability that the 8 mg/dl difference between the means is due to chance, the t value is determined according to the above equations. In this example: $\bar{x}$ = 149; $\bar{y}$ = 141; n_x = 6; n_y = 5; and SD_p = 3.54. The t value at 9 degrees of freedom equals 1.2, and the associated probability that the difference is due to chance, according to Table 3-6, is greater than 0.10. The null hypothesis is not rejected.

3. Student's t test for paired samples

a. Definition. Student's t test for paired samples compares the means of two small paired samples.

b. Uses. The uses and restrictions of Student's t test for paired samples are similar to those for other Student's t tests, except that this test is restricted to samples with matched pairs of less than 30 each.

c. Calculation. The t value for comparing the means from two paired samples is determined as:

$$t(df) = \frac{\bar{d}}{SD_p/\sqrt{n}}$$

with:

$$SD_p = \sqrt{\frac{\Sigma(d_i - \bar{d})^2}{n - 1}} \quad \text{or} \qquad \text{(E)}$$

$$SD_p = \sqrt{\frac{\Sigma d_i^2 - (\Sigma d_i)^2/n}{n - 1}}, \qquad \text{(F)}$$

where t(df) = the t value at the degrees of freedom; df = the number of degrees of freedom, which equals n − 1; d_i = the difference between each pair; $\bar{d}$ = the mean difference; and n = the number of pairs.

(1) The denominator of Student's t test is the standard error of the difference between the means.

(2) The pooled standard deviation is easier to calculate with equation F.

(3) The t value is used to determine the probability that the difference between the means of the pairs is due to chance at the calculated degrees of freedom (see Table 3-6).

d. Example. Eleven medical students are given separate tests on the subjects of internal medicine and general surgery. The two scores for each student represent a matched pair and are listed in Table 3-7. To determine the probability that the difference between each paired sample is due to chance, the t value is determined according to the above equations.

(1) The difference between each paired sample is calculated.

(2) The arithmetic mean of the differences is calculated and is 302 divided by 11, or 27.5.

(3) The squares of the differences are calculated, and the sum of the squares is 21,294.

(4) The square of the sum of the differences (91,204) divided by the number of pairs (11) equals 8291, which is subtracted from the sum of the squares (21,294). The resulting difference (13,003) is divided by the number of degrees of freedom (10), which yields the variance (1300).

(5) The standard deviation (36.1), which is the square root of the variance, is divided by the square root of the number of samples (3.3) to yield the standard error (10.9).

(6) The t value equals the mean difference between the samples (27.5) divided by the standard error (10.9) and equals 2.5.

(7) For 10 degrees of freedom, according to Table 3-6, a t value of 2.23 is associated with a

Table 3-7. The Association between Internal Medicine and General Surgery Test Scores for 11 Students

Medical Student Number	Internal Medicine Score	General Surgery Score	Difference between Scores	Square of Difference
1	75	90	−15	225
2	85	10	+75	5625
3	93	20	+73	5329
4	55	55	0	0
5	79	60	+19	361
6	86	30	+56	3136
7	90	70	+20	400
8	76	85	−9	81
9	89	25	+64	4096
10	54	75	−21	441
11	92	52	+40	1600
Total	874	572	+302	21,294

probability that the difference between the means of two samples is due to chance is 0.05. In this example, the t value indicates a probability between 0.05 and 0.01.

(8) With a 0.05 cutoff for rejecting the null hypothesis, the internal medicine and general surgery test scores are significantly different for these students. The null hypothesis is rejected.

G. The standard error and confidence limits

1. Standard error of the mean

a. Definition

(1) The **standard error** of a measure is based on a sample of a population and is the estimate of the standard deviation of the measure for the population.

(2) The **standard error of the mean**, one of the most commonly used types of standard error, is a measure of the accuracy of the sample mean as an estimate of the population mean. In comparison, the standard deviation is a measure of the variability of the observations.

(a) When studying a population, many different samples can be chosen, and the value of the mean of a characteristic for each sample may be different. Often, the means of the samples follow a normal distribution, even if the original population was not normally distributed. The **distribution of the means** of the samples has a standard deviation around the population mean, and the standard error of the mean from one sample is an estimate of this standard deviation.

(b) The standard error of the mean is based on the standard deviation of the sample and the sample size. As the sample size increases, the sample better reflects the total population, the sample mean more closely estimates the population mean, and the standard error of the mean from that sample decreases.

b. Uses

(1) The standard error of the mean is used to construct confidence limits around a sample mean (see section III G 2).

(2) Standard errors are used in Student's t test (see section III F).

c. Calculation. The standard error of the mean (SEM) is determined as:

$$\text{SEM} = \frac{\text{SD}}{\sqrt{n}},$$

where n = the number of observations in the sample.

d. Example. The mean weight of 100 randomly selected medical students is 140 lb, with a standard deviation of 28 lb. The standard error of the mean of the weights equals 28 lb divided by the square root of 100, which is 2.8 lb. Therefore, 2.8 lb is the estimate of the standard deviation of the population from which the sample was taken.

2. Confidence limits of a mean

a. Definition

(1) Confidence limits. The upper and lower confidence limits define the range of probability, that is, the **confidence interval** for a measure of the population based on a measure of a sample and the measure's standard error. Confidence intervals are expressed in terms of probability based on the α error. A $(1 - \alpha)$ confidence interval indicates that there is a $1 - \alpha$ probability that the population mean lies within the upper and lower confidence limits and an α probability that it lies outside these limits.

(2) The **confidence limits of a mean** define the confidence interval for the population mean based on a sample mean.

(a) For large samples, confidence limits are based on the critical ratio for the associated probability.

(b) For small samples (less than 30), confidence limits are based on the t value for the number of degrees of freedom and the associated probability.

b. Uses

(1) Confidence limits of a mean are used to estimate a population mean based on a sample from the population.

(2) The most commonly used confidence limits are 95% confidence limits, which indicate that there is a 95% probability that the population mean lies within the upper and lower confidence limits and a 5% probability that it lies outside these limits.

(3) Confidence intervals can be used in analyzing the binomial and Poisson distributions.

c. Calculation

(1) For large samples, the confidence limits of a mean are determined as:

$$(1 - \alpha) \text{ confidence limits} = \bar{x} \pm z_\alpha \text{ SEM or} \quad \text{(G)}$$

$$P(\bar{x} - z_\alpha \text{ SEM} \le \bar{\mu} \le \bar{x} + z_\alpha \text{ SEM}) = 1 - \alpha, \quad \text{(H)}$$

(2) And for small samples, the confidence limits of a mean are determined as:

$$(1 - \alpha) \text{ confidence limits} = \bar{x} \pm t_{df,\alpha} \text{ SEM or} \quad (I)$$

$$P(\bar{x} - t_{df,\alpha} \text{ SEM} \leq \bar{\mu} \leq \bar{x} + t_{df,\alpha} \text{ SEM}) = 1 - \alpha, \quad (J)$$

where $\bar{x} - z_\alpha$ SEM or $\bar{x} - t_{df,\alpha}$ SEM = the lower confidence limit; $\bar{x} + z_\alpha$ SEM or $\bar{x} + t_{df,\alpha}$SEM = the upper confidence limit; P = the probability that the population mean ($\bar{\mu}$) lies within the confidence limits; α = the type I error; n = the sample size; z_α = the critical ratio; and $t_{df,\alpha}$ = the t score at n − 1 degrees of freedom. When a smaller α error is accepted, the confidence interval is wider, and the probability that the population mean lies within the confidence limits is greater.

d. **Example.** Consider again the 100 medical students whose mean weight is 140 lb, with a standard error of 2.8 lb.

(1) For 95% confidence limits, α = 0.05 and z = 1.96 (sometimes approximated by 2).
  (a) The 95% lower confidence limit is 140 − (1.96) (2.8) = 134.5 lb.
  (b) The 95% upper confidence limit is 140 + (1.96) (2.8) = 145.5 lb.
  (c) Therefore, there is a 95% probability that the mean weight of the population of medical students from which the sample is drawn is between 134.5 lb and 145.5 lb, inclusive.

(2) For 99% confidence limits, α = 0.01 and z = 2.576.
  (a) The 99% lower confidence limit is 140 − (2.576) (2.8) = 132.8 lb.
  (b) The 99% upper confidence limit is 140 + (2.576) (2.8) = 147.2 lb.
  (c) The 99% confidence interval is between 132.8 lb and 147.2 lb, inclusive.

(3) If the sample size were 20, the calculations would be the same except that the t values for 19 degrees of freedom (2.09 for 95% confidence limits and 2.86 for 99% confidence limits) would be substituted for the critical ratio values.

H. Chi-square tests

1. r × c chi-square test

a. Definition

(1) The r × c chi-square test determines the extent that a single observed series of proportions differs from a theoretical or expected distribution of proportions or the extent that two or more series, proportions, or frequencies differ from one another, based on the **chi-square probability distribution**.

(2) The chi-square distribution is a continuous asymmetric distribution based on a normal approximation of the binomial distribution. The chi-square distribution at 1 degree of freedom is identical to the distribution of the squares of the critical ratio.

b. Applications and characteristics

(1) The r × c chi-square test is used to determine the extent that an observed distribution differs from a theoretical or expected distribution, or that two or more distributions differ from each other.

(2) The categories of data used in chi-square tests must be mutually exclusive and discrete.

(3) Only actual counts of the variables can be employed in chi-square tests.

(4) The r × c chi-square test can be used only if the theoretical or expected value of each variable is equal to or greater than 5. Observed values can be less than 5.

(5) Chi-square tests do not take into account whether the categories of data are ordered.

(6) Probability values are derived from the chi-square value and the number of degrees of freedom by using a chi-square table. For each degree of freedom, a row of increasing chi-square values corresponds to a row of decreasing probabilities for accepting the null hypothesis. (Table 3-8 is an abbreviated chi-square table.)

c. **Goodness of fit test** is one type of r × c chi-square test, which is used for a contingency table with only one row or one column. The value of the chi-square is determined as for other r × c contingency tables, but the number of degrees of freedom is calculated differently (see section III C 2 c).

d. Yates correction factor.

(1) Because the chi-square is based on a normal approximation of the binomial distribution, a correction for continuity, called **Yates correction factor**, often is included in the chi-square test equation.

(2) A chi-square symbol with the correction (c) subscript indicates that the chi-square value was calculated with the correction for continuity. Unless otherwise stated, a chi-square symbol without the correction subscript indicates that the chi-square value was calculated without the correction.

(3) The Yates correction factor is used for small samples.

(4) The Yates correction factor decreases the chi-square value and makes the probability estimate greater than it would have been without the correction.

Table 3-8. Chi-square table (abbreviated)

Degrees of Freedom	Probability		
	0.10	**0.05**	**0.01**
1	2.71	3.84	6.64
2	4.61	5.99	9.21
3	6.25	7.82	11.35

Reprinted from Centers for Disease Control: *Analytic Statistics: Statistical Methods—Testing for Significance*. Washington DC, US Department of Health and Human Services, Public Health Service, May, 1981.

(5) The Yates correction factor tends to decrease the likelihood of a type I error, that is, the null hypothesis is less often rejected.

e. Calculation. The chi-square value is determined as:

$$\chi^2_c(df) = \frac{(|O_i - E_i| - ½)^2}{E_i},$$

where $\chi^2_c(df)$ = the chi-square value that reflects the correction for continuity at the calculated degrees of freedom; O_i = the observed frequency or count for each variable or cell; E_i = the theoretical or expected frequency or count for each variable or cell; and the ½ in the numerator is Yates correction factor.

f. Example. Over a 4-year period, 95 individuals are electrocuted in bathtubs. The deaths are distributed by season as shown in Table 3-9. The probability that the seasonal distribution differs from what would be expected if there were no seasonal distribution (the null hypothesis) is calculated as follows.

(1) The expected number of deaths in each season is calculated as 24.

(2) The number of deaths that deviated from the expected number is calculated ($O_i - E_i$), Yates correction factor is subtracted, and this value is squared.

(3) Each of the squared deviates is divided by the respective expected number of deaths for that season.

(4) The sum of these values is the value of the chi-square (8.87).

(5) The number of degrees of freedom is 3.

(6) The probability is determined from a chi-square table (see Table 3-8). For 3 degrees of freedom and a chi-square value of 8.87, the probability is between 0.05 and 0.01 that the seasonal distribution observed is due to chance.

(7) If an arbitrary cutoff of 0.05 is accepted for statistical significance, that is, to reject the null hypothesis, then the seasonal distribution is significantly different from the distribution expected due to chance alone. The null hypothesis is rejected.

2. 2 × 2 chi-square test

a. Definition. The 2 × 2 chi-square test, a type of r × c chi-square test, is specific for fourfold or 2 × 2 contingency tables. The 2 × 2 chi-square always has 1 degree of freedom.

b. Applications. The uses and restrictions of the 2 × 2 chi-square test are the same as for the r × c chi-square test, except that it is restricted to fourfold table data analysis.

c. Calculation. The 2 × 2 chi-square value is determined using the same general chi-square equation as the r × c chi-square value. It is also determined more simply as:

$$\chi^2_c = \frac{N(|ad - bc| - N/2)^2}{(a+b)(c+d)(a+c)(b+d)}.$$

The symbols are the same as for the fourfold contingency table (see section III C 1 and Table 3-3). N/2 is the Yates correction factor.

Table 3-9. Calculating the Chi-square Value for Bathtub-Related Electrocutions by Season

Season	Observed Frequency (O_i)	Expected Frequency (E_i)	$O_i - E_i$	$(\|O_i - E_i\| - 0.5)^2$	$\frac{(\|O_i - E_i\| - 0.5)^2}{E_i}$
Winter	33	24	+9	72.25	3.01
Spring	30	24	+6	30.25	1.26
Summer	14	24	−10	90.25	3.76
Fall	19	24	−5	20.25	0.84
Total	96	96	0	. . .	8.87

d. Example. The chi-square value for the distribution of eye color and sex among 50 children discussed above and listed in Table 3-4C can be calculated in two ways.

(1) The chi-square can be calculated by first determining the expected number in each cell. The expected number of boys with blue eyes is (20)(15) divided by 50, which equals 6. The expected number in each of the other cells is calculated similarly or is determined from the expected fourfold contingency table, which has the same marginal values as the observed fourfold table. The expected number of girls with blue eyes is 9, of boys with brown eyes is 14, and of girls with brown eyes is 21.

(2) Since the observed and expected values for all four cells are known, the corrected chi-square value is calculated using the r × c chi-square test equation (see section III H 1 e) and equals 0.10.

(3) Alternatively, the corrected chi-square value can be calculated using the 2 × 2 chi-square equation, which yields:

$$\chi^2_C = \frac{50[|(5)(20) - (10)(15)| - 50/2]^2}{(15)(35)(20)(30)}$$

$$= \frac{50(25)^2}{315{,}000}$$

$$= 0.10.$$

(4) The two methods yield approximately equal results.

(5) The probability is determined from the chi-square table (see Table 3-8). For 1 degree of freedom and a chi-square value of less than 2.7, the probability is greater than 10% that the distribution of eye color and sex among the 50 children is due to chance.

3. The McNemar test

a. Definition. The McNemar test, a type of 2 × 2 chi-square test, is specific for comparisons of variables from matched pairs and uses information only from discordant pairs.

b. Applications and characteristics

(1) Except that the variables being compared are from matched pairs and are not independent, the uses and restrictions of the McNemar test are the same as those for the 2 × 2 chi-square test.

(2) The null hypothesis tested is that the expected frequencies for the discordant pairs are equal.

(3) The McNemar test is more appropriate for testing matched pairs than the simple chi-square test, because it tends to decrease the likelihood of a type I error (i.e., the null hypothesis is less often incorrectly rejected).

(4) In a McNemar test, there is 1 degree of freedom because, with the marginal values constant, one of the values in the discordant pair automatically determines the other value.

c. Calculation. The chi-square value for matched-pair analysis using the McNemar test is determined as:

$$\chi^2_C = \frac{(|f - g| - 1)^2}{f + g},$$

where f and g are the values of the discordant pair in the matched pair fourfold contingency table (Table 3-10).

d. Example. Two hundred individuals with the acquired immunodeficiency syndrome [AIDS] (patients) are matched with two hundred individuals without AIDS (controls) to determine risk factors. Table 3-11 lists the results of the investigation concerning the prior use of inhalant stimulants. In 18 pairs, the patients had used inhalant stimulants and the controls had not; in 9 pairs, the controls and not the patients had used inhalant stimulants. In the remaining pairs, both the cases and controls had the same history, with 32 pairs having used inhalant stimulants and 141 pairs having not used them. Using the McNemar test, the

Table 3-10. Fourfold Table for Matched-Pair Analysis

	Sample A		
Sample B	**Positive**	**Negative**	**Total**
Positive	e	f	e + f
Negative	g	h	g + h
Total	e + g	f + h	N

Table 3-11. Prior Use of Inhalant Stimulants among 200 Patients with AIDS and 200 Matched Controls

	Patients with AIDS		
Controls	**Used Stimulants**	**Did Not Use Stimulants**	**Total**
Used stimulants	32	9	41
Did not use stimulants	18	141	159
Total	50	150	200

probability that the difference between the patients and controls with respect to the use of inhalant stimulants is due to chance is determined as follows.

(1) The chi-square value is calculated as $(|9 - 18| - 1)^2/(9 + 18)$, which equals $8^2/27$, or 2.4.

(2) The probability is determined from the chi-square table (see Table 3-8). For 1 degree of freedom and a chi-square value of less than 2.7, the probability is greater than 10% that the differences in the use of inhalant stimulants by patients and controls is due to chance.

I. Fisher's exact test

1. Definition. Fisher's exact test determines the exact probability due to chance of an association between the two characteristics being analyzed in a fourfold table. This probability does not rely on the chi-square probability distribution.

2. Application and characteristics

a. Fisher's exact test is used to determine the exact probability that an observed distribution is due to chance for a fourfold table in which any of the expected values is less than 5.

b. To determine the probability that an observed distribution (fourfold table) is due to chance, the exact probabilities are calculated for the observed distribution and for more extreme distributions, and the calculated probability values are added together using the additive rule (see section III A 6 a).

3. Calculation. Probability using Fisher's exact test is determined as:

$$P = \frac{(a+b)!\ (c+d)!\ (a+c)!\ (b+d)!}{N!\ a!\ b!\ c!\ d!},$$

where P = the exact probability that the association between the two characteristics is due to chance in the distribution being tested; and the other symbols are as noted for the fourfold contingency table (see section III C 1).

4. Example. Of 30 individuals at a meeting, 13 became ill with gastrointestinal symptoms within 24 hours. The only foods consumed at the meeting were soda or milk. Everyone had either soda or milk, but no one had both. The distribution of individuals by presence of illness and type of drink consumed is depicted in Table 3-12*A*.

a. In this example, Fisher's exact test and not a chi-square test is used to test the association between illness and type of drink consumed because the smallest expected value—determined by multiplying the smallest columnar total (10) by the smallest row total (13) and dividing by the grand total (30)—is 4.3, which is less than 5.

b. The exact probability that the observed distribution is due to chance is (13!17!20!10!)/(30!11!2!9!8!), which equals 0.06311 (for factorials, see section III D).

c. The exact probability of each of the more extreme distributions is calculated by the smallest cell value from the observed fourfold table diminished by 1, with the other cells adjusted accordingly, until the smallest value in a cell is 0.

(1) The exact probability of the more extreme distribution in Table 3-12*B* is (13!17!20!10!)/(30!12!1!8!9!), which equals 0.01052. (Note that because the margins remain the same and only the cells change, the numerator used for each of the extreme distributions is the same as the numerator for the observed distribution.)

(2) The exact probability of the most extreme distribution in Table 3-12C is (13!17!20!10!)/(30!13!0!7!10!), which equals 0.00065.

d. The total probability of seeing the observed distribution or one even more extreme is the sum of the probabilities for each distribution—0.06311 + 0.01052 + 0.00065—which equals 0.07428.

e. With an arbitrary cutoff of 0.05 for statistical significance, the difference between the illness attack rates for those who drank soda and milk is not significant, and the null hypothe-

Table 3-12. Distribution of 30 Individuals by Gastrointestinal Illness and Beverage Consumed

Illness	Beverage Consumed: Milk	Soda	Total
	A. Observed Distribution		
Yes	11	2	13
No	9	8	17
Total	20	10	30
	B. More Extreme Distribution		
Yes	12	1	13
No	8	9	17
Total	20	10	30
	C. Most Extreme Distribution		
Yes	13	0	13
No	7	10	17
Total	20	10	30

sis is not rejected. [Although the difference is not statistically significant, other factors may incriminate the milk as the causative agent of illness (see Chapter 1, section VI).]

J. Correlation

1. Definition. Correlation is a measure of mutual correspondence between two variables and is denoted by the **coefficient of correlation**.

2. Applications and characteristics

a. The simple correlation coefficient, also called the **Pearson's product-moment correlation coefficient**, is used to indicate the extent that two variables change with one another in a linear fashion.

b. The correlation coefficient can range from −1 to +1.

(1) When the correlation coefficient approaches −1, a change in one variable is more highly or strongly associated with an inverse linear change (i.e., a change in the opposite direction) in the other variable (Fig. 3-10*A*).

(2) When the correlation coefficient equals 0, there is no association between the changes of the two variables (Fig. 3-10*B*).

(3) When the correlation coefficient approaches +1, a change in one variable is more highly or strongly associated with a direct linear change in the other variable (Fig. 3-10*C*).

c. A correlation coefficient can be calculated validly only when both variables are subject to random sampling [see section I B 2 a (2)] and each is chosen independently.

d. Although useful as one of the determinants of scientific causality, correlation by itself is not equivalent to causation. For example, two correlated variables may be associated with another factor that causes them to appear correlated with each other.

e. A correlation coefficient may be strong, but insignificant, because of a small sample size.

3. Calculation. The correlation coefficient is determined as:

$$r = \frac{CoV_{x,y}}{\sqrt{V_x V_y}} = \frac{CoV_{x,y}}{(SD_x)(SD_y)} \text{ or} \quad \text{(K)}$$

$$r = \frac{\Sigma(x_i - \bar{x})(y_i - \bar{y})}{\sqrt{\Sigma(x_i - \bar{x})^2 \, \Sigma(y_i - \bar{y})^2}} \text{ or} \quad \text{(L)}$$

$$r = \frac{\Sigma x_i y_i - (\Sigma x_i)(\Sigma y_i)/n}{\sqrt{[\Sigma x_i^2 - (\Sigma x_i)^2/n]\,[\Sigma y_i^2 - (\Sigma y_i)^2/n]}}, \quad \text{(M)}$$

where r = the correlation coefficient; $CoV_{x,y}$ = the sample covariance between variables x and y; V_x = the variance of the x variable; V_y = the variance of the y variable; and n = the

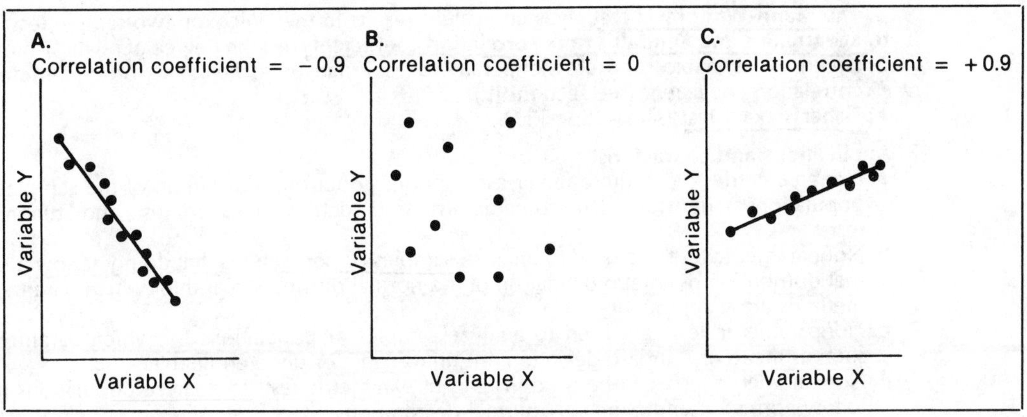

Figure 3-10. Correlation—the mutual correspondence between two variables—is measured by the correlation coefficient.

number of paired observations. The correlation coefficient is easier to calculate using equation M.

4. **Example.** Using equation M, the following steps are taken to determine the correlation coefficient between age and the number of prior arrests for 5 drunk drivers (Table 3-13).
   a. The product of the age and the number of prior arrests for each individual ($\Sigma x_i y_i$) is calculated, and the total equals 155.
   b. The product of the sum of the ages and the sum of the prior arrests for each individual is calculated and then divided by the number of paired observations [$(\Sigma x_i)(\Sigma y_i)/n$], which equals (100)(7)/5, or 140.
   c. The numerator is calculated by subtracting 140 from 155, which equals 15.
   d. The denominator is the square root of the respective sums of the squares of the deviations from each of the means. For age, the sum of the squares of the deviations equals 54 (see section II B 2 d for an example of calculation). For prior arrests, the sum of the squares of the deviations from the mean is similarly calculated and equals 15 minus the quotient 7^2 divided by 5, which equals 5.2
   e. The product of the two sums of the squares of the deviations from the respective means is (54)(5.2) or 280.8, the square root of which is 16.76. This is the denominator.
   f. The correlation coefficient is equal to the numerator (15) divided by the denominator (16.76) and in this example is +0.9. The age and the number of prior arrests for each individual are highly correlated. (Note, however, that the age does not cause the number of arrests nor does the number of prior arrests cause the age.)

K. Nonparametric tests

1. **Definition.** Nonparametric or **distribution-free** methods of statistical analysis test the null hypothesis or determine confidence limits for samples and populations regardless of the underlying population distribution.

2. **Types**
   a. The **Wilcoxon signed rank sum test** is for paired or matched data and is a nonparametric alternative to Student's t test for paired samples (see section III F 3).
   b. The **Wilcoxon two-sample test** is for unpaired data and is a nonparametric alternative to Student's t test for independent samples (see section III F 2).

Table 3-13. Calculating the Correlation Coefficient between Age and Number of Prior Arrests for Five Individuals

Case Number	Age (years)	Age Squared	Number of Prior Arrests	Number of Arrests Squared	Age × Number of Arrests
1	17	289	1	1	17
2	18	324	0	0	0
3	18	324	1	1	18
4	21	441	2	4	42
5	26	676	3	9	78
Total	100	2054	7	15	155

c. The **Mann-Whitney U test** gives equivalent results to the Wilcoxon two-sample test.
d. **Spearman's and Kendall's rank correlation coefficients** test the degree of relationship between two variables and are nonparametric alternatives to Pearson's product-moment correlation coefficient (see section III J).
e. **Fisher's exact test** (see section III I).

3. **Applications and characteristics**
   a. Nonparametric tests require fewer assumptions about the distribution of the samples or populations under study than do parametric tests such as chi-square tests and Student's t tests.
   b. Nonparametric tests are used to analyze samples or populations that do not follow a normal distribution or an approximation of the normal distribution and for which parametric methods are inappropriate.
   c. Nonparametric tests are used to analyze samples or populations for which parameters such as mean or standard deviation are unavailable or undeterminable.
   d. Nonparametric tests can be used instead of parametric tests to analyze populations that follow normal or approximately normal distributions.

4. **Example.** The internal medicine and general surgery test scores of the 11 medical students that were analyzed by Student's t test for paired samples in section III F 3 d can be reanalyzed by a nonparametric test. The scores are listed in Table 3-14. The association between the students' scores for the two tests is determined using the **Wilcoxon signed rank sum test** for pairs.
   a. The difference between the internal medicine and general surgery scores is calculated for each student.
   b. The absolute value for each of the calculated differences is determined.
   c. The absolute values are ranked by magnitude from 1 to 10. Differences of 0 are discounted and not included in the ranking.
   d. Each rank is assigned the sign of the calculated difference for that pair.
   e. The like-signed ranks are added together. The sum of the positive ranks equals +47; the sum of the negative ranks equals −8. The smaller signed rank sum, which in this example is 8, is used to determine the probability that the two scores are associated.
   f. A table of probability values for the Wilcoxon test on paired samples shows that for 10 pairs, a smaller rank sum of 8 is associated with a two-tailed probability of 0.05. Therefore, for these students, the internal medicine and general surgery test scores are significantly different, if the cutoff for rejecting the null hypothesis is 0.05.
   g. The conclusions reached using the parametric and nonparametric tests are the same.

5. Information on other nonparametric tests and tables for using nonparametric tests can be found in any standard statistics textbook (see Bibliography).

IV. SCREENING

A. Basic concepts

1. **Screening**
   a. Screening is the initial examination of an individual to detect disease not yet under medical care.

Table 3-14. Calculating the Wilcoxon Rank Sum Test for Pairs to Test the Association between Internal Medicine and General Surgery Test Scores for 11 Students

Medical Student Number	Internal Medicine Score	General Surgery Score	Difference between Scores	Absolute Value of Difference	Rank of Absolute Value	Signed Rank
1	75	90	−15	15	2	−2
2	85	10	+75	75	10	+10
3	93	20	+73	73	9	+9
4	55	55	0	0	. . .	. . .
5	79	60	+19	19	3	+3
6	86	30	+56	56	7	+7
7	90	70	+20	20	4	+4
8	76	85	−9	9	1	−1
9	89	25	+64	64	8	+8
10	54	75	−21	21	5	−5
11	92	52	+40	40	6	+6

b. Screening separates apparently healthy individuals into groups with either a high or low probability of developing the disease for which the screening test is being used.
c. Screening may be concerned with many different types of diseases, including:
(1) Acute communicable diseases (e.g., rubella).
(2) Chronic communicable diseases (e.g., tuberculosis).
(3) Acute noncommunicable diseases (e.g., lead toxicity).
(4) Chronic noncommunicable diseases (e.g., glaucoma).
d. Screening may be concerned with a single disease or with many diseases called **multiphasic screening.**

2. Case finding
a. Case finding is performed on patients who have sought medical care for a health problem.
b. Case finding is the examination of an individual for a disease unrelated to the health problem for which medical care was sought.

3. Diagnostic testing
a. Diagnostic testing is performed on ill or diseased patients.
b. Diagnostic testing is undertaken to explain or to determine the etiology of a patient's illness or disease.

4. Treatment testing
a. Treatment testing is performed on a patient who has received or is receiving therapy for a disease.
b. Treatment testing is designed to evaluate the patient's response to and the effectiveness of the therapy.

B. Screening programs are a major focus of efforts to promote health and to prevent disease. To be effective, however, a screening program should meet certain basic conditions.

1. The population being screened should be at a relatively high risk for the undiagnosed disease.
2. The undiagnosed disease should be of sufficient concern to the community being screened.
3. The undiagnosed disease should be more amenable to treatment or control than the disease that would be if diagnosed at a later stage in a symptomatic patient.
4. The screening test should have the following characteristics.
a. Test parameters should be high; the test should be sensitive and specific (see sections IV C 1, 2).
b. The test should be applicable to a large number of individuals.
c. The test should be easily and quickly accomplished.
d. The test should not cause harm to the individual being tested.
e. The test should be inexpensive.
5. Individuals for whom the screening test is positive should be assured follow-up evaluation.

C. Screening test parameters measure the clinical usefulness of the test. To determine these parameters, a fourfold table is used, in which the screening test results are tabulated according to the person's true disease status, which generally is determined by a "gold-standard" diagnostic test (Table 3-15).

Table 3-15. Results of a Screening Test for a Disease in a Population with Known Disease Status

	True Diagnosis		
Screening Test	**Diseased**	**Not Diseased**	**Total**
Positive	a*	b†	a + b
Negative	c‡	d§	c + d
Total	a + c	b + d	N‖

*a = the number of diseased persons with a positive screening test (the true-positives).
†b = the number of persons not diseased, but with a positive screening test (the false-positives).
‡c = the number of diseased persons with a negative screening test (the false-negatives).
§d = the number of persons not diseased and with a negative screening test (the true-negatives).
‖N = the total number of persons studied (a + b + c + d).

1. Sensitivity

a. Definition

(1) Sensitivity is the test's ability to identify correctly those individuals who truly have the disease.

(2) Sensitivity is the ratio of the number of individuals with the disease whose screening tests are positive to the total number of individuals with the disease under study. Sensitivity usually is expressed as a percentage.

(3) Sensitivity is independent of the disease prevalence in the population being tested (see Chapter 1, section IV B 2 b).

b. Calculation. The sensitivity of a test is determined as:

$$\text{sensitivity (\%)} = \frac{a}{a + c} \times 100,$$

where a = the number of individuals with the disease whose screening tests are positive (true-positives); c = the number of individuals with the disease whose screening tests are negative (false-negatives); and a + c = the total number of individuals with the disease (see Table 3-15).

c. Example. A new screening method for measuring diastolic blood pressure is compared to the standard method (sphygmomanometry) in a trial with 300 members of a community center (Table 3-16). Of the 45 persons with known diastolic hypertension, 36 have hypertension detected by the new method. The sensitivity of the test is 36/45, or 80%. Therefore, in 80% of the individuals who have hypertension as diagnosed by the standard method, the new screening test also detects the disease.

2. Specificity

a. Definition

(1) Specificity is the test's ability to identify correctly those individuals who truly do not have the disease.

(2) Specificity is the ratio of the number of individuals without the disease whose screening tests are negative to the total number of individuals without the disease under study. Specificity usually is expressed as a percentage.

(3) Specificity is independent of the disease prevalence in the population being tested.

b. Calculation. The specificity of a test is determined as:

$$\text{specificity (\%)} = \frac{d}{b + d} \times 100,$$

where b = the number of individuals without the disease whose screening tests are positive (false-positives); d = the number of individuals without the disease whose screening tests are negative (true-negatives); and b + d = the total number of individuals without the disease (see Table 3-15).

c. Example. In the trial of the new blood pressure screening method, 230 of the 255 persons without diastolic hypertension have normal blood pressure by the new method. The specificity of the screening test is 230/255, or 90%. Therefore, 90% of the individuals who do not have hypertension have negative results with the new screening test.

3. Positive predictive value

a. Definition

(1) The positive predictive value is the test's ability to identify those individuals who truly have the disease (true-positives) among all those individuals whose screening tests are positive.

(2) The positive predictive value is the ratio of the number of individuals with the disease whose screening tests are positive to the total number whose screening tests are positive. Positive predictive value usually is expressed as a percentage.

Table 3-16. Results of a New Screening Method for Measuring Diastolic Blood Pressure among 300 Members of a Community Center

	Known Diastolic Hypertension		
Screening Test	**Yes**	**No**	**Total**
Positive	36	25	61
Negative	9	230	239
Total	45	255	300

(3) The predictive value of a positive test increases with increasing disease prevalence.

b. **Calculation.** The positive predictive value of a test is determined as:

$$\text{PPV (\%)} = \frac{a}{a+b} \times 100,$$

where PPV = positive predictive value; and a + b = the total number of individuals with a positive screening test (see Table 3-15).

c. **Example.** In the trial of the new blood pressure screening method, 36 of the 61 individuals with a positive test have known diastolic hypertension. The positive predictive value of the test is 36/61, or 59%. Therefore, 59% of the individuals who have a positive screening test actually have hypertension.

4. Negative predictive value

a. **Definition**

(1) The negative predictive value is the test's ability to identify those individuals who truly do not have the disease (true-negatives) among all individuals whose screening tests are negative.

(2) The negative predictive value is the ratio of the number of individuals without the disease whose screening tests are negative to the total number whose screening tests are negative. Negative predictive value usually is expressed as a percentage.

(3) The predictive value of a negative test decreases with increasing disease prevalence.

b. **Calculation.** The negative predictive value of a test is determined as:

$$\text{NPV (\%)} = \frac{d}{c+d} \times 100,$$

where NPV = negative predictive value; and c + d = the total number of individuals with a negative screening test (see Table 3-15).

c. **Example.** In the trial of the new blood pressure screening method, 230 of the 239 individuals with a negative test do not have diastolic hypertension, but 9 actually do have hypertension. The negative predictive value of the test is 230/239, or 96%. Therefore, 96% of the individuals who have a negative screening test do not have hypertension.

5. Bayes theorem

a. **Definition**

(1) Bayes theorem is a statement of the conditional probability of a disease for an individual with a positive screening test.

(2) The probability of disease if the test is positive is related to the sensitivity and specificity of the test and the prevalence of disease in the population from which the individual came.

(3) The probability of disease given a positive test increases with increasing disease prevalence in the population.

b. **Calculation.** The probability of disease given that the test is positive is determined as:

$$P(+D \mid +T) = \frac{[P(+D)][P(+T \mid +D)]}{[P(+D)][P(+T \mid +D)] + [P(-D)][P(+T \mid -D)]},$$

where $P(+D \mid +T)$ = the probability of disease for an individual given that the test is positive; $P(+D)$ = the probability of disease in the population (the disease prevalence); $P(+T \mid +D)$ = the test sensitivity; $P(-D) = 1 - P(+D)$; and $P(+T \mid -D)$ = the probability of a positive test among those without disease (the false-positive rate), which is equal to 1 − the specificity.

c. **Example.** The prevalence of diastolic hypertension in the population screened above is 15%, or 0.15. The false-positive rate of the test is 25 divided by 255, or 0.10. The probability of an individual having diastolic hypertension if the screening test is positive is (0.15)(0.80)/[(0.15)(0.80) + (0.85)(0.10)], which equals 0.59, or 59%.

BIBLIOGRAPHY

Arkin H, Colton RR: *Tables for Statisticians*, 2nd ed. New York, Barnes and Noble, 1963

Colton T: *Statistics in Medicine*. Boston, Little, Brown, 1974

Department of Clinical Epidemiology and Biostatistics, McMaster University Health Sciences Centre: How to read clinical journals. *Can Med Assoc J* 124:555, 703, 869, 985, 1156, 1981

Fleiss JL: *Statistical Methods for Rates and Proportions*, 2nd ed. New York, John Wiley, 1981

Kahn HA: *An Introduction to Epidemiologic Methods*. New York, Oxford University Press, 1983

Last JM: *A Dictionary of Epidemiology*. New York, Oxford University Press, 1983

Swinscow TDV: *Statistics at Square One*, 7th ed. London, British Medical Association, 1980

STUDY QUESTIONS

Directions: Each question below contains five suggested answers. Choose the **one best** response to each question.

1. An analysis of the race of patients who visit an emergency room reveals that 40% are white, 35% are black, 20% are Hispanic, and 15% are Asian. These data would best be depicted graphically with a

(A) Venn diagram
(B) cumulative frequency graph
(C) normal curve
(D) histogram
(E) pie chart

Questions 2–4

In preparation for a national examination, 200 medical students completed 100 questions in a practice test. Each student answered between 35 and 59 questions correctly. The arithmetic mean number of correct answers was 47, with a standard deviation of 4. The number of correct answers per student was distributed normally.

2. The range of questions correctly answered is

(A) 12
(B) 24
(C) 36
(D) 65
(E) 94

3. The percentage of students who correctly answered 43 to 51 questions is about

(A) 8%
(B) 24%
(C) 34%
(D) 68%
(E) 95%

4. The percentage of students who answered at least 55 questions correctly is about

(A) 2%
(B) 5%
(C) 8%
(D) 11%
(E) 14%

(end of group question)

5. True statements concerning Student's t test and t distribution include all of the following EXCEPT

(A) the Student's t test is appropriate for sample sizes of fewer than 30
(B) as the sample size increases, the t value approaches the value of the critical ratio
(C) the t distribution reflects less variation due to chance than does the normal distribution
(D) the probability value derived from a t value depends on the number of degrees of freedom
(E) proportions can be used in calculating the t value

6. In a 3 × 4 contingency table, the number of degrees of freedom equals

(A) 1
(B) 5
(C) 6
(D) 7
(E) 12

7. True statements concerning chi-square tests and chi-square values include all of the following EXCEPT

(A) the categories of data used must be mutually exclusive
(B) chi-square values are useful in calculating confidence intervals
(C) chi-square tests do not take into account the ordering of data categories
(D) the probability value derived from a chi-square value depends on the number of degrees of freedom
(E) proportions cannot be used in calculating the chi-square value

8. Measures of dispersion include all of the following EXCEPT

(A) mode
(B) range
(C) variance
(D) standard deviation
(E) coefficient of variation

Directions: Each question below contains four suggested answers of which **one or more** is correct. Choose the answer

A if **1, 2, and 3** are correct
B if **1 and 3** are correct
C if **2 and 4** are correct
D if **4** is correct
E if **1, 2, 3, and 4** are correct

9. True statements concerning Fisher's exact test include which of the following?

(1) It is used instead of the chi-square test if the observed value in any cell of the fourfold table is less than 5
(2) It is used instead of the chi-square test if the expected value in any cell of the fourfold table is less than 5
(3) It requires that the probability value determined be adjusted according to the number of degrees of freedom
(4) It requires calculating probability values for the fourfold table under study and for tables that are more extreme

10. The standard error of the mean is calculated from the

(1) median
(2) sample size
(3) range
(4) standard deviation

11. Two variables, X and Y, are studied for a population, and the simple correlation coefficient (r) is equal to +0.80. The correlation coefficient indicates that

(1) variable X and variable Y have the same unit of measure
(2) variable X and variable Y are causally related
(3) there is an inverse linear relationship between variable X and variable Y
(4) variable X and variable Y are strongly associated

12. Nonparametric tests can be used to compare two populations when

(1) each population is unimodal
(2) both populations have equal numbers
(3) each population is independent
(4) each population is distributed normally

13. True statements concerning the chi-square test include which of the following?

(1) It requires that the expected value in each cell be at least 5
(2) It requires that the observed value in each cell be at least 5
(3) It depends on both the observed and expected values in each cell
(4) It depends on the arithmetic mean of the series under study

14. Tests based on the chi-square distribution include the

(1) Wilcoxon two-sample test
(2) Fisher's exact test
(3) Student's t test
(4) McNemar test

Directions: The groups of questions below consist of lettered choices followed by several numbered items. For each numbered item select the **one** lettered choice with which it is **most** closely associated. Each lettered choice may be used once, more than once, or not at all.

Questions 15–18

A fourth-year medical student has completed five elective rotations, which are weighted equally. The student is graded in each rotation on a scale of 1 to 10, as follows:

Skiing surgery	2
Cross-cultural pharmacology	3
Literary medicine	6
Introductory bartering	7
Diving medicine	7

For each descriptive statistic listed below, select the numerical value that is most appropriate.

(A) 3
(B) 4
(C) 5
(D) 6
(E) 7

15. Median
16. Mode
17. Mean
18. Range

Questions 19–23

The table below is a fourfold table, in which screening test results for disease Y are tabulated in relation to the true disease status of the population being tested.

	Disease Y		
Screening Test	**Yes**	**No**	**Total**
Positive	200	100	300
Negative	50	600	650
Total	250	700	950

Match each screening test parameter listed below to the appropriate numerical value.

(A) 250/950 or 26%
(B) 200/300 or 67%
(C) 200/250 or 80%
(D) 600/700 or 86%
(E) 600/650 or 92%

19. Sensitivity
20. Specificity
21. Positive predictive value
22. Negative predictive value
23. Disease prevalence

ANSWERS AND EXPLANATIONS

1. The answer is E. (*II C 1*) A pie chart is the most appropriate figure of those listed to represent a population by the proportional distribution of a discrete characteristic, which in this example is race. A bar chart would also be appropriate. A Venn diagram is used to show two or more characteristics within a population or one characteristic within two or more populations. A cumulative frequency graph is used for continuous data. A normal curve is a symmetrical curve of continuous and ordered data. A histogram is a special form of bar chart used for continuous and ordered data.

2. The answer is B. (*II B 1*) The range is the spread between the highest and lowest values in a series. It is calculated by subtracting the lowest value, which in this example is 35, from the highest value, 59. The result is 24.

3. The answer is D. (*III E 2*) A normal distribution curve can be characterized by the arithmetic mean and the standard deviation. In a normal distribution, about 68% of the population lies within 1 standard deviation of the mean, and 95% lies within 2 standard deviations of the mean. Conversely, 5% of the population lies outside 2 standard deviations of the mean. In this example, the mean (47) minus 1 standard deviation (4) equals 43 and the mean (47) plus 1 standard deviation (4) equals 51. Therefore, the percentage of students who correctly answered 43 to 51 questions is 68%.

4. The answer is A. (*III E 3*) In a normal distribution, about 95% of the population lies inside and about 5% lies outside 2 standard deviations of the mean. About half of those lying outside 2 standard deviations are greater than the mean plus 2 standard deviations, and an equal number are less than the mean minus 2 standard deviations. In this example, 55 correct answers represents the mean (47) plus 2 standard deviations (each standard deviation is 4). Therefore, about 2% of the students answered at least 55 questions correctly.

5. The answer is C. (*III F 1*) Student's t tests analyze small samples based on the t distribution, which allows for greater variation due to chance than does the normal distribution. As the sample size increases, the sample more closely approximates the population and the t value approaches the value of the critical ratio. The probability value derived from a t value depends on the number of degrees of freedom, which in turn is based on the sample size. Either actual counts or proportions can be used in calculating the t value.

6. The answer is C. (*III C 2*) The number of degrees of freedom is the number of variables in a distribution that can be assigned values freely, when the sum of the values is fixed. In a contingency table with 3 rows and 4 columns, the number of degrees of freedom is equal to the product of the number of rows minus 1 and the number of columns minus 1, which is 2×3, or 6.

7. The answer is B. (*III H 1*) The chi-square test determines the extent an observed distribution differs from a theoretical or expected distribution, regardless of the order of the categories of data. The probability value derived from a chi-square value depends on the number of degrees of freedom, which in turn is based on the sample size. The chi-square value is calculated on actual counts, not proportions. Chi-square values are not used in calculating confidence intervals.

8. The answer is A. (*II B*) Measures of dispersion include the range, variance, standard deviation, and coefficient of variation, which are summary measures for a sample or population that describe the scatter of the series. Measures of central tendency include the mode, median, and mean, which are summary measures for a sample or population that describe the middle or most frequently occurring values.

9. The answer is C (2, 4). (*III I*) Fisher's exact test determines the exact probability due to chance of an association between two variables that are being analyzed in a fourfold table. Fisher's exact test is used instead of the chi-square test if an expected value in any of the cells is less than 5, regardless of the observed value. The test yields the exact probability for the observed distribution and for more extreme distributions. No adjustment is necessary for varying degrees of freedom. (There is always only 1 degree of freedom in a fourfold table.)

10. The answer is C (2, 4). (*III G 1 c*) The standard error of the mean is an estimate of the standard deviation of the population based on the standard deviation of a sample. The standard error of the mean is equal to the standard deviation of the sample divided by the square root of the sample size.

11. The answer is D (4). (*III J 2*) The correlation coefficient is used to indicate the extent that two variables change with one another in a linear manner. The two variables can have the same or different units of measure. Correlation coefficients range from − 1 to + 1 and are unitless. A − 1 value indicates a strong inverse linear association (an increase in one variable is associated with a decrease in the other), while + 1 indicates a strong direct linear association. Causality cannot be determined from the correlation coefficient, because the two variables may be associated through a third variable rather than directly.

12. The answer is E (all). (*III K 1*) Nonparametric tests are analytic tests of the null hypothesis for samples and populations regardless of their size or the underlying distribution. The populations being compared may be dependent or independent.

13. The answer is B (1, 3). (*III H 1*) The chi-square test determines the extent that an observed distribution differs from a theoretical or expected distribution. Although the expected value in each cell must be at least 5 for the test to be valid, observed values can be less than 5. The chi-square value is independent of the arithmetic mean.

14. The answer is D (4). (*III H 3*) The McNemar test is based on the chi-square distribution, as are the goodness-of-fit test and the r × c chi-square test. Student's t test is based on the t distribution. The Wilcoxon two-sample test and Fisher's exact test are distribution-free nonparametric tests.

15–18. The answers are: 15-D, 16-E, 17-C, 18-C. (*II A 1–3, B 1*) The median is the value that divides a series of values into two equal parts. Because the number of test scores greater than 6 equals the number of scores less than 6, the median test score equals 6. The mode is the value that occurs most frequently in a series. In this distribution, the mode is 7. The mean is the sum of all the values in a series (25) divided by the number of values (5) and, therefore, in this example is 5. The range is the spread between the highest and lowest values in a series, which is determined by subtracting the lowest value (2) from the highest value (7). In this example, then, the range is 5.

19–23. The answers are: 19-C, 20-D, 21-B, 22-E, 23-A. (*IV C*) Screening test parameters are measures of the clinical usefulness of the test when compared with a definitive diagnostic test.

Sensitivity is a test's ability to identify correctly those persons who truly have the disease. In this example, the sensitivity (80%) is calculated by dividing the number of persons with the disease who screen positive (200) by the total number of persons with the disease (250).

Specificity is a test's ability to identify correctly persons who do not have disease. In this example, the specificity (86%) is the number of persons who do not have the disease and who screen negative (600) divided by the total number of persons who do not have the disease (700).

Positive predictive value is a test's ability to identify those persons who truly have the disease from among all those persons whose screening tests are positive. In this example, the positive predictive value (67%) is the number of persons with disease who screen positive (200) divided by the total number of persons who screen positive (300).

Negative predictive value is a test's ability to identify those persons who truly do not have disease from among all those persons whose screening tests are negative. Here, the negative predictive value (92%) is the number of persons who do not have disease and who screen negative (600) divided by the total number of persons who screen negative (650).

Other screening test parameters include the false-positive rate, which is the proportion of persons without disease who screen positive among all persons without disease, and the false-negative rate, the proportion of persons with disease who screen negative among all persons with disease.

The prevalence of a disease is the proportion of people who have the disease in the population. In this example, the prevalence is equal to 250 divided by 950, or 26%. Sensitivity and specificity are independent of the prevalence of the disease, while positive and negative predictive values vary with disease prevalence.

4

Epidemiology and Prevention of Selected Acute Illnesses

Robert G. Sharrar

I. INTRODUCTION. This chapter will discuss some communicable diseases of public health importance, emphasizing the various recommendations for controlling the spread of these diseases. Each section will present important epidemiologic features of the disease, the infectious disease process, and current recommendations for control.

II. GENERAL METHODS OF CONTROL

A. Agent

1. **Eliminate the agent** that causes disease.
   a. **Chemotherapeutic or chemoprophylactic agents** kill biologic agents internally so that they cannot infect others.
   b. **Disinfectants** kill organisms outside of the body. Blood spills are cleaned with detergent and water and the area disinfected with a 1:10 dilution of household bleach, which inactivates hepatitis B virus (HBV) and human immunodeficiency virus (HIV), the virus that causes acquired immune deficiency syndrome (AIDS).
   c. **Chlorination** of the water supply prevents the spread of many microorganisms.
   d. **Heat** is used to pasteurize milk or to destroy certain bacteria, like *Salmonella*, which are part of the food chain, and to inactivate botulinal toxin in contaminated food.
2. **Prevent the organism from multiplying** to the level at which it can cause disease.
   a. **Proper temperatures for storing and serving food** should be used so that the small number of organisms that frequently contaminate food are not able to multiply to a sufficient number (**inoculum**) to cause disease.
   b. **Chlorinating air cooling towers** can prevent *Legionella pneumophilia*, which is responsible for Legionnaires' disease, from reaching a sufficient inoculum to cause disease.
3. **Eliminate the reservoir** so that the agent has no natural place to multiply. Certain agents, like measles and smallpox, die out when there are no susceptible hosts in which to live. The virus that causes smallpox has been eradicated from the general population in this way.

B. Reservoir

1. **Human**
   a. **Isolation or quarantine.** The object is to isolate the agent that causes disease not the patient.
      (1) **Total physical isolation** is rarely indicated. It is used in special circumstances, such as hospitalized patients, and for certain diseases that are highly contagious, usually by the airborne route.
      (2) **Limited physical isolation** is used to restrict certain actions of the patients. Individuals with certain infections, such as *Salmonella*, *Shigella*, or acute hepatitis A virus (HAV) are not allowed to work in occupations that prepare or serve food for public consumption.
   b. **Chemotherapeutic agents.** Elimination of the organism from the carrier state or from symptomatic individuals can be accomplished with chemotherapeutic agents. Rifampin is used to eliminate the pharyngeal carriage of *Neisseria meningitidis* and *Hemophilus influenzae*. Proper antituberculosis therapy can eliminate *Mycobacterium tuberculosis* from symptomatic patients.
   c. **Immunization.** Prevention of the carrier state is accomplished with active immunizations. Dentists who receive HBV vaccine will not become infected with HBV or become chronic carriers of the hepatitis B surface antigen (HBsAg).

2. Animals

a. Avoid contact (bites) by potentially dangerous (rabid) animals. Rabies infection is known to be endemic in certain wild animals, such as skunks, raccoons, bats, and foxes. These animals should not be helped in emergency situations as injured animals may be rabid and not fed by individuals inexperienced in handling them.

b. Only certain animals are appropriate as household pets, and these pets should be properly immunized and seen regularly by a veterinarian. Raccoons and skunks should not be kept as pets, since some of these animals become rabid. Pet dogs should be examined periodically for the presence of ticks.

3. Environment

a. Certain environmental factors can serve as a breeding ground for agents or vectors of disease. *Histoplasma capsulatum* can grow in certain bird droppings, and stagnant water can serve as a breeding ground for mosquitoes. Areas containing bird droppings should be decontaminated with a formaldehyde solution before they are cleaned. Many communities have vector control programs that prevent the breeding of mosquitoes.

b. Adequate separation of the water supply from the sewage system has prevented the spread of many enteric diseases, such as HAV and polio.

C. Portal of exit. Since microorganisms exit the human and animal reservoirs in normal body functions, such as breathing and defecating, the portal of exit cannot be blocked. Percutaneous exit can be prevented by avoiding needle sticks and insect bites. When the environment is the reservoir, any changes, such as construction activity, may cause dissemination of organisms.

D. Mode of transmission

1. Direct

a. The transfer of organisms directly from one person to another can be blocked by simple processes, such as washing hands, wearing protective clothing, and using a condom.

(1) Hand washing is the most important procedure for preventing the spread of most infections.

(a) The microbial flora of the skin consists of resident microorganisms, which are not virulent, and transient microorganisms, which are acquired from colonized or infected patients or from the individual's own gastrointestinal tract. These transient microorganisms may be pathogens capable of causing serious systemic disease.

(b) Most routine, brief patient-care contacts do not require hand washing. However, hand washing should be done:

(i) Before performing invasive procedures.
(ii) Before touching susceptible or immunocompromised patients or open wounds.
(iii) Between contact with patients in high-risk areas.
(iv) After touching wounds.
(v) After touching body fluids, secretions, or excretions.
(vi) After touching potentially contaminated environmental items.

(c) Good hand-washing technique consists of a vigorous rubbing together of all surfaces of lathered hands for at least 10 seconds, followed by thorough rinsing under a stream of water. Plain soap can be used in routine situations, but antimicrobial hand-washing products should be used when handling newborns or touching immunocompromised patients.

(2) Protective apparel may include masks, gowns, gloves, protective eyewear, and in some instances, boots and hats. Protective garments should be worn only once and then discarded in appropriate receptacles.

(a) Masks are used primarily to prevent airborne transmitted diseases; however, they also protect against those diseases spread by direct contact or transfer between mucous membrane surfaces by preventing personnel from touching the mucous membranes of their eyes, nose, and mouth until after they have washed their hands and removed their masks. High-efficiency disposable masks, which cover the nose and mouth, are more effective than cotton gauze or paper tissue masks. Masks become ineffective after they become moist.

(b) Gowns should be worn when individuals will be exposed to blood, body fluids that might contain blood, or infective secretions or excretions. Sterile gowns should be worn when changing dressings on extensive wounds or burns.

(c) Gloves are used to prevent the transfer of organisms from the patient to the staff and vice versa and to prevent personnel from becoming transiently colonized by pathogenic organisms. Gloves should also be used when examining all mucous membrane surfaces.

(d) **Protective eyewear** should be used by dentists who are exposed to aerosols of saliva and blood because of the high-speed drills that are used. They should also be used by other indivduals who might come in contact with aerosols of infectious material.

(3) **Use of condoms** can prevent the transfer of most sexually transmitted diseases (STDs), including herpes simplex virus (HSV), *Chlamydia*, syphilis, gonorrhea, and AIDS.

b. Organisms that spread by the large airborne droplets can be blocked by teaching patients to cover their mouths when coughing or sneezing and by using disposable tissues.

2. **Indirect**

a. **Diseases transmitted by arthropod vectors**, such as mosquitoes, mites, and ticks, can be prevented by avoiding bites from these insects.

(1) **Protective screening** of a residence can prevent insects from entering.

(2) **Protective clothing**, such as long pants and long sleeve shirts, should be worn when exposure is expected.

(3) **Insect repellents** on exposed skin surfaces, preferably repellents containing over 30% active ingredient of N,N diethyl metatoluamide (deet), should be used.

(4) **Remove ticks** from the body immediately, with tweezers if possible. Gentle, steady traction should be used to avoid leaving mouth parts in the skin. The tick that causes Rocky Mountain spotted fever must be attached to the body for several hours to allow transmission of the rickettsial organism.

b. **Diseases spread by common vehicle** can be prevented by eliminating the vehicle or by preventing significant contamination.

(1) **Disposable patient-care equipment** should be used when possible and properly discarded. Articles contaminated with infective material should be discarded or bagged and labeled before being sent for decontamination and reprocessing.

(2) **Screen blood** for serologic markers of biologic agents that cause disease. Those units that are positive should not be used for transfusion purposes. The American Red Cross screens every unit of blood with the following tests for specific diseases:

(a) Rapid plasma reagin (RPR) test for syphilis

(b) HBsAg for HBV

(c) HIV antibodies for AIDS

(d) Hepatitis B core antibody (anti-HBc) and alanine aminotransferase as surrogate markers for non-A, non-B hepatitis

(e) Blood screening for cytomegalovirus (CMV) antibodies, (If antibodies are found, the blood should not be given to neonates because of the severity of CMV infection in the perinatal period.)

(3) **Proper canning, preparation, serving, and storage of food** can prevent contamination of food or prevent a small bacterial inoculum from multiplying to the point at which it can cause disease.

(a) Canning requires a processing temperature of 250°F (120°C) or higher (steam under pressure) to destroy the spores of *Clostridium botulinum*.

(b) Poultry, which is frequently contaminated with *Salmonella*, must be heated to an internal (core) temperature of 165°F (75°C).

(c) Steam serving tables should maintain a minimum temperature of at least 140°F (60°C).

(d) Food should be refrigerated at temperatures below 45°F (8°C). Many foods require lower temperatures.

(e) Food contaminated with *Staphylococcus* enterotoxin must be discarded, since the enterotoxin cannot be inactivated by heat.

c. **Diseases spread by the airborne route** are much more difficult to control. The droplet nuclei remain suspended in the air and can be widely dispersed by air currents. Ultraviolet lights and isolation of patients in well-ventilated rooms have been used.

E. **Portal of entry.** Since most microorganisms enter the host through normal body functions, such as breathing and eating, the portal of entry is difficult to block. Percutaneous entry can be prevented by using sterile needles, by avoiding insect bites, and by covering open cuts or sores.

F. **Susceptible host**

1. **Good health habits** like rest, exercise, and a balanced diet may protect a person from certain diseases. While no one has proven that good health habits are effective, no one has proven that they are not. Studies have shown that excessive alcohol intake interferes with serum bactericidal properties and white cell function. Tobacco smoke interferes with the ciliary motion lining the respiratory tract and leads to anatomic changes, which can result in chronic bronchitis and recurrent episodes of bacterial and viral pneumonias.

2. **Prevention of skin breakdown** is important since skin is an effective barrier against all biologic agents.
3. **Natural immunity** is acquired immunity. All children are born with some antibody protection, which they acquire from their mother. This passive immunity lasts about 6 months. When the maternal protection disappears, the infant must develop his or her own immunity. This naturally acquired immunity occurs when the child is exposed to biologic agents as he or she begins the socialization process. This may begin when the child is exposed to other children in school or day-care centers, or when the child is exposed to older siblings who attend schools or day-care centers. Unfortunately, socialization brings exposure and exposure brings disease. However, children handle many diseases better than adults.
4. **Artificially acquired immunity** occurs when individuals are immunized with vaccines. It is artificial since it is caused by a man-made vaccine. It is acquired since the individual makes his or her own antibodies. Vaccines make susceptible hosts resistant to circulating organisms. They have been used to eradicate smallpox from the globe and to eliminate measles and polio from most parts of the United States. As the proportion of immune (immunized plus previously infected) individuals increase, the amount of wild virus in the population decreases, and the amount of clinical disease decreases since there are fewer susceptible people exposed to the biologic agent.
5. **Chemoprophylaxis** can temporarily protect a susceptible host during periods of intense exposure. Chloroquine phosphate is used to prevent malaria in individuals traveling in malarious areas. Isoniazid is used to protect household or close contacts of patients with pulmonary tuberculosis until their tuberculin skin test can accurately be determined (3 months after exposure) and until the index case is no longer communicable.

III. IMMUNOBIOLOGIC AGENTS

A. Introduction

1. **Definitions**
   a. **Vaccine** is a suspension of attenuated live or killed microorganisms (bacteria or viruses) administered to induce immunity, thereby preventing an infectious disease. Commonly used vaccines include:
      (1) **Live attenuated viral vaccines**, such as measles, mumps, rubella, polio, and yellow fever vaccines.
      (2) **Killed or fractionated viral vaccines**, such as influenza, hepatitis B, polio, and rabies vaccines.
      (3) **Killed or fractionated bacterial vaccines**, such as *H. influenzae* type b, meningococcal or pneumococcal polysaccharide vaccines, and cholera or typhoid vaccines.
   b. **Toxoid** is a modified bacterial toxin that has been rendered nontoxic but that retains the ability to stimulate the formation of antitoxin. Commonly used toxoids include diphtheria and tetanus toxoids.
   c. **Immune globulin (IG)** is a sterile solution of human antibodies prepared by cold ethanol fractionation of large pools of blood plasma. It is primarily used for passive immunization against measles and hepatitis A and for routine maintenance of certain immunodeficient individuals.
   d. **Specific immune globulin** is a special sterile solution of human antibodies prepared from donor pools preselected for a high antibody titer content against a specific disease. Commercially available preparations include:
      (1) Hepatitis B immune globulin (HBIG).
      (2) Rabies immune globulin (RIG).
      (3) Tetanus immune globulin (TIG).
      (4) Varicella zoster immune globulin (VZIG).
   e. **Antitoxin** is a solution of antibodies derived from the serum of animals immunized with specific antigens. Antitoxins are used to provide passive immunity as treatment for certain bacterial infections or poisonous snakebites. Examples of antitoxins include:
      (1) Botulism antitoxin.
      (2) Diphtheria antitoxin.
      (3) *Crotalus* antitoxin against the venom of rattlesnakes.
2. **Disease prevention.** Immunobiologic agents were created to prevent:
   a. **Common diseases**, which cause a great deal of illness. In the era before vaccines, almost every child experienced measles, mumps, and rubella.
   b. **Serious diseases** with significant sequelae, including:
      (1) **Measles**, which can cause pneumonia, encephalitis, mental retardation, and death.
      (2) **Rubella**, which can cause congenital birth defects.

(3) Polio, which can cause paralysis and death.

c. Untreatable or difficult to treat diseases, such as:

(1) Viral infections, which cause cell destruction.

(2) Toxogenic infections, such as diphtheria and tetanus, which still have a high case fatality rate. Even with penicillin therapy, pneumococcal pneumonia is fatal in 5% of cases.

B. Recommendations for use of immunobiologic agents. Since no vaccine is completely safe or completely effective and since scientific data concerning all possible circumstances are incomplete, the decision to administer an immunobiologic agent must lie with the clinician who has some understanding of these vaccines and who knows the patient. The balance between benefits (prevention of a disease) and risks (side effects of the vaccine), which may be significant, must be considered in each instance.

1. Sources of vaccine information include:

a. Recommendations of the Advisory Committee on Immunization Practices (ACIP), which are issued by the Public Health Service (PHS), Centers for Disease Control (CDC) and periodically updated in the *Morbidity and Mortality Weekly Report (MMWR)*.

b. Report of the Committee on Infectious Diseases of the American Academy of Pediatrics, which is published in the "red book" and periodically updated in *Pediatrics*. The most recent edition of the red book (20th edition) was published in 1986.

c. Package inserts, which are also published in the *Physician's Desk Reference (PDR)*.

d. Technical Bulletin of the American College of Obstetricians and Gynecologists, which contains information about immunizing pregnant women.

e. Health Information for International Travel, which is published annually by the CDC as a guide to requirements and recommendations for specific immunizations and health practices for travel to various countries.

f. Advisory memoranda, which are published periodically by the CDC and advise international travelers about specific outbreaks of communicable diseases abroad.

g. Recommendations of ACIP, Adult Immunizations. *MMWR* suppl. vol. 33, no. 1S, 1984.

2. General guidelines for administration. For information about manufacturing, nature, and content of immunobiologic agents; route; dosage; contraindications; side effects; and storage, the package insert should be consulted.

a. Split doses or intradermal administration should not be done unless specifically recommended.

b. Multiple doses or periodic reinforcements are necessary for full protection by some vaccines.

(1) It is not necessary to restart or add extra doses to an interrupted series of an immunobiologic agent. Just continue the immunization schedule as if it were not interrupted.

(2) Doses given at less than recommended intervals should not be counted as part of the primary series. For example, two polio immunizations given a week apart should only be counted as one polio immunization.

c. Simultaneous administration of several immunobiologic agents

(1) Most of the widely used vaccine antigens can safely and effectively be given simultaneously.

(a) Inactivated vaccines can be administered simultaneously at separate sites.

(b) Live attenuated viral vaccines can be given on the same day, or else they should be given at least 1 month apart.

(c) Inactivated and live attenuated vaccines may be administered at the same time.

(2) Administration of immune globulin (IG) and vaccines

(a) Inactivated vaccines have a large antigenic load, do not require multiplication in the body, and can be given anytime after IG. When administered simultaneously, they should be given at different sites.

(b) Live attenuated viral vaccines have a small antigenic load, require multiplication in the body, and cannot be given with IG.

(i) A live vaccine should not be given for at least 6 weeks and preferably 3 months after the administration of IG.

(ii) If IG has to be given less than 14 days after administration of a live vaccine, the vaccine should be repeated 3 months after the IG.

(iii) Preliminary data suggest that IG may not interfere with oral polio or yellow fever immunizations.

d. Reactions to vaccine components

(1) Some vaccines (e.g., yellow fever, measles, mumps, and influenza) are grown in embryonated chicken eggs.

(a) Yellow fever vaccine should not be given to individuals with a known egg hypersensitivity.
(b) Any vaccine grown on embryonated eggs should not be given to anyone with a known anaphylactic hypersensitivity to eggs.
(c) If an individual can eat eggs without adverse effects, then he or she can be immunized with measles, mumps, or influenza vaccines.

(2) Some vaccines contain preservatives, such as thimerosal (a mercurial) or trace amounts of an antibiotic (neomycin). They should not be given to individuals who have had anaphylactic reactions to these agents.
(3) No currently recommended vaccine contains penicillin or its derivatives. Therefore, a history of penicillin allergy is not a contraindication to immunization.
(4) A live attenuated viral vaccine should not be given to individuals who are immunocompromised. Since recipients of oral polio vaccine (OPV) excrete the vaccine strain in their stools, OPV should not be given to individuals who live in households with immunocompromised hosts.
(5) Individuals with severe febrile illnesses should not be immunized until they have recovered primarily to avoid blaming a vaccine for a manifestation of the underlying illness. However, minor colds or respiratory infections should not be used as excuses to avoid immunizations.
(6) Adverse events following immunizations may or may not be related to the vaccine. All temporally associated events severe enough to require medical attention should be reported to local or state health officials and to the vaccine manufacturer.

e. Vaccination during pregnancy

(1) Although there are no studies showing teratogenic effects, live attenuated viral vaccines should not be given to pregnant women or to those likely to become pregnant within 3 months of receiving the vaccine.
(2) Pregnant women at substantial risk of exposure may receive a live viral vaccine. When possible, it should be given during the second or third trimester.
(3) Children of pregnant women should receive age-appropriate immunizations. There is no evidence that children given measles, mumps, or rubella vaccine can transmit them.
(4) There is no evidence that inactivated vaccines or IG pose any risk to the fetus.

C. Vaccines available for routine immunizations

1. Diphtheria, tetanus toxoids, and pertussis (DTP) vaccine. Diphtheria and tetanus toxoids (DT) vaccine is used for children under 7 years of age. Tetanus and diphtheria toxoids (Td) vaccine is used for individuals 7 years of age and older. Single antigen preparations are also available.

a. Diphtheria

(1) Diphtheria is a rare disease in the United States with less than 5 reported cases each year.
(2) Immunization does not eliminate *Corynebacterium diphtheriae* in the nasopharynx or on the skin.
(3) Results of serosurveys suggest that many adults are not protected against diphtheria.
(4) Diphtheria infection may not confer immunity since some strains that cause disease are nontoxicogenic. Active immunization should be initiated at the time of recovery.

b. Tetanus

(1) There are less than 100 reported cases of tetanus each year.
(2) In 1983, 57% of the cases were over 60 years of age. Serosurveys show that over 50% of individuals over 60 years of age have inadequate levels of antitoxin.
(3) In 1982 and 1983, 6% of tetanus cases had no history of a wound. An additional 17% of the reported cases had nonacute skin lesions, such as ulcers or abscesses.
(4) Clinical tetanus does not confer immunity. Active immunization should be instituted at the time of recovery.
(5) For tetanus prophylaxis in wound management, the physician must:
(a) Determine if the patient has completed a primary series (two doses). Individuals who have had military service since 1941 have received at least one dose. Uncertain immunizations should not be counted.
(b) Administer Td or DT to anyone who has not completed his or her primary series or if more than 10 years have passed since the last dose.
(c) Give Td or DT for certain wounds, such as those contaminated with dirt, feces, soil, saliva, and for puncture wounds, avulsions, and wounds resulting from missiles, crushing, burns, or frostbite if more than 5 years have passed since the last dose.
(d) Use TIG in individuals who have not had a primary series who have wounds as described in (c) above.

c. Pertussis

(1) Approximately 2 to 3000 cases are reported each year.

(2) Over 50% of the reported cases and almost all of the deaths occur in individuals less than 1 year of age. In 1982–1983, 43% of the patients were less than 6 months old.

(3) Serious reactions (and frequency of occurrence), which can occur following DTP immunizations, represent an absolute contraindication for further immunizations with a vaccine containing pertussis. These reactions are:

(a) Persistent, inconsolable crying lasting 3 hours or more (1/100 doses) or an unusual, high-pitched cry occurring within 48 hours (1/900 doses).

(b) Fever of 105°F (40.5°C) or greater within 24 hours (1/330 doses).

(c) Collapse or shock-like state (hypotonic-hyporesponsive episode) within 48 hours (1/1750 doses).

(d) Convulsions with or without fever occurring within 3 days (1/1750 doses). Children who get convulsions within 4–7 days should be carefully evaluated before receiving additional DTP immunizations.

(e) Acute encephalopathy within 7 days, including severe alterations in consciousness with generalized or focal neurologic signs (1/110,000 doses).

(f) Permanent neurologic deficit occurring within 7 days (1/310,000 doses).

(4) Children or infants with an evolving neurologic disorder should not receive pertussis vaccine. These disorders include:

(a) Uncontrolled epilepsy.

(b) Infantile spasms.

(c) Progressive encephalopathy.

(5) Children with stable conditions such as cerebral palsy, developmental delay, controlled seizures, or with corrected neurologic disorders may be immunized with a pertussis vaccine.

2. Oral, attenuated poliovirus vaccine (OPV) [containing poliovirus types 1, 2, and 3] and **inactivated poliovirus vaccine (IPV)**.

a. Poliomyelitis is rare in the United States today. Fewer than 12 cases of paralytic polio are reported each year. Most of these are in vaccinates or their contacts. In 1954, more than 18,000 cases of paralytic disease were reported. In the era before vaccine when polio came to town, parents would not allow their children to go to swimming pools, movie theaters, or play with children on the next block. Almost everyone knew someone who was paralyzed from this dreadful disease. When IPV was licensed in 1955, parents wept with joy and had their children immunized.

b. Wild polioviruses have diminished markedly. Inapparent infection with wild strains early in life no longer play a significant role in establishing immunity. Universal immunization of all infants and children with polio vaccine is a necessity.

c. OPV immunization

(1) The primary series of OPV consists of three doses.

(2) Breastfeeding does not interfere with successful OPV immunizations.

(3) OPV has been associated with paralytic disease in vaccine recipients and their close contacts. The risk is 1 case for every 3.2 million doses administered.

(4) OPV should not be given to immunodeficient patients or to household contacts of immunodeficient patients.

d. IPV immunization

(1) The primary series of IPV consists of four doses. Additional supplementary doses should be given every 5 years.

(2) IPV is used to immunize susceptible adults and immunodeficient patients.

(3) IPV is used to immunize children who cannot be isolated from immunodeficient household contacts.

e. Routine immunization of adults (18 years old or older) residing in the United States is not recommended. However, certain adults who are at risk of exposure to wild poliovirus should be immunized, including:

(1) Travelers to areas where poliomyelitis is epidemic or endemic.

(2) Members of communities or specific population groups with disease caused by wild polioviruses.

(3) Laboratory workers handling specimens that may contain polioviruses.

(4) Health care workers in close contact with patients who may be excreting polioviruses.

3. Live attenuated measles, mumps, and rubella virus (MMR) vaccine. Measles-rubella, mumps-rubella, and single antigen vaccines are also available.

a. Measles (see section IV A)

(1) Individuals born before 1957 usually have immunity from measles as a result of infection with the natural disease and do not need to be immunized. Everyone else who has not received a live measles vaccine after his or her first birthday, or anyone who was

immunized before 1967 with an unknown type should receive the measles vaccine.
(2) Booster immunizations are not recommended.

b. Mumps

(1) Vaccine for mumps became commercially available in 1967.
(2) Clinical vaccine efficacies have ranged from 75%–90%.
(3) Only about 3000 cases of mumps are reported each year, which represents a 98% decrease in reported cases since the vaccine was licensed.

c. Rubella

(1) About 600–700 cases are reported each year, which represents a 98% decline in reported cases since the vaccine was licensed in 1969. There has also been a marked decrease in the reported cases of congenital rubella syndrome.
(2) Because of a theoretical risk to the fetus, rubella vaccine should not be given to pregnant women, and women should not become pregnant for 3 months after vaccination. However, the risk of teratogenicity from rubella vaccine is quite small, and rubella immunization during pregnancy is not a reason to recommend interruption of the pregnancy.
(3) Rubella immunization of a woman who has no history of vaccination is justifiable without serologic testing.

4. *H. influenzae* type b (Hib) polysaccharide vaccine

a. *H. influenzae* is the most common cause of bacterial meningitis in children under 5 years of age. An estimated 12,000 cases occur each year. The mortality rate is 5%, and one-third of these children have permanent neurologic sequelae.

b. Hib disease is more common in certain high-risk groups, such as:
(1) Native Americans.
(2) Blacks.
(3) Individuals of low socioeconomic status.
(4) Patients with certain medical problems such as:
(a) Asplenia.
(b) Sickle cell disease.
(c) Hodgkin's disease.
(d) Antibody deficient syndromes.
(5) Children who attend day-care centers.

c. All children should be immunized with Hib at 24 months of age; however, children who attend day-care centers should be immunized at 18 months of age.

d. Children who have had Hib disease under 24 months of age or children who were immunized under 24 months of age should be immunized or reimmunized. An immunologic response to either natural disease or immunization under 24 months is not considered sufficient to prevent future disease.

5. Influenza vaccine (see section IV B 3 b)

6. Hepatitis vaccine (see section VI B 3 d)

7. Pneumococcal polysaccharide vaccine

a. Pneumococcal polysaccharide vaccine contains purified capsular materials of the 23 types of *Streptococcus pneumoniae* responsible for 87% of recent bacteremic pneumococcal diseases in the United States.

b. Booster doses are not recommended.

c. Patients who received the earlier pneumococcal polysaccharide vaccine containing 14 types of *S. pneumoniae* should not be reimmunized with the newer vaccine.

d. This vaccine can be given to everyone. However, vaccination is particularly recommended for:
(1) Adults:
(a) With chronic illnesses involving the heart or lungs.
(b) With chronic illnesses associated with an increased risk of pneumococcal disease or its complications, including:
(i) Splenic dysfunction or anatomic asplenia.
(ii) Hodgkin's disease.
(iii) Multiple myeloma.
(iv) Alcoholism and cirrhosis.
(v) Renal failure.
(vi) Cerebrospinal fluid leaks.
(vii) Immunosuppressive disorders.
(c) Over 65 years of age.
(2) Children 2 years of age or older with chronic illness specifically associated with increased risk for pneumococcal disease or its complications, including:
(a) Anatomic or functional asplenia, such as sickle cell disease or splenectomy.

(b) Nephrotic syndrome.
(c) Cerebrospinal fluid leaks.
(d) Conditions associated with immunosuppression.

D. Immunization schedules (Table 4-1). Every patient-physician encounter requires an evaluation of a patient's immunization status. No one in the twentieth century should ever develop a vaccine-preventable illness because of lack of immunization. All immunizations administered should be well documented on the medical record and on the patient's permanent, personal, comprehensive immunization record. The record should contain the type of vaccine administered, the lot number, manufacturer, and the month, day, and year of administration. The patient should be instructed to keep this record in a safe place so it is accessible when needed. Individuals who are traveling abroad and need additional immunizations should consult their local or state health departments for current recommendations.

IV. MEASLES AND INFLUENZA

A. Measles (rubeola)

1. Epidemiologic features

a. Pre-vaccine era (before 1963)

(1) Measles was a common disease of childhood. From 1950–1962, over 500,000 cases were reported annually.
(2) Communitywide outbreaks were common and tended to occur every couple of years. Large families often had several children ill at the same time.
(3) Outbreaks were most likely to occur in the late winter or early spring.
(4) Age distribution
(a) Ninety percent of reported cases occurred in individuals less than 10 years of age.
(b) An estimated 95% of Americans had measles by 15 years of age.
(c) Over 50% of the cases occurred in schoolchildren between 5–9 years of age.

b. Post-vaccine era

(1) Measles is now an uncommon disease of childhood. In 1985, only 2700 cases were reported.
(2) Communitywide outbreaks are rare. Focal outbreaks have occurred in communities or on college campuses, primarily in unimmunized or improperly immunized individuals. In 1985, 56% of the reported cases occurred in such individuals.
(3) Cases are most likely to occur in the late winter or early spring.
(4) The age distribution of reported cases has shifted upwards.
(a) Over 60% of the reported cases are now occurring in individuals 10 years of age and older.
(b) In 1984 and 1985, 5% of the reported cases were over 25 years of age.
(c) Over 50% of the cases now occur in schoolchildren between 10–14 years of age.
(5) Encephalitis with resulting brain damage and mental retardation occurs in 1 of every 2000 reported cases.

Table 4-1. Immunization Schedules

Recommended Age	Vaccine
Normal Infants and Children	
2 months	DTP and OPV
4 months	DTP and OPV
6 months	DTP
15–18 months	MMR, DTP, and OPV
24 months	Hib
4–6 years	DTP and OPV
14–16 years	Td
Normal Adults	
> 18 years	Td every 10 years
Born after 1956	Measles vaccine
Women in their reproductive years	Rubella vaccine
High-risk adults*	Hepatitis vaccine
	Pneumococcal vaccine
	Influenza vaccine

Note.—DTP = diphtheria-tetanus-pertussis; OPV = oral poliovirus; MMR = measles-mumps-rubella; Hib = *H. influenzae* type b; and Td = tetanus and diphtheria.
*See appropriate sections for a description of these groups.

(6) Death from respiratory or neurologic complications occur in 1 of every 3000 reported cases.

2. Infectious disease process

a. Agent. A RNA virus, which is classified as a paramyxovirus, is the agent.

b. Reservoir. Man with clinical disease is the reservoir for measles.

(1) Subclinical cases do not occur, or they are extremely rare. There is no carrier state.

(2) The patient is communicable from just before the prodromal period to about 4 days after the onset of rash. The peak period of communicability is during the prodromal period.

c. Portal of exit is via respiratory secretions.

d. Mode of transmission is by direct contact with infectious droplets. Airborne transmission also occurs.

e. Portal of entry is via the respiratory tract. Entry via the conjunctiva has also been postulated.

f. Susceptible host

(1) Everyone is susceptible. The onset of disease can occur from 6–18 days after exposure.

(2) Clinical disease confers lifelong immunity.

(3) Immunity is acquired by immunization with a live attenuated measles vaccine.

(4) Clinical disease is more severe in malnourished individuals.

3. Control strategies

a. Measles vaccine

(1) From 1963–1967, a killed measles vaccine was available. Approximately 1.8 million doses were distributed, and an estimated 600,000–900,000 individuals received this vaccine. However, this vaccine was discontinued because it was not effective and because it was associated with atypical measles, which occurred after exposure to natural measles.

(2) From 1963–1974, a live attenuated measles vaccine (Edmonston B strain) was available. Approximately 19 million doses were distributed. Since this vaccine caused a rectal temperature of 103°F (39.5°C) in 30%–60% of recipients, a dose of IG was administered with it.

(3) In 1965 and 1968, further attenuated strains (Schwartz and Moraten) of measles vaccine were marketed.

b. Recommendations concerning vaccine usage

(1) In 1963, the recommendations were to administer the vaccine at 9 months of age when maternal antibodies were presumably absent.

(2) In 1965, the age for administering measles vaccine was raised to 12 months because maternal antibodies were shown to persist to 11 months.

(3) In 1976, the age for administering measles vaccine was raised to 15 months because of better seroconversion.

c. Programs of the PHS for controlling measles

(1) In 1966, a National Measles Eradication Program was initiated. Measles could be eradicated if the following four essential conditions were met; however, eradication efforts failed because it was not possible to satisfy the four essential conditions.

(a) Routine immunization of all infants at approximately 1 year of age

(b) Immunization of all susceptible children on entry to school or other places of congregation to raise the immune threshold, which would prevent the occurrence of epidemics

(c) Improved surveillance of the disease to identify all cases

(d) Prompt epidemic control when cases or outbreaks are first recognized to eliminate the measles virus from the population so that there would be no reservoir in which the virus could survive

(2) In 1977, the Childhood Immunization Initiative was undertaken because it was estimated that 20 million American children under 15 years of age lacked adequate protection against the vaccine preventable diseases of childhood. The goals of this program were:

(a) To ensure that at least 90% of the nation's children under 15 years of age had received needed vaccines by October 1, 1979. School health records were reviewed to identify children who needed immunizations and to make certain that these children were either immunized in special school programs or referred for immunizations.

(b) To develop a permanent system to maintain this level of protection. State or local health departments were encouraged to develop and enforce regulations requiring immunizations or proof of immunity as a condition for entering or continuing in school.

(3) In 1978, attempts were made to eliminate indigenous measles from the United States by October 1, 1982. Imported measles cases and all cases resulting from such importation in the following two generations were excluded. The strategy included:
(a) Achieving and maintaining high immunization levels.
(b) Effective surveillance.
(c) Aggressive outbreak control.

d. Results of control strategies. Figure 4-1 shows the reported measles cases in the United States from 1950–1981.
(1) Since 1981, the number of reported cases has ranged from 1500–3200 cases per year. This represents a decrease of over 99% as compared to the era before vaccine.
(2) In 1985, almost 30% of the reported cases occurred in the preschool age population who also had the highest incidence rate of 4.7 per 100,000 population. Immunization of preschoolers at the proper age has always been difficult, especially in the lower socioeconomic segments of the population in urban areas.
(3) The current measles vaccine has an efficacy of around 95%. Therefore, some cases of measles will occur in properly immunized persons.
(4) A booster measles immunization is not required.

B. Influenza is not a very interesting disease to medical students as it is nothing more than a febrile upper respiratory illness. To house officers and clinicians, it is frustrating because viral pneumonias are untreatable. To an epidemiologist and a virologist, influenza is absolutely fascinating.

1. Epidemiologic features

a. Influenza occurs as sporadic cases, localized outbreaks, epidemics, and pandemics.

b. Influenza outbreaks have a characteristic pattern. The virus normally seeds the population with isolated sporadic cases. The actual epidemic begins abruptly, spreads quickly so that peak activity occurs in 2–3 weeks, and is over in 5–6 weeks, depending on the size of the community. The amount of influenza activity in a community is measured by:
(1) Increased absenteeism in schools and industries.
(2) Increased visits to emergency rooms for upper respiratory illness symptoms.
(3) Increased hospitalizations for penumonia.
(4) Increased pneumonia-influenza mortality. This excess mortality normally occurs 2 or more weeks after the epidemic has peaked, and it is considered an index of the severity of the outbreak.

c. Nationwide epidemics occur every 2–3 years; worldwide epidemics occur at longer intervals and are normally preceded by a major change in the antigenic structure.

d. In temperate zones, epidemics occur in the winter months, but in the tropics, they can occur at any time.

e. Attack rates during epidemics range from 10%–50%. Although the highest clinical attack rates are in the school age population, the highest case fatality rates are in the older or more debilitated segments of the population.

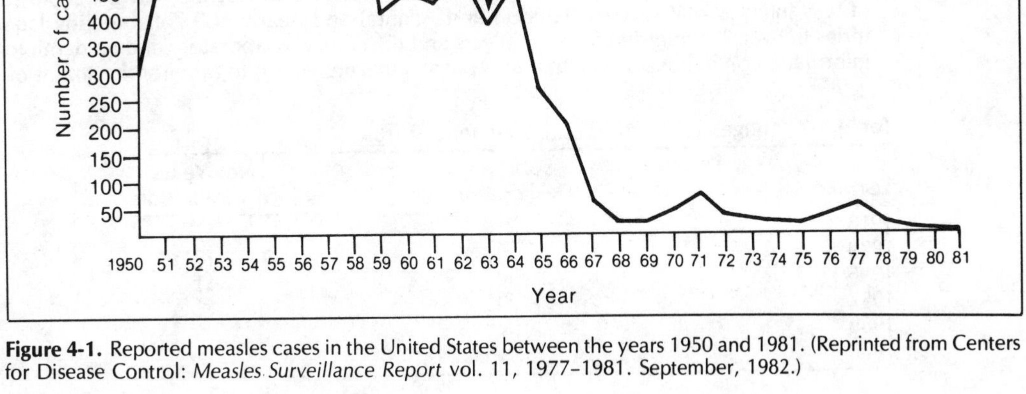

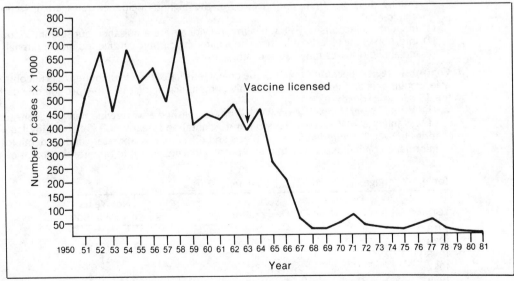

Figure 4-1. Reported measles cases in the United States between the years 1950 and 1981. (Reprinted from Centers for Disease Control: *Measles Surveillance Report* vol. 11, 1977–1981. September, 1982.)

f. During an outbreak, several different strains of influenza virus may circulate at the same time, although one strain is normally predominant. It is difficult to isolate an influenza virus between epidemic periods.

g. In interpandemic years, widespread influenza activity and excess mortality normally occurs in January through March. In pandemic years, widespread influenza activity and excess mortality normally occurs between October and December.

2. Infectious disease process

a. Agent

(1) Influenza is caused by a RNA virus, which can be divided into three distinct types—A, B and C. Types A and B cause widespread epidemics, while type C causes local outbreaks of mild disease.

(2) The surface of the virus has two main antigenic structures:

(a) Hemagglutinin (H) spike, which is the site for attachment of the virus to host cell.

(b) Neuraminidase (N) spike, which may play a role in releasing virus particles from the cell.

(3) The H and the N antigens undergo antigenic variation. This is particularly true for type A.

(a) Antigenic drift refers to minor changes that continuously occur within a subtype.

(b) Antigenic shift refers to major changes that occur periodically. The new virus has very little or no serologic relationship with previous strains of influenza virus. Pandemic years are normally preceded by a major antigenic shift.

(c) In this century, five new H and two N antigens have appeared (Table 4-2). Since 1977, a variety of H_1N_1 and H_3N_2 strains have been circulating simultaneously.

(d) Because of the antigenic variations that occur, influenza isolates have a special nomenclature. The strain designation consists of the virus type, geographic origin, laboratory reference number, and year of occurrence. The antigen description follows in parentheses and describes the antigenic character of the hemagglutinin and the neuraminidase. The strains that were used in the 1986–1987 vaccine were A/Chile/1/83(H_1N_1), A/Mississippi/1/85(H_3N_2), and B/Ann Arbor/1/86.

b. Reservoir. Man is the reservoir for the strains that cause disease in humans. Animal strains of influenza viruses do exist.

c. Portal of exit is via the respiratory tract. The period of communicability begins at the onset of clinical disease and persists for about 5 days.

d. Mode of transmission is by the airborne route. Infected individuals cough out large numbers of virus particle aerosols, less than 10 μ in size. The explosive nature of most epidemics suggest that a single infected person can infect a large number of individuals in a relatively short period of time.

e. Portal of entry is via the respiratory tract.

f. Susceptible host

(1) Everyone is susceptible to a new strain of influenza virus.

(2) Since antigenic types of H and N tend to recirculate periodically, and since some immunity develops from prior exposure, the highest incidence rates are in schoolchildren.

(3) Influenza infections in young healthy individuals are a nuisance but seldom serious.

(4) Infection in the elderly or in those debilitated by chronic cardiac, pulmonary, renal, or metabolic diseases may cause death.

3. Control strategies. Because of the unique characteristics of the virus, influenza is uncontrollable. Pneumonia and influenza are the only communicable diseases that are still one of the top 10 causes of death.

a. The World Health Organization (WHO) has established a worldwide network, consisting of two international centers (London and Atlanta) and nearly 100 collaborating laboratories in over 70 countries, which collects and disseminates laboratory and epidemiologic information on influenza. The main purpose of this network is to monitor the strains of in-

Table 4-2. Antigenic Variation of the Influenza Virus

Year	Subtype Designation	No. Years in Circulation
1918	$H_{sw1}N_1$	11
1929	H_oN_1	17
1946	H_1N_1	11
1957	H_2N_2	11
1968	H_3N_2	9
1977	H_1N_1	. . .

fluenza viruses in circulation and to detect any significant antigenic changes that may precede a pandemic. The information is also used to update the formulation of influenza vaccines.

b. Control programs have been directed at high-risk individuals and consist of immunizations with an inactivated influenza vaccine or of chemoprophylaxis with amantadine.

(1) The PHS recommends that immunizations be offered to:

(a) Adults and children with chronic disorders of the cardiovascular or pulmonary system that require regular medical evaluation.

(b) Residents of nursing homes.

(c) Individuals over 65 years of age.

(d) Adults and children with other chronic disorders.

(e) Medical personnel who can transmit an influenza infection to their high-risk patients.

(f) Anyone who wants the vaccine.

(2) The antigenic components of the vaccine are based upon the types of influenza viruses that were circulating in the community in the previous year. Consequently, the vaccine is almost always at least a year behind.

(3) Chemoprophylaxis with amantadine:

(a) Interferes with the uncoating step in the virus replication process and reduces viral shedding.

(b) Is only effective against type A.

(c) Must be taken throughout the influenza season.

V. SEXUALLY TRANSMITTED DISEASES (STDs)

A. Introduction. The term STD, which describes the mode of transmission rather than the site of infection, came into common use during the 1970s as the medical community became aware of the large number of infections spread from person to person during sexual contact. Since these diseases were no longer restricted to the genital tract and since many of them were of a systemic nature, the term STD has gradually replaced the term venereal disease.

1. Diagnostic laboratory tests. The development of better and more rapid diagnostic laboratory tests has helped to define the problem and its many ramifications. STDs comprise more than 50 different disease entities, including 25 different syndromes, and are caused by more than 21 different organisms. The list includes hepatitis, cytomegalovirus (CMV), enteric infections, and ectoparasites, to name only a few.

2. Incidence. There has been a marked increase in the total number of cases and in the incidence of many of these diseases.

a. There are approximately 12,000,000 cases of STDs each year, including:

(1) 3.0 million cases of *Chlamydia*.

(2) 3.0 million cases of trichomoniasis.

(3) 1.8 million cases of gonorrhea.

(4) 1.2 million cases of urethritis (nongonococcal and nonchlamydial).

(5) 1.0 million cases of mucopurulent cervicitis (nonchlamydial).

(6) 1.0 million cases of human papillomavirus (HPV).

(7) 200,000–500,000 cases of HSV.

(8) 200,000 cases of HBV.

(9) 90,000 cases of syphilis.

b. Approximately 2.5 million teenagers are affected with STDs annually.

c. Approximately 65% of all cases occur in individuals under 25 years of age.

3. The population at risk of acquiring an STD has increased, as a result of demographic, sociologic, and behavioral changes that have occurred over the past 20 years.

a. The number of people in the 15–34-year-old age group has grown from 42 million in 1970 to an estimated 61 million by 1985, a 45% increase. This population is also sexually active at an earlier age than the previous generation.

(1) The percent of urban teenage girls experiencing premarital intercourse increased from 30% in 1971, to 43% in 1976, and to 50% in 1979.

(2) Individuals who become sexually active early are more likely to have multiple partners. The percent of sexually experienced unmarried teenagers with multiple partners increased from 39% in 1971 to 50% in 1976.

b. Sexually active adults are either remaining single or postponing marriage. In 1980, 28% of 25-year-old women and 43% of 25-year-old men were single as compared to 10% and less than 20% in 1970, respectively.

c. There has also been a change in the pattern of contraceptive practices in the United States.

Women now use oral contraceptives to protect against pregnancy, which may have caused a corresponding increase in sexual activity as well as a decrease in the use of condoms and other barrier contraceptive methods, which are thought to be somewhat protective against STDs.

4. **Human casualties.** The extent of human suffering caused by STDs has been recognized by health officials and clinicians. Women and newborn children have the most significant complications of these diseases.
   a. Perhaps the most severe complications in women is pelvic inflammatory diseases (PID).
      (1) PID occurs in 10%–20% of women infected with the gonococcus. It can also be caused by other organisms such as *Chlamydia* and *Mycoplasma*.
      (2) Approximately 4% of women become infertile following a single episode of PID, 33% after the second episode, and 60% after the third episode.
      (3) Over 1 million cases of PID are diagnosed and treated each year. Over 276,000 women are hospitalized, and almost 40,000 have hysterectomies each year as a result of PID.
   b. Officials estimate that between 100,000 to 150,000 women become sterile each year because of pelvic infection due to STDs. The percent of couples 20–26 years of age classified as infertile increased from 3.6% in 1965 to 10.6% in 1982.
   c. The number of ectopic pregnancies in the United States has nearly quadrupled since 1970 with almost 70,000 cases in 1983.
      (1) Studies have shown that 6% of pregnancies occurring in women with a previous history of PID were ectopic.
      (2) Women with a history of PID are 10 times more likely to experience an ectopic pregnancy than those without such a history.
   d. At least four viruses (i.e., HSV, HPV, HBV, and CMV) have been associated with cancer, including:
      (1) Cervical intraepithelial neoplasia (HSV and HPV).
      (2) Carcinoma of the cervix (HSV).
      (3) Vulvar carcinoma (HSV).
      (4) Penile carcinoma (HPV and HSV).
      (5) Anal carcinoma (HPV).
      (6) Hepatocellular carcinoma (HBV).
      (7) Kaposi's sarcoma (CMV).
   e. The impact of STDs on the fetus and newborn can be devastating. Syphilis, HSV, CMV, and *Chlamydia* all cause significant morbidity and mortality including miscarriages, stillborns, neonatal deaths, mental retardation, neonatal conjunctivitis, and pneumonia.

5. **Costs.** The tremendous economic costs of STDs to society have been recognized by health officials. The total cost of STDs is estimated to exceed $3 billion annually. The total (direct and indirect) cost of PID and its complications of infertility and ectopic pregnancies exceeded $2.6 billion in 1985.

B. Syphilis

1. **Epidemiologic features**
   a. Syphilis ranks as the third reportable communicable disease in the United States. Other diseases like chicken pox and other STDs like *Chlamydia*, HSV, HPV, and trichomoniasis occur more frequently but are not reportable to health departments. In fiscal year 1985, there were 67,000 reported cases of syphilis (all stages), including 27,000 primary and secondary cases.
   b. In fiscal year 1985, 55% of the reported cases came from the 26% of the nation's population who live in the 63 cities with populations greater than 200,000.
   c. Highest case rates are in the 20–29-year-old age group; it is two to three times higher in men as compared to women.
   d. Syphilis is more common in homosexual men.
   e. Congenital syphilis is most likely to occur in the newborn infants of young, unmarried women who have not received proper prenatal care.
   f. Untreated syphilis infection can cause blindness, psychosis, or cardiovascular disease.

2. **Infectious disease process**
   a. **Agent.** *Treponema pallidum* is a spirochete that causes syphilis; it is indistinguishable from the spirochetes that cause pinta or yaws.
      (1) *T. pallidum* is 6–15 μm in length and 0.15 μm in width.
      (2) It can only be seen with darkfield microscopy, which shows a rotary motion with flexion and back-and-forth motion.
      (3) It is extremely fragile and can be destroyed by soap, antiseptics, and drying.
      (4) It is sensitive to penicillin and a number of other antimicrobial agents.

b. Reservoir of infection is man who is most likely to transmit the infection during the first years of infection when cutaneous lesions are present (primary and secondary stages). Communicability may persist for several years. Untreated women may infect their fetuses for many years; however, this risk declines and may no longer be present after 8 years.

c. Portal of exit is:

(1) Percutaneously through cutaneous lesions, such as a chancre, mucous patch, condyloma latum, and the lesions of secondary syphilis.

(2) Transplacental from mother to child.

(3) By a sanguineous nasal discharge (snuffles), which contains spirochetes. This may be the earliest sign of congenital syphilis.

d. Mode of transmission

(1) Direct contact with infectious exudates from moist mucosal or cutaneous lesions is the most common mode of transmission.

(a) The risk of getting syphilis from a sexual partner with early syphilis is estimated to be around 30% with a range of 10%–60%.

(b) The prevalence of syphilis among contacts with prolonged and repeated exposure (marital partners) may approach 90%.

(2) Transplacental transmission has been documented as early as the ninth week of pregnancy.

(3) Transmission by blood transfusions no longer occurs.

(4) Transmission by accidental needle sticks is highly unlikely.

e. Portal of entry is believed to be through tiny abrasions produced during sexual intercourse. Although the organisms cannot enter through intact skin, they can probably penetrate unbroken mucous membranes. However, they can enter directly into the bloodstream by the transplacental route.

f. Susceptible host

(1) Everyone is susceptible.

(2) There is no natural or acquired immunity.

(3) Reinfection is common. No vaccine is available.

(4) The antibody response that is invoked can be used for diagnostic purposes.

(a) A fourfold rise in the RPR test—a nontreponemal titer test—can be used to diagnose a recent infection that requires retreatment.

(b) The fluorescent treponemal antibody absorption (FTA-ABS) test remains positive for life and, therefore, cannot be used to diagnose repeat infections.

3. Control strategies

a. Routine screening with serologic tests for syphilis should be done on:

(1) All individuals with multiple sex partners.

(2) Any individual with another STD.

(3) All pregnant women as a means of preventing congenital syphilis. Women who have positive serologies should be rescreened during the third trimester or at the time of delivery.

b. Routine premarital testing or **testing all hospitalized patients** is probably not a cost-effective way of controlling syphilis.

c. Case investigation and contact tracing by experienced investigators has been shown to interrupt the transmission of syphilis. All identified sexual contacts during the communicable stage must be located and treated epidemiologically. For primary, secondary, and early latent syphilis, the periods of concern are 3 months, 6 months, and 1 year, respectively.

d. A control program conducted by federal, state, and local health officials has been in effect since the early 1940s. The success of this program can be documented.

(1) The number of reported cases of all stages of syphilis has decreased by 89%.

(2) Reported cases of congenital syphilis have declined by 98%, and infant deaths directly related to syphilis have decreased by 99%. However, over the past several years, the number of cases of congenital syphilis has increased dramatically.

(3) First admissions to mental hospitals with the diagnosis of syphilis psychosis (general paresis) have declined by 98%.

C. Gonorrhea

1. Epidemiologic features

a. Gonorrhea ranks as the number one reportable communicable disease in the United States.

b. The number of reported cases tripled between fiscal year 1965 (325,000 cases) and fiscal year 1976 (over 1,000,000 cases). During the early 1980s, the number of reported cases declined somewhat but now appears to be on the rise again.

c. There are an estimated 1 to 1.5 million cases that are not reported.

d. The highest case rates are in the 15–24-year-old age group, particularly among men rather than women. The incidence rate in cities with over 200,000 population is twice the rate of smaller cities and rural areas.

e. In certain venereal disease clinics, 40% of infected patients return within 12 months, and 20% of these reinfections return within 6 weeks.

f. Penicillinase-producing *Neisseria gonorrhoeae* was first detected in the United States in 1976 when 98 cases were reported from 17 states. Most of these cases could be traced to military personnel or civilians who acquired the disease in the Far East and transmitted it to their sexual partners in the United States. By 1982, penicillinase-producing *N. gonorrhoeae* had been documented in every state. During fiscal year 1985, 6454 cases were reported with 64% of these cases occurring in Florida, Los Angeles, and New York City. This increase has been caused by the continued importation of the Asian/Pacific strain and the African strain and from sustained domestic transmission.

2. Infectious disease process

a. Agent

(1) *N. gonorrhoeae*, the cause of gonorrhea, is a gram-negative diplococcus organism.

(2) There are many different strains that can be distinguished on the basis of:

(a) Nutritional requirements (auxotyping).

(b) Antibiotic sensitivity patterns.

(c) Antigenic diversity.

(d) Plasmid analysis.

(3) Different strains circulate in different segments of the population and have different clinical characteristics.

(a) One strain, which is more sensitive to penicillin and tetracycline and which is more common in whites than blacks, is more likely to cause an asymptomatic urethral infection in men and also accounts for most of the cases of disseminated gonococcal infection.

(b) Another strain, which is more resistant to antibiotics and fecal lipids, is more common in homosexual men.

(c) Strains resistant to penicillin, tetracycline, and spectinomycin have been isolated. Penicillin resistance can be caused by a plasmid (β-lactamase positive–penicillinase-producing *N. gonorrhoeae*) or it could be chromosomally mediated (β-lactamase-negative).

b. Reservoir of infection is man who may be symptomatic or asymptomatic. (Asymptomatic carriage may persist for many months.) The exact proportion of asymptomatic infections probably varies from area to area.

(1) About 5% of men with urethral infections are asymptomatic.

(2) About 10% of homosexual men with rectal infections are asymptomatic.

(3) Asymptomatic infections in women range from 25% to 80%.

(4) Over 90% of pharyngeal infections are asymptomatic.

c. Portal of exit. The organism, which can only infect columnar and transitional epithelium, is already on the surface of the body and can easily be dislodged.

d. Mode of transmission

(1) Most cases are transmitted through sexual activity when mucous membrane surfaces come into contact with infected exudates.

(a) The risk of a male acquiring the gonococcus from a single exposure to an infected female is estimated to be around 18%–25%. Multiple exposures increase the risk.

(b) The risk of a female acquiring the gonococcus from an infected male is unknown, but it is felt to be high (maybe 75% or higher).

(c) Transmission of the organism from pharyngeal carriage to other sites is uncommon.

(2) Nonvenereal transmission may occur between an infected mother and her newborn.

(3) Transmission by fomites or by nonsexual personal contact over the age of 1 probably occurs infrequently or not at all.

e. Portal of entry is via the mucous membrane surfaces of the body lined by nonsquamous epithelium.

f. Susceptible host

(1) Everyone is susceptible.

(2) There is no natural or acquired immunity. No vaccine is available.

(3) Reinfection is common.

(4) Prepubertal women with columnar or transitional vaginal epithelium may develop a vulvovaginitis, while adult women with squamous epithelium will not.

(5) Women using intrauterine contraceptive devices have a high risk of developing salpingitis.

(6) Complement-deficient individuals are more likely to develop bacteremia.

3. Control strategies

a. Appropriate and multiple cultures should be performed on individuals being evaluated in sexually transmitted disease clinics.

(1) Women should have endocervical and rectal cultures.

(2) Homosexual men should have urethral and rectal cultures.

(3) Individuals who have oral sex should have pharyngeal cultures.

b. Every individual with a positive gonococcal culture should be properly treated with an approved antimicrobial regimen.

c. All gonococcal isolates should be tested for β-lactamase production.

d. A test of cure should be done on all patients, especially women who may be asymptomatic, 4–7 days after completion of therapy. These isolates should be tested further for antibiotic sensitivity.

e. Although it is not possible to interview or do contact tracing on all infected individuals, it should be done on:

(1) Women with PID. Studies have shown that 50% of the male contacts of women with PID have gonorrhea. Since multiple episodes of PID lead to sterility, reinfection must be prevented.

(2) Individuals with a recurrent gonorrhea infection.

(3) Patients with penicillinase-producing *N. gonorrhoeae*. Health officials are concerned about this strain of gonorrhea because the cost of treating it is more than ten times as expensive as the corresponding regimen for a penicillin-sensitive organism.

f. All identified sexual contacts of a known case of gonorrhea should be treated epidemiologically even before their culture results are known.

g. Because of the high number of asymptomatic gonorrhea infections in women, screening gonorrhea cultures are recommended for certain sexually active women. Screening takes place in health department clinics, hospitals, emergency rooms, family planning clinics, student health centers, correction centers, and in certain obstetrics and gynecology clinics. In fiscal year 1985:

(1) A total of 7.4 million culture specimens were obtained from women as part of a nationwide screening program.

(2) Of these, 301,500 (4.1%) were positive for gonorrhea, and 286,400 (95%) of these women were located and treated.

h. Every state has regulations requiring the prophylactic instillation of a 1% silver nitrate solution or an erythromycin (0.5%) or tetracycline (1.0%) ophthalmic ointment in the eyes of newborn infants to prevent gonococcal conjunctivitis.

i. The national program to control gonorrhea, which was implemented in 1972, has been moderately successful.

(1) Between 1965–1975, the gonorrhea morbidity rate increased at an annual rate of 12%.

(2) Between 1976–1984, the number of reported cases of gonorrhea leveled, and the rates actually declined.

(3) However, the number of reported cases and gonorrhea rates increased during fiscal year 1985 by 6.8% and 5.8%, respectively (Fig. 4-2). These data are remarkable when one considers the fact that various demographic pressures should have driven the case count even higher.

D. Acquired immune deficiency syndrome (AIDS)

1. Epidemiologic features

a. AIDS is a new disease that began to occur in the United States in the late 1970s but was not identified as a syndrome until the summer of 1981.

b. The number of reported cases continues to rise. As of October 1986, there were approximately 25,000 reported cases with a doubling time every 12–14 months.

c. AIDS primarily occurs in young men of all racial and ethnic groups between 20–49 years of age. Only 7% of the reported cases are women. Nationally, 60% have been white, 24% have been black, 15% have been Hispanic, and 1% are of unknown ethnic origin.

d. The disease has been reported in certain high-risk groups, including:

(1) Homosexual and bisexual men who account for 68% of cases. The risk is increased for homosexual men who:

(a) Have had multiple sexual partners.

(b) Have had anonymous contacts.

(c) Practice certain sexual acts like receptive anal intercourse.

(2) Homosexual and bisexual intravenous drug users who account for 8% of cases.

(3) Intravenous drug users who account for 17% of the total cases and for over 50% of the cases in the heterosexual population.

(4) Patients with hemophilia or other coagulation disorders who account for 1% of cases.

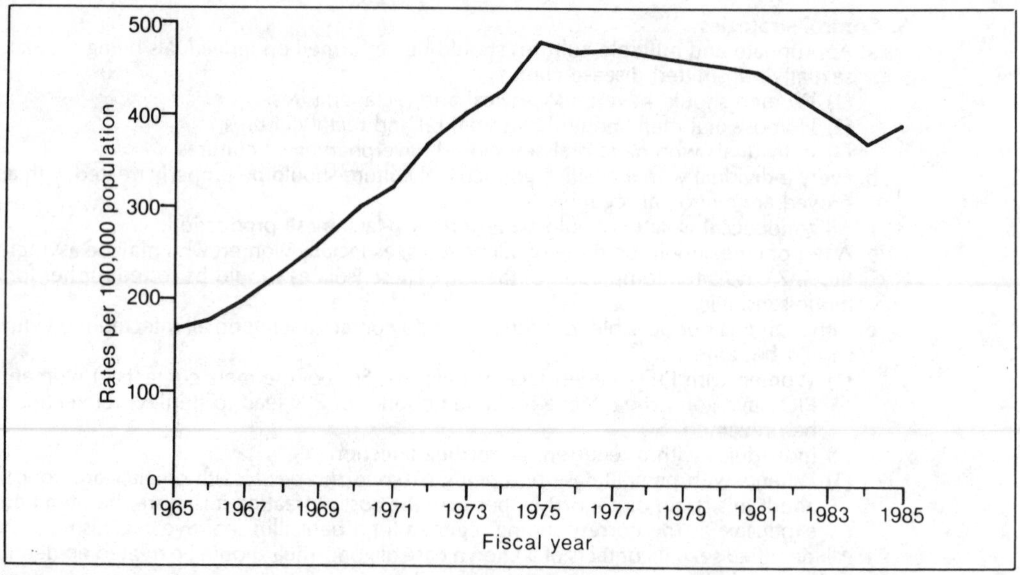

Figure 4-2. Gonorrhea case rates per 100,000 population in the United States between 1965 and 1985. (Reprinted from Centers for Disease Control: *Division of Sexually Transmitted Diseases and STD Laboratory Annual Report*. Fiscal year, 1985.)

They contract AIDS through infected plasma products (clotting factor concentrates), which are used to treat their coagulation disorders.

(5) Heterosexual contacts of patients with AIDS or individuals in the high-risk groups who account for 2% of cases.
- **(a)** Approximately 80% of these cases are women whose sexual partners had AIDS or were in the high-risk groups, such as bisexual men, intravenous drug users, or hemophiliacs.
- **(b)** Only 20% were men who said they contracted the disease from infected women contacts who were primarily intravenous drug users.

(6) Individuals transfused with infected blood products who account for about 2% of cases.

(7) Individuals without a known cause who account for 5% of reported adult cases. These cases can be further subdivided.
- **(a)** Forty percent of these cases have occurred in individuals who have immigrated from countries where AIDS is not associated with the aforementioned risk factors.
- **(b)** Thirty percent of these cases are still under epidemiologic investigation and may be reclassified as additional information is obtained.
- **(c)** Twenty percent of these cases either died before adequate information could be obtained, were lost to follow-up, or refused to answer questions.
- **(d)** Ten percent of these cases, or less than 1% of the total, cannot be explained. Many of these individuals have serologic evidence of other sexually transmitted diseases, such as syphilis or HBV, suggesting that they probably contracted the disease from sexual activity.

(8) Pediatric patients, including:
- **(a)** Children born to parents who belong to a high-risk group (79%).
- **(b)** Children who have had blood transfusions (14%).
- **(c)** Hemophiliacs (4%).
- **(d)** Children in an unknown category (3%). There are insufficient data on both parents to classify them.

e. The disease has *not* been reported in certain close contacts, including:

(1) Health care workers
- **(a)** Approximately 1500 health care workers who had close contact with AIDS patients were examined for serologic evidence of HIV infection, and 26 were positive. Of these:
  - **(i)** Twenty-three individuals belonged to a well-established risk group.
  - **(ii)** Two individuals gave a history of having stuck a needle in their hand after drawing blood from an AIDS patient.
  - **(iii)** One individual was tested anonymously, and no additional information is available.

(b) There have been no known health care worker anywhere in the United States who developed AIDS from routine exposure to AIDS patients.

(2) Household contacts

(a) Over 350 household contacts have been serologically evaluated for evidence of HIV infection. The only household contacts found to be infected were sexual partners or infants born to infected mothers.

(b) There are no known instances of household spread of AIDS from one adult to another or from one child to another through normal casual (nonsexual) contact.

f. AIDS had been documented in all 50 states, the District of Columbia, the three United States territories, and in at least 92 countries on 6 continents. In the United States, almost 75% of all of the reported cases have occurred in 5 states—New York, California, Florida, New Jersey, and Texas. These are the areas of the country that have a large number of individuals in the high-risk groups. They are also the areas that have had the disease for the longest periods of time.

2. Infectious disease process

a. Agent

(1) Human immunodeficiency virus (HIV), the cause of AIDS, is a RNA retrovirus that requires an enzyme, reverse transcriptase, to multiply. Reverse transcriptase permits viral replication by forming DNA from viral RNA. Humans do not have reverse transcriptase. This virus was formerly called the human T-lymphotrophic virus type III/lymphadenopathy associated virus (HTLV-III/LAV).

(2) The antigenic structure of the surface of the virus undergoes continuous change. This change takes place inside the patient so that antigenically different viruses can be isolated at different times.

(3) The virus attacks and destroys the T_4 (helper) lymphocyte. It can also live in certain nerve cells.

(4) HIV is fragile outside of the body and can be inactivated by a number of disinfectants, including a 1:10 dilution of household bleach, gluteraldehyde, hydrogen peroxide, isopropyl alcohol, and ethyl alcohol to name a few. Under laboratory conditions and using high concentrations of HIV, the virus can live for several days in the wet or dry state outside the body. However, these concentrations are not achieved in normal body fluids, so this fact does not appear to be of any epidemiologic significance.

b. Reservoir of infection is humans in both the symptomatic and asymptomatic state. Based on seroprevalence data in high-risk groups and on estimates of the number of people in these groups, the PHS estimates that between 1–2 million Americans have been infected with this virus.

c. Portal of exit. The portals of exit for this virus are the percutaneous route (blood), the genital tract (semen and vaginal secretions), and the transplacental route. The virus has also been isolated in saliva, tears, breast milk, and urine.

d. Mode of transmission

(1) The documented modes of transmission include:

(a) Sexual transmission, which includes both male homosexual transmission and heterosexual men-to-women and women-to-men transmission. Rectal and vaginal intercourse carry the highest risks of transmission.

(b) Percutaneous exposure to contaminated blood, such as sharing needles in intravenous drug abuse or receiving contaminated blood or blood products. Blood donors are not at risk by donating blood.

(c) Transmission from mother-to-child either in utero, at the time of delivery, or shortly thereafter.

(2) Since there has been no documented spread to health care workers through routine exposure or to household contacts through casual (nonsexual) exposure and since there has been no significant spread to individuals not in the well-defined risk groups, it can be argued that this disease cannot be transmitted by:

(a) **Airborne route.** AIDS cannot be contracted by being in the same room with an AIDS patient.

(b) **Casual contact.** It appears that AIDS cannot be transmitted by saliva or tears.

(c) **Foodborne route.** AIDS cannot be contracted by eating food prepared by an individual infected with the AIDS virus.

(d) **Vectors.** AIDS cannot be transmitted by mosquito or other insect bites.

e. Portal of entry. The virus enters the body through breaks in the skin or mucosal surfaces.

f. Susceptible host

(1) Individuals of every age, both sexes, and all racial, ethnic, and socioeconomic groups are susceptible.

(2) No cofactors have been identified as being necessary for this disease.

(3) There is no scientific evidence that exercise, rest, or good nutrition can prevent the progression of this disease.

(4) Infection with the HIV virus may be a lifelong problem. At least some of the currently infected asymptomatic individuals will develop the full-blown clinical syndrome at some time in the future. Others may remain asymptomatic for life.

3. Control strategies. Although there is no current treatment for HIV infection and no vaccine for preventing HIV infection, this disease can be controlled. Some control measures have already been implemented, and other educational programs for behavior modification have been developed.

a. Blood screening. Control measures that make the blood supply safe have already been implemented.

(1) Individuals who should not donate blood include:

(a) Any man who has had sexual contact with another man since 1977.

(b) Present or past abusers of intravenous drugs.

(c) Individuals from countries where AIDS is common (Central Africa and Haiti) and not associated with any known risk factors.

(d) Sexual partners of the above groups.

(e) Any man who has had sex with a prostitute in the past 6 months.

(2) Every unit of blood that is collected is screened for antibodies against the AIDS virus, and the positive units are discarded. The current positivity rate is about 3–4 per 10,000 units screened.

(3) The manufacturing process for factor VIII concentrate is now subjected to heat treatment, which inactivates the AIDS virus.

b. Educational programs for behavior modification for homosexual men and intravenous drug users have been developed in some parts of the country.

(1) For safe sex recommendations, see section V F. Many homosexual men have adopted these recommendations as indicated by the declining incidence of rectal and pharyngeal gonorrhea. Safe sex recommendations include:

(a) Limiting the number of sexual partners.

(b) Avoiding the transfer of body fluids from one partner to the other by using condoms. Do not engage in unprotected vaginal or rectal intercourse.

(c) Hugging and touching activities, which will not transmit HIV.

(2) The recommendations for intravenous drug users is, "Do not use drugs or do not share your equipment." The impact of this message on drug users is unknown.

c. Other control strategies have yet to be developed. It is important to emphasize that since AIDS is a new disease, it might take new strategies for control and that society may be forced into doing things that have not been done previously.

E. *Chlamydia*

1. Epidemiologic features

a. Although health officials do not keep statistics on the number of cases that occur, *Chlamydia* is believed to be the most common sexually transmitted bacterial pathogen in the United States today. An estimated 3–4 million cases occur each year.

b. Infection is more common in urban areas in low socioeconomic groups, particularly those individuals under 20 years of age with multiple partners.

c. Prevalence rates

(1) Adult heterosexual men—2%–31%

(2) Homosexual men—5%–10%

(3) Heterosexual women—3%–27%

2. Infectious disease process

a. Agent. *Chlamydia trachomatis*, the causative agent, is classified as a bacteria and has the following characteristics.

(1) It grows only intracellularly.

(2) It contains both DNA and RNA.

(3) It divides by binary fission.

(4) It has cell walls similar to gram-negative bacteria.

b. Reservoir of infection is man in both the clinical and asymptomatic state. Most women with cervical infections, most homosexual men with rectal infections, and as many as 30% of heterosexual men with urethral infections have few or no symptoms.

c. Portal of exit. The organism mainly infects the squamocolumnar-columnar epithelial cells lining mucosal surfaces. These cells are destroyed as a result of the infection and are discarded with the inflammatory debris.

d. Mode of transmission
(1) Most cases are transmitted through sexual activity when a mucous membrane surface comes into contact with infected exudates.
(2) An infant can acquire a chlamydial infection coming through the birth canal.
e. Portal of entry is the mucous membrane surfaces of the body.
f. Susceptible host
(1) There is no natural or acquired immunity.
(2) Approximately 45% of gonorrhea cases have coexisting chlamydial infections.
(3) *Chlamydia* causes:
(a) Approximately 50% of the nongonococcal urethritis and acute epididymitis in men.
(b) Mucopurulent cervicitis and approximately 40% of pelvic inflammatory disease (PID) in women.
(c) Inclusion conjunctivitis and afebrile interstitial pneumonia in infants born to infected mothers.

3. Control strategies
a. Certain patients should receive empirical treatment for chlamydial infection, including those with:
(1) Certain clinical conditions caused by *Chlamydia*, such as nongonococcal urethritis, acute epididymitis, mucopurulent cervicitis, and PID.
(2) Gonococcal infections.
(3) Sexual partners of the above-mentioned groups.
b. Since *Chlamydia* organisms are very sensitive to tetracycline and erythromycin, test of cure cultures are not necessary.
c. *Chlamydia* infections can now be diagnosed by culture or by two different antigen tests.
(1) Culture is the preferred method, but it takes several days and is costly.
(2) Direct smear fluorescent antibody test can be done quickly, but it takes trained personnel and high-quality equipment. Only a limited number of tests can be done because it is a labor-intensive process.
(3) Enzyme-linked immunoabsorbent assay can be used to test large numbers of specimens, but it takes about 4 hours to complete.
(4) Other tests will undoubtedly be developed in the coming years.
d. Certain populations should be screened for *Chlamydia* infection including:
(1) Individuals attending an STD clinic who would not otherwise receive therapy for *Chlamydia*.
(2) Health care facilities that may have a high prevalence of infections, such as adolescent and family planning clinics.
(3) Young, urban individuals of low socioeconomic status who have multiple sex partners and who would not otherwise receive therapy for *Chlamydia*.
(4) Certain groups of pregnant women, including:
(a) Adolescents ($<$ 20 years of age).
(b) Unmarried women.
(c) Married women who may be at high risk because of multiple sex partners or a history of other STD.
e. Gonococcal and chlamydial ophthalmia can be prevented by instilling either erythromycin (0.5%) ophthalmic ointment or tetracycline (1%) ointment into the eyes of all neonates. This should be done as soon as possible after birth and never later than 1 hour. Single-use tubes or ampules are preferable to multiple-use tubes.

F. Primary prevention of STDs. It is important to prevent the acquisition of certain STDs because they are either untreatable (e.g., herpes and AIDS), difficult to treat (e.g., human papillomavirus), or because they cause a destructive process in the subclinical state (e.g., latent and congenital syphilis).

1. Modification of sexual activity, which would decrease the likelihood of exposure to or contact with infectious agents.
a. Engage in mutually monogamous relationships.
b. Limit the number of sexual partners.
c. Inspect and question new partners.
d. Avoid certain sexual practices involving anal or fecal contact.

2. Barrier methods of contraception (i.e., condoms, diaphragms, and spermicides) provide protection against STDs.
a. The advantages of a condom, which must be properly used at all times, include:
(1) It protects both partners.
(2) It prevents the transfer of infected body secretions from one individual to another.

(3) It prevents mucosal surfaces from coming into contact with infected lesions.

b. Diaphragms cover the cervix and would, therefore, block an important portal of entry for many infectious agents. When used with a spermicide, they may decrease a woman's risk of acquiring a sexually transmitted disease. However, there is no evidence that a diaphragm protects a man from acquiring an STD.

3. The only STD that can be prevented with a vaccine is HBV. However, it is expensive, requires three injections, and does not work well in immunosuppressed individuals.

4. Prophylactic antibiotics taken before or after exposure should not be done because:
   a. No single antibiotic covers all potential STDs.
   b. Allergic reactions may occur.
   c. They may lead to the emergence of resistant organisms.

5. There is no evidence that postcoital urination, washing, or douching prevents the acquisition of an STD.

VI. VIRAL HEPATITIS

A. Hepatitis A virus (HAV)

1. Epidemiologic features

a. Infection with HAV (**infectious hepatitis**) has a worldwide occurrence with high seroprevalence rates in very early life in developing countries where sanitation is inadequate and at a later age in developed countries.

b. In the United States, most cases occur in individuals under 15 years of age during the winter and spring.

c. Epidemics have occurred in institutions, day-care centers, rural areas where sanitation may be poor, and where people are crowded together.

d. About 21,500 cases are reported in the United States each year. The actual number of cases is probably several times the reported number, most of which have no identifiable risk factors. Identifiable risk factors include contact with:
(1) Individuals with an HAV infection.
(2) Homosexual individuals.
(3) Foreign countries.
(4) Children who attend day-care centers.

2. Infectious disease process

a. **Agent**
(1) HAV is a small (25–29 mm), nonenveloped, RNA-containing virus (picornavirus).
(2) Only one antigenic class has been identified.
(3) The virus remains stable at 4°F (−20°C) for long periods of time and at 140°F (60°C) for at least 39 minutes. In some outbreaks, the virus appears to have survived brief steaming or cooking and in refrigerated clams or oysters for 48 hours.
(4) HAV has been found in blood and stools but not in urine and other body fluids.

b. **Reservoir**
(1) Humans are the primary reservoir, although nonhuman primates have been infected.
(2) There are no chronic carriers. There is a brief period of viremia, which precedes the onset of hepatic disease.
(3) HAV appears to be maintained in nature by serial transmission during the incubation period.
(4) The patient is communicable from about 2 weeks before the onset of clinical disease to about 1 week after. The greatest period of infectivity is before the onset of jaundice.

c. **Portal of exit**
(1) HAV multiplies in the hepatocytes and reaches the intestinal tract by way of the bile duct.
(2) It is then excreted in large quantities (10^8 particles/g) via the stool. Peak virus excretion occurs during last half of the incubation period rather than during acute illness.
(3) The amount of virus shed in the stool appears to be unrelated to the severity of clinical illness.
(4) Percutaneous transmission, which exits from needle sticks during the brief periods of viremia, are possible, but documented instances of percutaneous transmission or transfusion-related infections are very rare.

d. **Mode of transmission** is primarily by direct person-to-person transmission via the fecal-oral route or by common vehicle via contaminated food or water.
(1) Transmission is facilitated by:
(a) Poor personal hygiene.
(b) Poor sanitation.

(c) Intimate (intrahousehold or sexual) contact.

(2) Sharing utensils (i.e., drinking out of the same cup) or cigarettes or kissing do not transmit the infection.

(3) Foodborne outbreaks are almost always caused by:

(a) Foods that are not cooked.

(b) Foods touched by infected human hands after cooking.

(c) Ingesting raw shellfish, such as clams and oysters, which have been harvested from sewage-contaminated waters.

e. Portal of entry is almost always by ingesting the virus.

f. Susceptible host

(1) Infection is related to age and socioeconomic status. Approximately 20% of Americans are infected by age 20 and 50% by age 50. Incidence appears to be declining. In developing countries, over 90% of individuals have antibodies by adulthood.

(2) The incubation period is 15–50 days with an average of 28–30 days.

(3) Young children are more likely to have subclinical infections while adults are more likely to have overt disease. Less than 20% of children in day-care centers are believed to develop clinical disease, while over 80% of infected adults probably become symptomatic.

(4) Infection confers lifelong immunity.

3. Control strategies for HAV infection include good personal hygiene, removal of known cases from occupations that prepare or serve food for public consumption, and the postexposure prophylactic administration of human immune serum globulin (IG).

a. Strict isolation of the patient is not necessary if the following precautions and hygienic practices are instituted:

(1) All cases and household contacts should wash their hands with soap and water before eating and after using the toilet.

(2) Toothbrushes, washcloths, and towels should not be shared.

(3) Eating utensils should be carefully washed with soap and water.

(4) Bathroom facilities may be shared by all household members.

b. IG should be given in the standard single intramuscular dose (0.02 ml/kg) as soon as possible after exposure but not later than 2 weeks. Serologic confirmation of HAV in an index case is recommended, but not necessary, before treatment of contacts. IG may either prevent infection altogether, or it may modify the severity of the disease.

(1) IG is recommended:

(a) For all household and sexual contacts of persons with HAV.

(b) For controlling HAV infections in day-care facilities.

(i) In day-care centers with children in diapers, IG should be given to all children and staff if one case of HAV occurs in either a child or in an employee or if cases occur in two or more of the children's households. If cases occur in three or more families, IG should also be administered to household members of the children's families.

(ii) In day-care centers without diapered children, IG should only be given to classroom contacts of an index case.

(c) For food handlers who work in a restaurant or cafeteria where another food handler has been diagnosed as having HAV. Although IG is not usually recommended for patrons, it may be given to patrons when:

(i) The infected person handled food that was not cooked before it was eaten.

(ii) The hygienic practices of the infected food handler are deficient.

(iii) Patrons can be identified and treated within 2 weeks of exposure.

(d) For preventing HAV infection in travelers to tropical areas or developing countries. This is especially true for tourists who travel to out-of-the-way places where they may be exposed to infected persons or contaminated food and water. The actual dose of IG depends on body weight and length of stay.

(e) For controlling outbreaks after an epidemiologic investigation has identified individuals at risk.

(2) IG is not recommended:

(a) For casual contacts at work or school.

(b) For classmates of elementary or secondary schools after a single case.

(c) For hospital personnel caring for a patient.

(d) For individuals exposed to a common source (food) of HAV infection when cases begin to occur after the 2-week period at which point IG is ineffective.

B. Hepatitis B virus (HBV)

1. Epidemiologic features

a. Infection with HBV (**serum hepatitis**) has a worldwide occurrence with the highest incidence in Africa and Asia where infection may occur in infancy and childhood. In the United States, most cases occur in young adults in urban areas from 15–30 years of age. The disease is not evenly distributed in the population but is concentrated in certain segments, including:

(1) Asian refugees.
(2) Clients in institutions for the mentally retarded.
(3) Intravenous drug users.
(4) Household contacts of HBV carriers.
(5) Patients on hemodialysis.
(6) Homosexual men.
(7) Health care workers.

b. There are approximately 200,000 HBV infections in the United States each year. Approximately 50,000 will become symptomatic with jaundice, 10,000 will be hospitalized, and 250 will die of fulminant disease. The lifetime risk of developing HBV infection is 5%–10% for the general United States population but may be as high as 100% in certain groups. There are between 500,000 to 1,000,000 carriers in the United States.

c. Long-term sequelae of HBV infection include:

(1) Chronic hepatitis.
(2) Cirrhosis.
(3) Primary hepatocellular carcinoma.

2. Infectious disease process

a. Agent

(1) HBV is a 42 mm, double-shelled DNA virus. At one time, it was called the Dane particle. Other components include:

(a) HBsAg, which exists in a spherical (15–25 mm) or cylindrical (20 × 200 mm) form. There are four distinct subtypes (i.e., adr, adw, adyw, adyr), which vary geographically and thus, are useful in epidemiologic studies. The HBsAg appears 30–60 days after exposure and persists for various periods of time.

(b) Hepatitis B core antigen (HBcAg), which is the internal core of the virus.

(c) Hepatitis B e antigen (HBeAg), which is associated with HBV replication and high infectivity. It parallels the presence of DNA polymerase, which is associated with complete virons.

(2) The virus is apparently quite stable and can survive for hours and days outside the body.

(3) Serologic response to HBV infection includes:

(a) Antibody to HBsAg (anti-HBs) indicates past infection, immune response to HBV vaccine, or passive antibody from hepatitis B immune globulin (HBIG).

(i) The development of anti-HBs eliminates HBsAg and prevents the development of the carrier state.

(ii) Anti-HBs is also associated with long-term immunity. Infection with one subtype confers protection against infections with other subtypes.

(b) Antibody to HBcAg (anti-HBc) indicates past infection with HBV.

(c) IgM class antibody to HBcAg (IgM anti-HBc) indicates recent HBV infection and may persist for 4–6 months.

(d) Antibody to HBeAg (anti-HBe) suggests a low titer of HBV and a low degree of infectivity.

b. Reservoir

(1) Man is the only known reservoir.

(2) Carriers of HBV, who maintain the virus in nature, are defined as individuals who are HBsAg positive at least twice a minimum of 6 months apart. Certain groups, like patients on hemodialysis or clients in institutions for mentally retarded, are more likely to become chronic carriers; thus, other factors, such as immunocompetence, which allows for the establishment of chronic infections, are also important. The likelihood of developing the carrier state also depends upon the age at which infection occurs:

(a) Only 6%–10% of infected adults become chronic carriers of HBsAg.

(b) Approximately 90% of infants infected in the perinatal period become carriers.

(3) Table 4-3 shows the prevalence of HBV markers in various population groups.

(4) HBV has been found in almost all body secretions or excretions, including blood, serum, semen, vaginal fluid, saliva, breast milk, urine, and feces. The highest concentration of HBV is in blood and serous fluid.

c. Portal of exit

(1) HBV can leave the body via breaks in the skin from cuts, wounds, weeping lesions, or needle sticks, or it can exit via body fluids like semen, vaginal fluid, or saliva.

(2) Individuals who are HBeAg positive are more likely to shed higher numbers of organisms.

Table 4-3. Prevalence of Hepatitis B Virus (HBV) Serologic Markers in Various Population Groups

Population Group	Prevalence of Serologic Markers of HBV infection: HBsAg	All markers
High risk		
Immigrants and refugees from areas of high HBV endemicity	13%	70%–85%
Institutionalized mentally retarded individuals	10%–20%	35%–80%
Users of illicit parenteral drugs	7%	60%–80%
Homosexually active men	6%	35%–80%
Household contacts of HBV carriers	3%–6%	30%–60%
Hemodialysis patients	3%–10%	20%–80%
Intermediate risk		
Health care workers who have frequent blood contact	1%–2%	15%–30%
Prisoners (male)	1%–8%	10%–80%
Staff at institutions for the mentally retarded	1%	10%–25%
Low risk		
Health care workers with infrequent blood contact	0.3%	3%–10%
Healthy adults		
(first-time volunteer blood donors)	0.3%	3%–5%

Reprinted from *MMWR* 34(22):319, 1985.

d. Mode of transmission is primarily by direct person-to-person contact via infected body fluids or by common vehicle, such as a contaminated needle. Most clinical cases have had no known percutaneous exposure during the 6 months prior to their disease.

(1) Foodborne transmission of HBV has never been documented.

(2) Arthropodborne (mosquito) transmission of HBV has not been documented.

(3) Transmission is more likely to occur:

(a) In populations with overcrowding, lack of sanitation, and poor personal hygiene.

(b) When there is close contact between individuals who have high concentrations of virus in their blood. These high-risk and intermediate-risk groups are listed in Table 4-3. Epidemiologic studies have shown especially high transmission rates in families who adopt antigen-positive children and in sexual partners of infected adults.

(c) In infants born to HBsAg-positive mothers, especially those mothers who are also HBeAg positive. Only a minority of the infants born to these mothers are infected at birth; however, some become infected at the time of birth, and others become infected during the first year of life.

(d) In intravenous drug users who share contaminated needles.

e. Portal of entry of HBV occurs through breaks in the skin (percutaneous) or through permucosal exposure to infective body fluids.

f. Susceptible host

(1) All ages are susceptible, but clinical expression of disease occurs in only 10% of children infected and in 25%–50% of adults infected.

(2) The incubation period is 45–180 days with an average between 60–90 days.

3. Control strategies include good personal hygiene, screening blood, discarding all units positive for the HBsAg, avoiding contacts with blood or body fluids containing blood, and administering HBIG or HBV vaccine.

a. Good personal hygiene is the same as that described for HAV infection [see section VI A 3 a (1)–(4)] except that razors also should not be shared.

b. Avoid contact with blood by wearing gloves and gowns when handling or exposed to blood or body fluids containing blood. All blood spills should be cleaned with soap and water and disinfected with a 1:10 dilution of household bleach.

c. Administer IG or HBIG, which contains anti-HBs. IG has a titer of at least 1:100 by radioimmunoassay, while HBIG has a titer of higher than 1:100,000 by radioimmunoassay. HBIG is preferred for postexposure prophylaxis, but IG may be used in the same dose if HBIG is not available.

d. HBV vaccine was licensed in 1981 and is a suspension of 22 nm surface antigen particles that have been purified from human plasma and inactivated by biochemical procedures.

(1) Three intramuscular injections at 0, 1, and 6 months, respectively, in the deltoid (arm) have been shown to produce antibodies in over 90% of healthy adults. Field trials have shown an 80%–95% efficacy in preventing infection among susceptible individuals. Although some authorities recommend booster doses at 5-year intervals, this is not the recommendation of the PHS. The vaccine costs about $120 for the three doses.

(2) **No significant adverse reactions** have been related etiologically to the vaccine although severe illnesses have occurred after receipt of vaccine. These illnesses are probably not related to the vaccine. Administration of the vaccine to HBsAg carriers or to previously infected individuals have no therapeutic or adverse consequences.

(3) **Suboptimal responses** have occurred in dialysis patients and in individuals who received their immunization in the buttock. A postimmunization antibody titer may be indicated with reimmunization if necessary.

e. Pre-exposure immunization should be given to susceptible individuals who are at risk of acquiring HBV infection, including:

(1) Health care workers who are exposed to blood or blood products or potential accidental needle sticks. (Vaccinations should be completed while the health care worker is still in school.)
(2) Clients and staff who work closely with institutionalized mentally retarded individuals.
(3) Hemodialysis patients.
(4) Homosexually active men as soon as their homosexual activity begins.
(5) Users of illicit injectable drugs.
(6) Patients with clotting disorders who receive clotting factor concentrates.
(7) Household and sexual contacts of HBV carriers.
(8) Families adopting or providing foster care for HBsAg-positive children.
(9) Heterosexually active individuals with multiple sexual partners.
(10) International travelers who plan to visit areas with high levels of endemic HBV, particularly if they plan:
  (a) To have contact with blood.
  (b) To have sexual contact with residents.
  (c) To reside in these areas for more than 6 months.
(11) Prisoners in prisons and children in classrooms containing HBV carriers who behave aggressively or have special medical problems that increase the risk of exposure to their blood.
(12) Certain high-risk ethnic populations, such as Alaskan Eskimos, native Pacific Islanders, and immigrants from areas (Asia and Africa) that have high rates of HBV infection.

f. Post-exposure prophylaxis is indicated for infants born to HBsAg-positive mothers, for individuals who have had percutaneous or permucosal exposure to HBsAg-positive blood, or for sexual partners of an HBsAg-positive person.

(1) **Perinatal exposure** is one of the most efficient modes of HBV transmission. Infants born to HBsAg- and HBeAg-positive mothers have a 70%–90% chance of becoming infected and a 90% chance of becoming chronic HBV carriers.
  (a) High-risk pregnant women should be screened in the prenatal period. Table 4-4 lists these women.
  (b) HBIG and HBV vaccine should be given as soon as possible after delivery, preferably in the delivery room. HBIG given at birth should not interfere with the routine childhood immunizations at 2 months of age.
  (c) The currently recommended schedule consists of intramuscular injections at different sites of 0.5 ml HBIG and 0.5 ml HBV vaccine within 12 hours of birth. The HBV vaccine should be repeated at 1 and 6 months. This regimen has been shown to prevent the HBV carrier state in 85%–90% of infants.

Table 4-4. Women for Whom Prenatal HBsAg Screening Is Recommended

Women of Asian, Pacific Island, or Alaskan Eskimo descent, whether an immigrant or born in the United States
Women born in Haiti or sub-Saharan Africa
Women with histories of:
Acute or chronic liver disease
Work or treatment in a hemodialysis unit
Work or residence in an institution for the mentally retarded
Rejection as a blood donor
Blood transfusion on repeated occasions
Frequent occupational exposure to blood in medicodental settings
Household contact with an HBV carrier or hemodialysis patient
Multiple episodes of venereal diseases
Percutaneous use of illicit drugs

Reprinted from *MMWR* 34(22):330, 1985.

(d) The child should be tested for HBsAg and anti-HBs at 12–15 months to determine the success of the immunizations.

(2) Percutaneous or permucosal (ocular or mucous membrane) **exposure to HBsAg-positive blood** has been shown to transmit HBV infection. The risk of developing an HBV infection following a needle-stick injury with a needle contaminated with HBsAg blood is about 6%–30%. This risk can be decreased by 75% with two injections of HBIG: one immediately after exposure and the other, a month later. Since this type of exposure usually occurs in health care workers, the incident can be used to encourage immunizations (see Table 4-5).

(a) All nonimmunized individuals with a percutaneous or permucosal exposure to a patient's blood should receive the HBV vaccine series.

(i) If the source is known to be HBsAg positive, HBIG at a dose of 0.06 ml/kg should be given at a separate intramuscular site as soon as possible.

(ii) If the HBsAg status of the source is unknown and if the source is known to be at high risk of previous HBV infection, then the source should be tested for HBsAg. If positive, the exposed individual should receive HBIG as outlined above. In order to be effective, HBIG must be administered within 7 days of exposure.

(b) All previously completely immunized exposed persons to a known HBsAg source should be tested for anti-HBs unless they have been tested within the last 12 months. If anti-HBs are present, nothing else needs to be done.

(c) If the exposed person to a known HBsAg-positive source or to a high-risk source is incompletely immunized against HBV infection or has been shown to be a nonresponder, adminster one dose of HBIG (0.06 ml/kg) and either complete the vaccination schedule or administer a booster dose of vaccine.

(d) Nothing needs to be done to a previously immunized person exposed to a low-risk HBsAg-positive source or to an unknown source.

(3) Sexual partners of HBsAg-positive individuals should receive HBIG (0.06 ml/kg), provided that it can be given within 14 days of the last exposure. A second dose of HBIG should be given 3 months later if sexual contact is continuous and if the index patient remains HBsAg positive. Ninety percent of individuals with acute HBV infection become HBsAg negative within 15 weeks of diagnosis. Steady sexual contacts of HBsAg-positive carriers should receive HBV vaccine.

(4) Nonsexual household contacts of patients with acute HBV infection do not need post-exposure prophylaxis. However, household contacts of chronic HBsAg carriers need to be immunized with HBV vaccine.

Table 4-5. Recommendations for Hepatitis B Prophylaxis Following Percutaneous Exposure

	Exposed Individual	
Source	**Unvaccinated**	**Vaccinated**
HBsAg positive	HBIG × 1 immediately* Initiate HB vaccine series†	Test exposed individual for anti-HBs If inadequate antibody, administer HBIG (× 1) immediately plus an HBV vaccine booster dose
Known source		
High risk HBsAg positive	Initiate HB vaccine series Test source for HBsAg If positive, administer HBIG × 1	Test source of HBsAg only if exposed individual is a known vaccine nonresponder; if source is HBsAg positive, give HBIG × 1 immediately plus HBV vaccine booster dose
Low risk HBsAg positive	Initiate HBV vaccine series	Nothing required
Unknown source	Initiate HBV vaccine series	Nothing required

Reprinted from *MMWR* 34(22):331, 1985.

*HBIG dose, 0.06 ml/kg intramuscularly.

†HBV vaccine dose, 20 μg intramuscularly for adults, and 10 μg intramuscularly for infants or children under 10 years of age. First dose should be given within 1 week, and the second and third doses, 1 and 6 months later, respectively.

C. Non-A, non-B hepatitis

1. **Epidemiologic features.** There are at least two types of viral hepatitis caused by at least two unidentified agents.
   a. One type, similar to HAV infection, has occurred in epidemic and sporadic patterns in the Indian subcontinent and North Africa. Waterborne epidemics have occurred as well as person-to-person transmission via the fecal-oral route. The chronic carrier state does not appear to exist.
   b. Another type, similar to HBV infection, may be caused by several different agents. This type is transmitted primarily by percutaneous exposure to contaminated blood and is the most common cause of post-transfusion hepatitis in the United States. Close contact transmission has also been reported. A chronic carrier state exists.
2. **Control strategies** consist of good personal hygiene and not sharing intravenous needles. There are no vaccines, and IG has not been shown to have any protective effects.

D. Hepatitis D virus (HDV)

1. **Infectious disease process.**
   a. **Agent**
      (1) The delta agent of the HDV (delta hepatitis) is a defective virus, 35-37 nm in size, which consists of RNA genetic materials with an internal protein antigen (delta antigen) surrounded by a coat of HBsAg.
      (2) Since the delta agent requires the presence of HBV for synthesis, coinfection must take place for the clinical expression of the disease. Infection of a HBV carrier leads to a chronic delta infection and chronic active hepatitis. In the United States, 25%–50% of fulminant HBV cases have a concurrent delta agent infection.
   b. **Mode of transmission** is similar to HBV.
2. **Control strategies** consist of preventing HBV infections and of preventing the HBV carrier state. Superinfection of HBsAg carriers cannot be prevented with any known biologic agent.

VII. TUBERCULOSIS

A. Epidemiologic features

1. **Worldwide disease** has caused significant morbidity and mortality. Tuberculosis will continue to be a problem in the United States as long as it remains a worldwide problem.
2. **Infection with the tubercle bacilli** is determined by a positive skin test to an intradermal injection of 5 international units (IU) of the international standard of purified protein derivative (Mantoux test).
   a. In general, 10 mm of induration at 48–72 hours is considered positive for the general population. Household contacts are considered positive with a 5 mm induration.
   b. The reaction becomes positive about 2–10 weeks after infection and remains positive throughout life. It is a measure of tuberculous infection not tuberculous disease.
   c. Cutaneous anergy may occur in individuals with advanced tubercular disease or in immunosuppressed individuals.
   d. In individuals over 35 years of age, a booster phenonemon exists. When tuberculin skin tests are applied a week apart, the second test may show a marked increase in size of the reaction. The size of the induration in the second test should be the baseline reading for that patient.
3. **Tuberculosis disease** (i.e., clinical symptoms) can occur from a primary infection or from the reactivation of a latent infection. Pediatric cases usually represent a primary infection, and most adult cases occur from the reactivation of a latent infection, one that was acquired many years previously.
4. **Incidence.** In 1983, 24,000 cases of tuberculosis were reported. About 92% of these cases occurred from reactivation of a latent infection, and only 8% represented new infections. The overall case rate for the United States was 10 per 100,000 population in 1983.
5. **Prevalence** of tuberculosis infection as determined by positive tuberculin skin tests increases with increasing age. Most individuals born in the United States today remain tuberculin negative. However, high tuberculin positivity rates occur in certain segments of the population, such as the elderly, nonwhites, and in individuals with low socioeconomic status. Tuberculosis infection is also common in immigrants from Asia, Latin America, and the Caribbean. It is estimated that perhaps 50% of the people in developing countries are infected with the tubercle bacilli.

6. **Case rates** for tuberculosis parallels the prevalence rates of tuberculosis infection. Cases are more likely to occur in older (> 45 years of age) than younger age groups, in nonwhite races (more than five times higher in older age groups) than in whites, and in men than women. The racial differences may be related to socioeconomic factors, or there may be genetic differences in susceptibility. Tuberculosis morbidity is not evenly distributed in the United States.
   a. The highest case rates are along the southeastern seaboard, through the Appalachian mountain region, along the United States border with Mexico, and in scattered areas of the northwest containing many native Americans.
   b. The case rate per 100,000 population in 1981 ranged from 8.8 to 24.8 with an overall rate of 11.9. The higher case rates were in cities containing more than 100,000 population and increased as the population increased.
   c. Tuberculosis is not just an urban problem since 55% of the cases occurred in communities of fewer than 100,000 population.

B. Infectious disease process

1. **Agent.** The causative agent is *Mycobacterium tuberculosis* var. *hominis*.
   a. Drug resistant organisms often initially cause illness in certain population groups, such as Asians and Hispanics.
   b. Drug resistance can also develop while individuals are on therapy, either because they have not taken their medications properly or because therapy was inappropriate.
   c. Tubercle bacilli can be destroyed by direct sunlight, ultraviolet light, heat, and some disinfectants, such as phenol or tricresol solution.
   d. Organisms can remain viable in dried sputum for long periods of time. Droplet nuclei may remain infectious for 8–10 days. However, when exposed to sunlight, the organisms die more quickly.
2. **Reservoir** of infection is man.
3. **Portal of exit** is via the respiratory tract. The organism exits the body in respiratory secretions created by coughing, sneezing, talking, singing, or other respiratory action. Patients with cavitary pulmonary lesions with large numbers of organisms in their sputa are at greatest risk of spreading the disease. Extrapulmonary tuberculosis is noncommunicable.
4. **Mode of transmission** is by inhalation of droplet nuclei, the airborne route. These droplet nuclei can remain suspended in the air, float to all parts of a room, and infect people in other rooms via ventilating systems. However, transmission is not easily achieved. It normally requires prolonged exposure to an infectious case.
5. **Portal of entry** is via the respiratory tract. Most primary lesions in the lungs are found in the periphery, suggesting that the site of implantation is the alveoli.
6. **Susceptible host.** Once infection has occurred, the outcome for the individual depends on a number of factors.
   a. **Age at the time of infection** is important. Infants and adolescents are more likely to experience severe disease.
   b. **The risk of developing clinical disease** is greatest (around 5%) within the year following infection (i.e., conversion of skin test from negative to positive). However, the risk of developing acute disease never disappears as long as living tubercle bacilli are present in the host.
   c. **Reactivation of a latent infection** is more likely to occur in the elderly, in patients with diabetes or silicosis, and in immunosuppressed individuals.
   d. Clinical disease in patients with AIDS or HIV infection is normally extensive and presents with atypical manifestations. Extrapulmonary forms, such as lymphatic and disseminated (miliary) disease are more common, and pulmonary disease with mediastinal or hilar lymphadenopathy occurs in any lobe and without cavitation.

C. Control strategies. Morbidity and mortality from tuberculosis has been declining since the beginning of the twentieth century. Although improvements in diets, housing, and living conditions have contributed significantly to this decline, the advent of effective chemotherapy in the late 1940s and early 1950s has accelerated this decline. The objectives of a tuberculosis control program are to eliminate morbidity and mortality in infected individuals and to interrupt transmission of the tubercle bacilli in the community. Control programs can be divided into two components—surveillance and containment.

1. **Surveillance** refers to the process of identifying infected patients.
   a. **Medical care.** Many patients are identified because they either seek medical care for symptoms of tuberculosis or for other unrelated medical problems.

b. Contact investigation. Some cases are identified because of contact investigation around known cases. Since positive culture results may take 8 weeks, contact investigation should begin if the history, sputum smear, and chest x-rays are suggestive of tuberculosis and should be performed in widening concentric circles (starting with household contacts) until the level of infection (as determined by a tuberculin skin test) detected approximates the level of infection within the local community. The decision to evaluate a contact should be based on characteristics of the case, the environment, and the contact.

(1) Case characteristics should include an evaluation of the degree of infectiousness. Factors to consider include:

(a) The duration of respiratory symptoms, such as cough.

(b) The type of disease, such as pulmonary cavitary disease or tuberculous laryngitis.

(c) The number of acid-fast bacilli in the sputum smear.

(d) The characteristics of the sputum. High volume and watery sputum are regarded as risk factors.

(2) Environmental factors consist mainly of evaluating the concentration of droplet nuclei in the air shared by the case and contacts. This would include an evaluation of:

(a) The volume of air in the room.

(b) The ventilation of the room. In general, the concentration of infectious particles is increased in poorly ventilated rooms.

(c) Whether or not air is recirculated or subjected to ultraviolet radiation or filtration.

(3) Contact characteristics include:

(a) The amount of time spent with the case. In general, high-risk contacts are normally household contacts or individuals who have had close contact over a prolonged period of time.

(b) The physical proximity to the case. Transmission of tuberculous infection is unlikely with brief exposure to relatively small numbers of aerosolized particles.

(c) Whether or not the contact had prior infection with tuberculosis or was taking antituberculosis therapy.

c. Screening programs. A few cases are identified through screening programs. Routine screening of the general United States population is no longer recommended. Screening of some segments of the population is indicated to detect cases of tuberculosis so that further transmission can be prevented and so that chemoprophylaxis can be given.

(1) Screening consists of:

(a) The application of a two-step intermediate strength Mantoux test.

(b) A chest x-ray for individuals who:

(i) Have a positive skin test.

(ii) Are 65 years of age or older.

(iii) Have signs or symptoms of tuberculosis.

(2) Screening is indicated:

(a) In populations with a high rate of infection such as immigrants from Asia, Latin America, and the Caribbean.

(b) In institutions where transmission of tuberculosis is likely, such as health care facilities (i.e., nursing homes and mental hospitals) or correction institutions, or where a case of tuberculosis would pose a particular hazard to others (i.e., day-care centers and newborn nurseries). Initial screening of new personnel and clients should be done. The need for repeat screening of nonreactors should be determined by the individual institutions and should be based on the risk of acquiring new infection.

2. Containment refers to those methods of stopping the spread of infection and disease. Containment activities consist of:

a. Administration of proper antituberculosis chemotherapy for the proper duration of time. Because of the duration of therapy and side effects of the drugs, the physician must work with the patient to make certain that he or she takes the medication. The patient can proceed normally as long as the prescribed medication is taken properly. More than 95% of cases can be cured with initial treatment.

(1) Proper therapy consists of two or more drugs, preferably drugs that the patient has never received before. Never add one new drug at a time to a failing regimen or to a patient who has received previous therapy.

(2) Isoniazid (INH) and rifampin (RMP) for 9 months is the current recommendation for treating uncomplicated cases acquired in the United States. Over 90% of patients taking INH and RMP become sputum negative in 3 months.

(3) A third drug, such as ethambutol (EMB), should be given to patients who might have drug-resistant organisms. Foreign-born Latin Americans and foreign-born Asians have resistant organisms in 12% and 15% of cases, respectively. One of the three drugs can be discontinued when sensitivity results become available.

(4) Drug sensitivity studies should be used when treating patients who might have drug-resistant organisms. Until drug sensitivities are available, the patient should be placed on two drugs that he or she has never had before. Intermittent regimens have been developed to treat patients who require close supervision.

b. Administration of antituberculous chemoprophylaxis to infected individuals (those with a positive intermediate Mantoux skin test) **who are at risk of developing clinical disease.** PHS trials using INH have shown a 50% reduction in clinical disease over a 20-year period. The level of protection exceeded 90% in patients who took their medication properly.

(1) Groups that should benefit from preventive therapy include:

(a) Individuals whose skin test has converted from negative to positive in the previous 2 years. Many of these (5%–23%) may develop disease in a few years.

(b) Close contacts of newly discovered cases of tuberculosis.

(i) Tuberculin-positive reactors ($\geq$ 5 mm induration) have a 1.6% incidence of developing tuberculosis during the first year after contact.

(ii) Tuberculin-negative contacts, especially infants, children under 6 years of age, or persons with impaired immunity should also be given preventive therapy.

(iii) For tuberculin-negative adults, other factors such as degree of infectiousness of the index case, daily consumption of alcohol, and side effects of INH should be considered.

(iv) All tuberculin-negative contacts should be retested 12 weeks later, and if still negative and if exposure has ended, the preventive therapy can be discontinued. If positive, therapy should be continued for 12 months.

(c) Individuals with chest x-rays showing abnormalities suggestive of tuberculous parenchymal scarring (solitary calcified granulomas are excluded). The risk of developing disease ranges from 0.4%–3.5% each year.

(d) Individuals with certain conditions, including hematologic or reticuloendothelial malignant neoplasm, AIDS or HIV infection, silicosis, chronic renal insufficiency, diabetes mellitus, and heroin addicts.

(e) Individuals on immunosuppressive therapy or systemic corticosteroids in dosages greater than 15 mg prednisone per day.

(f) Individuals with nutritional deficiency and substantial weight loss, including gastrectomy and intestinal bypass.

(g) Tuberculin-positive individuals under 35 years of age. The rate of developing disease in this group is about 0%–1% per year, which could yield a significant lifetime risk.

(2) The only drug proven to be effective preventive therapy is INH. A dosage of 300 mg in adults and 10 mg/kg of body weight (up to 300 mg) in children should be taken as a single daily oral dose. The duration of treatment is 1 year. The cost of the drug for 1 year is around $5.00.

(a) Short courses of therapy may be used, but they are probably less effective. A 9-month course of chemoprophylaxis may be used in household contacts of a source case receiving a 9-month course of chemotherapy if the contact had a normal chest x-ray.

(b) Lapses in therapy of less than 1 month can probably be ignored in terms of calculating the total duration of treatment. If the patient has completed more than 6 months of therapy before a time lapse of 1 month, preventive therapy could be terminated. If the patient has not completed 6 months of therapy at the time of a 1 month lapse, therapy should be restarted with the goal of completing 6 subsequent months of therapy.

(c) Twice weekly supervised administration of INH at a dosage of 15 mg/kg of body weight (900 mg maximum) for 12 months may be considered.

(3) INH chemoprophylaxis should not be used:

(a) In the presence of clinical disease. Two drugs are needed.

(b) In individuals who were previously adequately treated.

(c) In individuals who have had previous adverse reactions to INH.

(d) In patients with unstable hepatic function.

(e) In pregnant women until after delivery unless strongly indicated (i.e., close contact or recent converter).

(f) In individuals taking significant amounts of other hepatotoxins (i.e., alcohol).

(4) Toxic effects from INH include:

(a) Hepatitis, which occurs in 2.1% of individuals over 50 years of age and is rare in persons under 20. Patients who are over 35 years of age should be followed with transaminase levels at 1, 3, 6, and 9 months. Clinical symptoms should also be monitored since enzyme elevations will occur.

(b) Peripheral neuropathy, mood changes, and hypersensitivity reactions. The peripheral neuropathy, which is more common in persons with diabetes, uremia, and alcoholism, can be prevented by daily administration of 10 mg of pyridoxine (vitamin B_6).

(5) Patients who are contacts of proven INH-resistant organisms and for whom the consequences of infection are likely to be severe may be given chemoprophylaxis with RMP at 10 mg/kg of body weight up to 600 mg a day in a single oral dose. This regimen has not been shown to be effective in clinical trials, but it is believed to be effective on a theoretical basis. The cost of RMP for a year at this dosage is approximately $250.

3. Control and eradication of tuberculosis can only be accomplished by the combined efforts of both the private and public sectors of the medical community.

a. The private medical community should be aware of and implement current national recommendations for chemotherapy and for chemoprophylaxis. In 1980, only 40% of all infected contacts identified received a complete course of preventive therapy. They should also report all cases of tuberculosis to the health department so that appropriate control procedures can be instituted.

b. State and local health departments have certain resources that can be helpful to physicians and that can be used to control tuberculosis, including:

(1) A case registry that contains clinical and laboratory data on all reported cases. This registry contains information about:

(a) The duration of illness.

(b) The type and extent of disease.

(c) Hospitalization.

(d) Sputum smear and culture results.

(e) Previous therapy and most recent sensitivity studies.

(2) Consultants trained in the treatment of tuberculosis who can:

(a) Help decide current therapy.

(b) Resolve difficult clinical problems.

(c) Advise on the feasibility of an intermittent therapy program.

(3) Free antituberculosis drugs so that patients have one less expense to worry about.

(4) Free clinics where the patient can be followed on a regular basis.

(5) An outreach program in which public health nurses or public health investigators can:

(a) Conduct appropriate contact investigations.

(b) Find patients who were lost to follow-up.

(c) Administer therapy so that it is convenient for the patient.

(6) A public health laboratory that can confirm the isolate and do appropriate sensitivity studies.

VIII. MENINGITIS.

No disease causes more concern among officials of schools and day-care centers or parents than spinal meningitis. Since viral meningitis is rarely fatal, parental and public anxieties can be controlled by education and assurances. This section will discuss only bacterial meningitis, which is a serious public health problem and which does require public health intervention. The three most common types of bacterial meningitis are *H. influenzae* meningitis, meningococcal meningitis, and pneumococcal meningitis. Almost 70% of the reported cases occur in children under 5 years of age.

A. *H. influenzae* meningitis

1. Epidemiologic features

a. *H. influenzae* is the most common cause of bacterial meningitis in children under 5 years of age. About 12,000 cases occur each year. It is one of the most common causes of preventable mental retardation.

b. It occurs primarily as isolated cases with some secondary spread. Widespread outbreaks have not occurred.

c. At least 50% of children have had at least one *Hemophilus* infection during the first year of life, and almost everyone has been infected by 3 years of age.

d. Peak incidence of meningitis is from 3 months of age to 2 years.

e. Secondary attack rate of household contacts in the month following disease is 0.3%, which is about 600 times higher than in the general population. Secondary household attack rate was 4% for children 2 years of age, 2% for children 2–3 years of age, 0.1% for children 4–5 years of age, and 0% for those over 6 years of age. Among household contacts, 64% of cases occurred within the first week, 20% during the second week, and 16% during the third and fourth weeks.

f. Secondary spread to day-care classroom contacts under 4 years of age is also high.

2. Infectious disease process

a. Agent. The causative agent is *H. influenzae*.

(1) *H. influenzae* exist in both the encapsulated and unencapsulated form. The encapsulated type can be subdivided into six capsular types—a, b, c, d, e, and f.

(2) The most invasive disease (i.e., meningitis and acute epiglottiditis) is caused by type b and is frequently referred to as Hib.

(3) Plasmid-mediated ampicillin-resistant strains have been occurring since 1974. Currently, about 12%–40% of isolates are resistant to ampicillin.

b. Reservoir. Humans are the reservoirs of infection. Nasopharyngeal carriage is common with colonization rates ranging from 0%–23% with a mean of 10%. During an 18-month period, 71% of toddlers and 48% of preschool children became colonized.

c. Mode of transmission is by direct contact with respiratory droplets from the nose and throat of infected individuals more often carriers than cases.

d. Portal of entry is the nasopharynx.

e. Susceptible host

(1) Newborns are protected by maternal antibodies during the first 3 months of life.

(2) Pharyngeal carriage throughout infancy and childhood stimulates a naturally acquired immunity. Invasive disease caused by a capsular strain of *Hemophilus* is rare in adults.

(3) Disease is more common in certain high-risk groups (see section III C 4 b)

3. Control strategies for invasive Hib disease (i.e., meningitis and acute epiglottiditis) consist of verifying the diagnosis, notifying the parents, chemoprophylaxis, and immunization with a polysaccharide vaccine (see section III C 4 c, d).

a. Verify the diagnosis.

b. Notify the parents and inform them that their child has had contact with a case of meningitis and that:

(1) Secondary spread to children over 6 years of age is uncommon.

(2) Their child should be monitored for signs of illness and that if their child develops fever, rash, headache, or stiff neck, he or she should be seen by a physician. (This is a good practice to follow even if the child has not been exposed to a case of meningitis.)

(3) In some instances, antimicrobial chemoprophylaxis or immunization might be indicated.

c. Antimicrobial chemoprophylaxis is the most effective preventive measure since many children are too young to respond to vaccine.

(1) Chemoprophylaxis should be offered to:

(a) All household contacts of a case of invasive Hib disease in which another child under 4 years of age resides.

(b) All classmates and staff in a day-care center classroom that has children under 2 years of age who have been exposed to invasive Hib disease. Some authorities feel that this recommendation should not be implemented unless two cases have occurred.

(c) All patients who were treated for invasive disease because antimicrobial therapy of invasive disease does not eradicate nasopharyngeal carriage.

(d) Children who have had the Hib vaccine or who have had previous Hib disease. Although these groups are felt to be at decreased risk of disease, the Hib vaccine does not affect nasopharyngeal carriage of the organism, which may be passed on to susceptible classmates.

(2) Nasopharyngeal cultures are not helpful in determining who should receive chemoprophylaxis and should not be done.

(3) The drug of choice for chemoprophylaxis is RMP.

(a) The dosage is 20 mg/kg by mouth once daily (maximum daily dose of 600 mg) for 4 days. In neonates under 1 year of age, the dosage is 10 mg/kg once daily for 4 days.

(b) RMP is not recommended for pregnant women.

(c) RMP turns urine and tears orange. The patient should not wear contact lenses while taking chemoprophylaxis.

(4) To be effective in day-care centers, at least 75% of the children must receive RMP. All classroom contacts should receive RMP at the same time. In public health practice, this is difficult to achieve.

(5) For the pediatric population unable to swallow RMP capsules, the drug may be mixed with several teaspoons of applesauce immediately before administration or a suspension of RMP may be freshly prepared.

(6) Chemoprophylaxis should be offered as soon as possible after the index case is identified but some benefit may be attained even if offered more than 14 days after the index case.

d. For information concerning immunization with a polysaccharide vaccine see section III C 4 c, d)

B. Meningococcal meningitis

1. Epidemiologic features

a. Meningococcal meningitis occurs in isolated cases, in small clusters, or in communitywide outbreaks. Large outbreaks due to serogroups A and C have occurred in recent years in the sub-Saharan region of Africa and in Brazil. The last major outbreak of group A meningitis in the United States occurred in 1945.

b. Meningococcal meningitis is the second most common bacterial meningitis in the United States with 3000 to 4000 cases reported each year.

c. The case fatality rate for meningococcal meningitis is 10% and 20% for meningococcemia.

d. Most cases occur in late winter and early spring.

e. Peak incidence is around 6–12 months of age with a smaller peak at 15–24 years of age. It is more likely to occur in newly aggregated young adults who are living in crowded conditions such as in institutions and barracks.

f. Close contacts of confirmed cases are about 1000 times more likely to develop meningococcal illness than the general population. One-third of these secondary cases occur within 4 days of the index case, and 0.3%–1.0% of close household contacts will develop disease in the month after the index case.

2. Infectious disease process

a. Agent. The causative agent is *Neisseria meningitidis*.

(1) Nine different serogroups—the most common of which are A, B, C, W-135, X, Y, and Z—have been identified on the basis of a specific capsular polysaccharide.

(2) Serogroup B accounts for 50%–55% of cases, serogroup C for 20%–25%, serogroup W-135 for 15%, serogroup Y for 10%, and serogroup A for 1%–2%.

(3) Some serogroups appear to be less virulent, although fatal infections and secondary spread have occurred with all types.

b. Reservoir of infection is man. Pharyngeal carriage is high and ranges from 5%–70%, depending on the population, age, season, and living conditions.

c. Mode of transmission is by direct contact with respiratory droplets from the nose and throat of infected persons, more often carriers than cases.

d. Portal of entry is the nasopharynx.

e. Susceptible host

(1) Newborns are protected by maternal antibodies during the first 3 months of life.

(2) Pharyngeal carriage throughout infancy, childhood, and early adulthood stimulates a naturally acquired immunity. Meningococcal disease in individuals over 25 is uncommon.

(3) Individuals who are complement deficient are at increased risk of disease and may actually have mutliple episodes of infection. Asplenic persons are at increased risk and also experience particularly severe infections.

3. Control strategies consist of verifying the diagnosis, notifying the parents, chemoprophylaxis, and immunization with a meningococcal polysaccharide vaccine.

a. Verify the diagnosis.

b. Notify the parents (see VIII A 3 b).

c. Antimicrobial chemoprophylaxis is the chief preventive measure in sporadic cases.

(1) It should be offered to:

(a) Household contacts.

(b) Day-care center contacts.

(c) Medical personnel who resuscitated, intubated, or suctioned the patients before antibiotics were instituted.

(d) Individuals who had contact with the patient's oral secretions through intimate contact or through the sharing of food and beverages.

(e) All patients who were treated for meningococcal disease before discharge from the hospital because antimicrobial therapy does not reliably eradicate nasopharyngeal carriage of *N. meningitidis*.

(2) The drug of choice for chemoprophylaxis is RMP, which has been shown to be 90% effective in eradicating nasopharyngeal carriage.

(a) RMP is given by mouth twice a day for 2 days. Dosage is 600 mg every 12 hours for adults, 10 mg/kg every 12 hours for children 1 month of age or older, and 5 mg/kg every 12 hours for children under 1 month of age.

(b) For additional comments, see VIII A 3 c (2), (3) (b), (c), (4)–(6).

d. Meningococcal polysaccharide vaccine

(1) In this country, there is a bivalent (serogroups A and C) vaccine and a quadrivalent (serogroups A, C, Y, and W-135) vaccine available.

(2) Military recruits currently receive the quadrivalent vaccine.

(3) Routine immunization of civilians in the United States is not recommended because:

(a) Risk of infection is low.

(b) A vaccine against serogroup B, the major cause of disease, is not available.

(c) Most disease occurs in children who do not respond to the vaccine.

(4) Vaccines may be helpful:
(a) In certain high-risk groups.
(b) For international travel.
(c) In aborting communitywide outbreaks.

C. Pneumococcal meningitis is caused by *Streptococcus pneumoniae* (see section III C 7).

BIBLIOGRAPHY

Advisory Committee on Immunization Practices (ACIP): Diphtheria, tetanus, and pertussis: guidelines for vaccine prophylaxis and other preventive measures. *MMWR* 34:405–414, 419–426, 1985

ACIP: General recommendations on immunization. *MMWR* 32:1–17, 1983

ACIP: Measles prevention. *MMWR* 31:217–224, 229–231, 1982

ACIP: Meningococcal vaccines. *MMWR* 34:255–259, 1985

ACIP: Poliomyelitis prevention. *MMWR* 31:22–26, 31–34, 1982

ACIP: Polysaccharide vaccine for prevention of *Haemophilus influenzae type b* disease. *MMWR* 34: 201–205, 1985

ACIP: Prevention and control of influenza. *MMWR* 35:317–325, 1986

ACIP: Recommendations for protection against viral hepatitis. *MMWR* 34:313–324, 329–335, 1985

ACIP: Update: prevention of *Haemophilus influenzae type b* disease. *MMWR* 35:170–174, 179–180, 1986

American Thoracic Society: Control of tuberculosis. *Am Rev Respir Dis* 128:336–342, 1983

Benerson AS (ed): *Control of Communicable Diseases in Man*, 14th ed. Washington, DC, Official Report of the American Public Health Association, 1985

Diagnosis and management of mycobacterial infection and disease in persons with human T-lymphotrophic virus type III/lymphadenopathy associated virus infection. *MMWR* 35:448–452, 1986

Farer LS: The current status of tuberculosis control efforts. *Am Rev Respir Dis* 134:402–407, 1986

Francis DP, Maynard JE: The transmission and outcome of hepatitis A, B, and non-A, non-B: a review. *Epidemiol Rev* 1:17–31, 1979

Garner JS, Favero MS: Guidelines for handwashing and hospital environmental control. Hospital Infections Program, Center for Infectious Diseases, Centers for Disease Control, Public Health Service, Department of Health and Human Services, 1985

Garner JS, Simmons BP: Guidelines for isolation precautions in hospitals. *Infect Control* 4:245–325, 1983

Holmes K, Mardh P, Sparling PF, et al: *Sexually Transmitted Diseases*. New York, McGraw-Hill, 1984

Last JM (ed): *Maxcy-Rosenau Public Health and Preventive Medicine*, 11th ed. New York, Appleton-Century-Crofts, 1973

Leman SM: Type A viral hepatitis: new developments in an old disease. *N Eng J Med* 313:1059–1065, 1985

Mandell GL, Douglas JRG, Bennett JE: *Principles and Practice of Infectious Diseases*. New York, John Wiley, 1979

Report of the Committee on Infectious Diseases, 20th ed. Evanston, IL, American Academy of Pediatrics, 1986

Stone KM, Grimes DA, Magder LS: Primary prevention of sexually transmitted diseases. A primer for clinicians. *JAMA* 255:1763–1766, 1986

Williams WW: Guidelines for infection control in hospital personnel. *Infect Control* 4:326–349, 1983

STUDY QUESTIONS

Directions: Each question below contains five suggested answers. Choose the **one best** response to each question.

1. All of the following statements about tuberculosis are true EXCEPT

(A) the risk of developing tuberculosis disease is greatest within the first year following infection
(B) most cases of tuberculosis occur as a result of primary infection
(C) isoniazid chemoprophylaxis may be given to selected high-risk patients over 35 years of age
(D) routine screening of the general United States population is no longer recommended
(E) most cases of tuberculosis can be successfully treated with two drugs

2. The most common cause of bacterial meningitis in children under 5 years of age is

(A) *Neisseria meningitidis*
(B) *Streptococcus pneumoniae*
(C) *Listeria monocytogenes*
(D) group B streptococci
(E) *Hemophilus influenzae* type b

3. Blood, which is used for transfusion purposes, is routinely screened for serologic markers for all of the following diseases EXCEPT

(A) hepatitis B
(B) herpes simplex
(C) syphilis
(D) cytomegalovirus
(E) acquired immune deficiency syndrome

4. Contraindications for administering a live attenuated viral vaccine include all of the following EXCEPT

(A) current febrile illness
(B) recent administration of immune globulin
(C) immunosuppressive disorder
(D) administration of another live vaccine
(E) pregnancy

Directions: Each question below contains four suggested answers of which **one or more** is correct. Choose the answer

A if **1, 2, and 3** are correct
B if **1 and 3** are correct
C if **2 and 4** are correct
D if **4** is correct
E if **1, 2, 3, and 4** are correct

5. The administrator of a day-care center reports that a child under his care has just been diagnosed as having meningitis. He is concerned about the other children in the center and wants to know what to do. In order to make recommendations, the physician must also know the

(1) number of children in the center
(2) age range of the children
(3) number of employees in the center
(4) type of meningitis

6. Documented spread of hepatitis B has occurred

(1) from mother to child in the perinatal period
(2) in household contacts
(3) among sexual contacts
(4) from eating food

7. Hepatitis A has which of the following epidemiologic characteristics?

(1) The virus is transmitted by poor personal hygiene, poor sanitation, and intimate household or sexual contacts
(2) The amount of virus shed in the stool appears to be related to the severity of clinical illness
(3) The administration of immune globulin within 2 weeks of exposure can prevent or modify illness
(4) The existence of a chronic carrier state has been identified

Directions: The groups of questions below consist of lettered choices followed by several numbered items. For each numbered item select the **one** lettered choice with which it is **most** closely associated. Each lettered choice may be used once, more than once, or not at all.

Questions 8–12

For each gonorrhea control strategy, select the characteristic of the disease that it is designed to prevent.

(A) Nonvenereal transmission
(B) Penicillin-resistant organisms
(C) Reinfection
(D) Asymptomatic infection
(E) None of the above

8. Multiple cultures should be taken on individuals being evaluated.

9. All gonococcal isolates should be tested for β-lactamase production.

10. Prophylactic eye drops should be instilled into the eyes of newborns to prevent gonococcal conjunctivitis.

11. Contact tracing and epidemiologic treatment of all identified contacts should be performed.

12. Gonorrhea cultures should be done on certain sexually active women.

Questions 13–17

Match each characteristic of hepatitis with the type of hepatitis that is most appropriate.

(A) Hepatitis A
(B) Hepatitis B
(C) Non-A, non-B hepatitis
(D) Delta hepatitis
(E) None of the above

13. It is the most common cause of post-transfusion hepatitis in the United States.

14. Coinfection must take place for the clinical expression of the disease.

15. It is a common problem in day-care centers and in families who have children attending day-care centers.

16. Chronic infection may lead to cirrhosis or primary hepatocellular carcinoma.

17. It can be prevented with a vaccine.

ANSWERS AND EXPLANATIONS

1. The answer is B. (*VII A 3, 4, B 6 b*) Most individuals infected with the tubercle bacilli handle the disease quite well. Although they get over the primary infection, the organism remains viable inside of the body. At any time in the future, the infection can reactivate causing tuberculous disease. Pediatric cases usually represent a primary infection, while most adult cases occur from the reactivation of a latent infection, one that was acquired many years previously. Of the 24,000 cases of tuberculosis that were reported in 1983, 92% occurred from reactivation of a latent infection, and only 8% represented new infections. This is why certain high-risk individuals should receive chemoprophylaxis with isoniazid to kill the viable organisms so that reactivation does not take place.

2. The answer is E. (*VIII A 1 a*) *Hemophilus influenzae* is not only the most common cause of bacterial meningitis in children under 5 years of age, but it is also one of the most common causes of preventable mental retardation. Because of the severity of this disease, a polysaccharide vaccine has been developed to prevent infection. Unfortunately, it is not effective under 18 months of age, and is only partially effective from 18–23 months.

3. The answer is B. [*II D 2 b (2)*] Blood is a common vehicle through which many diseases are transmitted; thus, blood is screened for serologic markers of biologic agents that cause disease. The American Red Cross screens blood for hepatitis B, syphilis, cytomegalovirus, and acquired immune deficiency syndrome. Blood containing cytomegalovirus antibodies is not given to neonates because of the severity of the disease in the perinatal period. Although blood is screened for syphilis, the chance of getting syphilis from a blood transfusion is extremely remote. Since herpes simplex is not transmitted via blood and since most individuals have had prior herpes infections, blood is not screened for this disease.

4. The answer is D. [*III B 2 c (1) (b), (2) (b), d (4), (5), e (1)*] Two live attenuated viral vaccines may be administered on the same day, or they must be separated by at least a month. Since these vaccines require multiplication of the antigen in the body, they should not be given to immunocompromised hosts who might have trouble eliminating the infection or to pregnant women because of a theoretical harmful effect on the developing fetus. The recent administration of immune globulin can also inactivate the vaccine and prevent the vaccine from stimulating an immune response. No immunization should be given to an individual with a current febrile illness.

5. The answer is C (2, 4). (*VIII A 3 a–c, B 3 a–c*) The most important fact to determine before recommendations can be made to the administrator of the day-care center is the type of meningitis that the child contracted. Thus, the physician must contact the physician who made the initial diagnosis or the laboratory who isolated the organism. The age range of the children is necessary to determine if antimicrobial chemoprophylaxis is required.

6. The answer is A (1, 2, 3). (*VI B 2 d*) The mode of transmission of hepatitis B (HBV) is primarily by direct person-to-person contact via infected body fluids or by common vehicle such as a contaminated needle. Thus, transmission is likely to occur in populations with overcrowding, lack of sanitation, and poor personal hygiene, among sexual partners of infected adults, in household contacts, and in infants born to infected mothers who become infected in the perinatal period. There has never been a documented foodborne outbreak of HBV. Carriers of the HBsAg are allowed to work in occupations that prepare or serve food for public consumption. HBV is inactivated in its passage through the gastrointestinal tract.

7. The answer is B (1, 3). (*VI A 2 b (2), (4), c (2), (3), d (1)–(3), 3 b*) Hepatitis A virus multiplies in the liver and, regardless of symptomatology, is excreted in the stool in large quantities. Consequently, it is transmitted by poor personal hygiene, poor sanitation, and intimate contact. Immune globulin can prevent or modify infection if given within 2 weeks of exposure. The chronic carrier state does not exist, and the infected person is only communicable from about 2 weeks before the onset of jaundice until about 1 week later. The greatest period of infectivity is before the onset of jaundice.

8–12. The answers are: 8-D, 9-B, 10-A, 11-C, 12-D. (*V C 2 a (3), d (2), 3 a, c, e–g*) Multiple cultures should be performed on individuals being evaluated in a sexually transmitted disease clinic. Women should have endocervical and rectal cultures taken, and homosexual men require urethral and rectal cultures. Pharyngeal cultures should be done on all individuals who have oral sex.

Testing gonococcal cultures for β-lactamase production determines whether or not the isolate is a penicillinase-producing *Neisseria gonorrhoeae* and, therefore, resistant to penicillin. However, the β-lactamase test will not pick up the organisms that have a chromosomally mediated penicillin resistance.

Nonvenereal transmission of gonorrhea from mother to child at birth causes a neonatal ophthalmia. This can be prevented with prophylactic eye drops.

Although it is not possible to do contact tracing on all cases, it should be done on selected cases, such as individuals with repeated infections and women with pelvic inflammatory disease, to prevent reinfection. Since the organism may be difficult to isolate, all identified contacts should be treated epidemiologically. Screening certain sexually active women would identify asymptomatic carriers.

13–17. The answers are: 13-C, 14-D, 15-A, 16-B, 17-B. [*VI A 1 c, B 1 c, 3 d, C 1 b, D 1 a (2)*] Non-A, non-B hepatitis is caused by at least two types of viruses and is the most common cause of post-transfusion hepatitis in the United States. Control strategies consist of good personal hygiene and not sharing intravenous needles. There are no vaccines, and IG has no protective effect.

Hepatitis B (HBV) vaccine can prevent HBV infection as well as the clinical expression of delta hepatitis (HDV), which requires an HBV coinfection for synthesis. HDV usually has a severe clinical course.

Since hepatitis A (HAV) is transmitted by the fecal-oral route, HAV is a common problem in day-care centers, institutions, rural areas where sanitation may be poor, and where people are crowded together. Patients are communicable from about 2 weeks *before* the onset of clinical disease to about 1 week *after*.

Chronic HBV infection has been associated with cirrhosis and heptocellular carcinoma.

5
Epidemiology and Prevention of Selected Chronic Illnesses

Donald J. Balaban
Gail K. Wright

I. INTRODUCTION. This chapter is intended to provide a background for clinicians on the prevalence and risk factors for selected chronic diseases in the United States population in the mid-1980s. Changes in incidence over time, population subgroups who are particularly at risk, and the financial burden to society are considered for each condition based on existing data. Detailed references are provided for the epidemiologic studies, cost estimates, and preventive strategies presented.

Recommendations for screening and preventive measures constantly change. At any point in time, specific recommendations for preventive strategies will not be accepted by all investigators; thus, this chapter presents areas of general consensus and emphasizes preventive strategies—whether primary, secondary, or tertiary—that are appropriate for primary care physicians.

Death rates and mortality rates for the diseases discussed in this chapter are given in Figures 5-1 and 5-2.

II. HEART DISEASE

A. Epidemiology

1. Mortality rate

a. The 1983 death rate from heart disease was 276.2 individuals per 100,000 population; these deaths comprised 38.2% of all deaths in the United States.

b. One-fourth of all individuals who succumb to cardiovascular disease are under the age of 65.

2. Prevalence

a. About 4.6 million Americans have coronary heart disease; over 37 million have serious hypertension.

b. Blacks are almost twice as likely to be hypertensive as whites. It has been reported that 36.2% of black men and 38.2% of black women are hypertensive.

c. White men are more likely than white women to suffer myocardial infarction and sudden death; the sex differential is much less prominent in nonwhite populations. Women have a greater risk of angina pectoris than men who have a greater risk of myocardial infarction and sudden death.

3. Time trends. Age-adjusted cardiovascular death rates in the United States for the decade ending in 1980 declined by about 30% over the previous decade. This recent decline in coronary mortality is related to:

a. Better diagnosis and treatment.

b. Improvements in life-style and related cardiovascular risk factor levels.

c. Increased efforts in primary and secondary prevention (see section II D).

B. Costs

1. The cost for the first year of treatment for heart disease was estimated to be $1.39 billion in 1975.

2. The cost of cardiac care, including cost output due to disability, was estimated to be $64.4 billion in 1984.

C. Causal and risk factors

1. Elevated blood pressure, as indicated by increasing levels of systolic or diastolic blood pressure, is a contributor to coronary heart disease risk.

2. High levels of serum cholesterol and low density lipoprotein (LDL) are tied to the frequency, mechanisms, and possible prevention of coronary heart disease. Longitudinal studies of

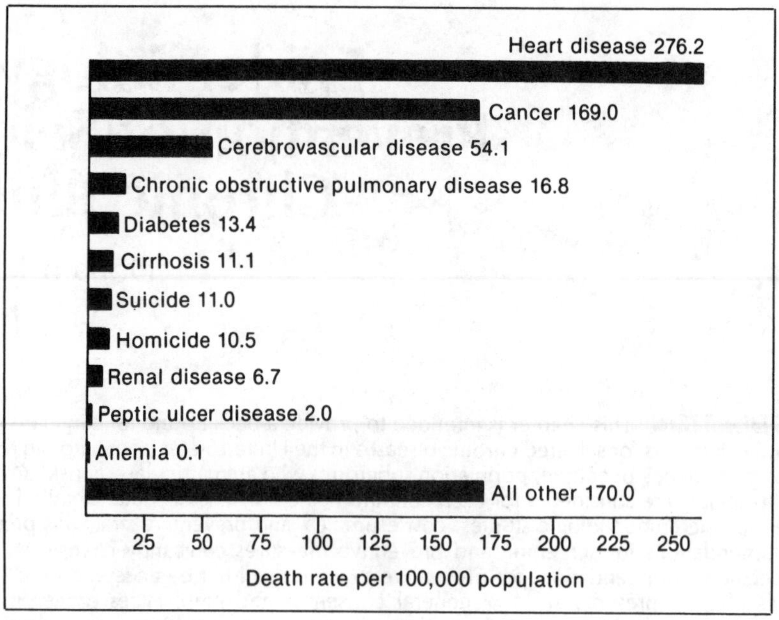

Figure 5-1. Mortality in the United States in 1983. (Adapted from Cancer statistics, 1986. *CA* 36:9–25, 1986.)

blood lipids in healthy adults show consistent and linear increases in individual risk of coronary heart disease, as indicated by high levels of total serum cholesterol and LDL, at least through middle age.

3. **Smoking** places individuals at an increased risk for developing and dying from coronary artery disease.

4. **Oral contraceptive use**, especially among women over age 35 and those who smoke, has been linked to an increased incidence of heart disease.

5. **Family history of early coronary heart disease** is a well-known risk factor.

6. **Obesity among sedentary individuals** is a contributory cause of heart disease.

D. Prevention

1. **Screening.** The Canadian Task Force recommends screening for hypertension at least every 5 years for men and women 16 to 64 years of age and every 2 years after age 65. The cost-effectiveness of widespread screening for coronary heart disease has yet to be determined.

2. **Primary care**
   a. **Hypertension control** is believed to contribute greatly to the decline in cardiovascular mortality, particularly the mortality attributable to stroke and cardiac failure. For example, a 2 mm Hg decrease in diastolic blood pressure in a population results in an estimated 8.7% decline in the population's risk of developing coronary heart disease.
   b. **Cholesterol control.** Decreased consumption of milk, butter, eggs, and animal fats results in lower cholesterol levels. For example, a daily decrease of 5 mg of cholesterol in a population results in an estimated 5% decline in the population's risk of developing coronary heart disease.

3. **Cessation of smoking.** Physicians should counsel their patients to stop smoking and provide support and motivation through regularly scheduled visits. The cessation must be immediate and total to be most effective. However, a 20% decrease in smoking in a population has been reported to result in an estimated 10.5% decline in the population's risk of developing coronary heart disease.

4. **Physical exercise.** Epidemiologic evidence suggests a protective effect against coronary death from regular, vigorous physical activity. However, it also suggests, that the protective effects of regular physical activity can be mitigated by the presence of other unfavorable sociocultural risk factors, such as hypercholesterolemia.

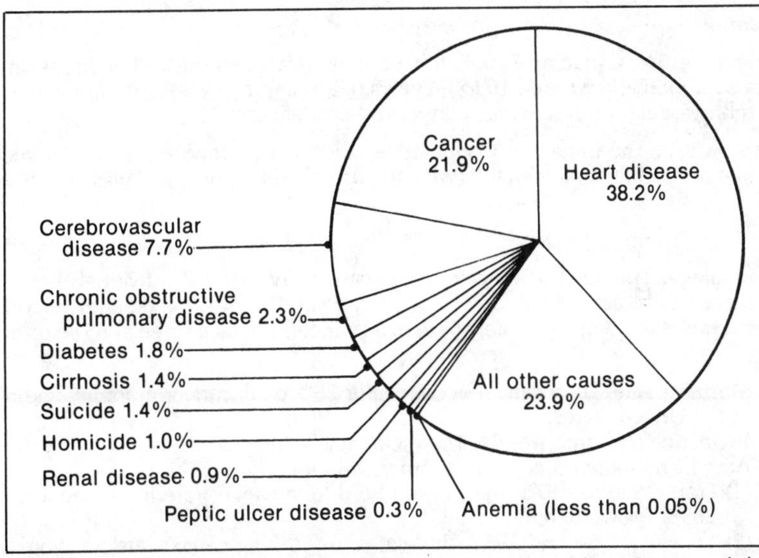

Figure 5-2. Death rates in the United States in 1983. (Adapted from Cancer statistics, 1986. *CA* 36:9–25, 1986.)

5. Education

a. In the early 1970s, the National High Blood Pressure Education Program formulated new educational objectives to raise patients' awareness of hypertension. Programs were developed to keep hypertensive patients on their appropriate therapy and to follow their physician's advice. Results suggest that the percentage of hypertensive subjects controlling their blood pressure more than doubled, from 16.5% to 34.1%, with the greatest increase coming since 1976.

b. Patient education should be targeted to high-risk groups (e.g., blacks who have both higher rates of hypertension and lower control rates).

III. CEREBROVASCULAR DISEASE

A. Epidemiology

1. Mortality rates

a. The 1983 death rate from cerebrovascular disease was 54.1 individuals per 100,000 population; these deaths comprised 7.7% of all deaths in the United States.

b. Cerebrovascular disease accounts for about 200,000 deaths per year in the United States.

2. Incidence and prevalence

a. There are approximately 500,000 new episodes of cerebrovascular disease each year.

b. The chances of suffering a stroke before the age of 70 are 1 in 20; the incidence doubles each successive decade after the age of 45.

3. Time trends

a. Stroke mortality declined by 46% between 1968 and 1981.

b. The decline in the rates for deaths attributable to hypertension and all cardiovascular diseases, with an increasing rate of decline since 1972, may reflect changes in disease classification, diagnostic customs, or coding rules but also may be due to increased awareness, detection, and treatment of hypertension.

B. Costs. The cost for the first year of treatment of stroke was estimated to be $1.53 billion in 1975.

C. Causal and risk factors

1. Hypertension increases the risk of stroke. Epidemiologic evidence is strong that hypertension is one of the causes of atherosclerosis, particularly in combination with hyperlipidemia.

2. Smoking also increases the risk of stroke. In fact, several case-control and cohort studies have shown a smoker:nonsmoker stroke mortality ratio of 1.2:1.5.

3. Oral contraceptive use, particularly by women who smoke, is associated with an increased risk of stroke.

D. Prevention

1. **Screening.** The Canadian Task Force recommends screening for hypertension at least every 5 years for men and women 16 to 64 years of age and every 2 years after age 65. Screening for cerebrovascular disease is not considered cost-effective.

2. **Aspirin use.** The Canadian Cooperative Study Group reported a 48% reduction in risk for stroke or death among men following the use of aspirin; no effect was established for women.

IV. CANCER

A. Epidemiology. The 1983 death rate for all cancers was 169.0 individuals per 100,000 population; these deaths accounted for 21.9% of all deaths in the United States, second only to heart disease (Table 5-1). Approximately 51% of all cancers are diagnosed at 65 years of age and older.

1. **Lung**
   a. **Mortality rate.** Lung cancer accounts for 25% of all cancer mortality and 5% of all deaths in the United States.
   b. **Incidence and time trends.** The incidence of lung cancer is now increasing faster among American women than among American men.
      (1) From 1950 to 1978, the age-adjusted lung cancer rate increased 192% for men and 263% for women.
      (2) Between 1950 and 1957, the age-adjusted lung cancer rate for women increased an average of 1% per year, but from 1968 to 1977, the rate increased almost 7% per year.
      (3) Between 1950 and 1957, the age-adjusted lung cancer rate for men climbed to an average of 6.7% per year, but from 1968 to 1977 the rate fell to a 4% average annual increase.

2. **Breast**
   a. **Mortality rate.** Breast cancer accounted for 9.2% of all cancer deaths in the United States from 1973 to 1977. The mortality rate for this period was 15.1 individuals per 100,000 population.
   b. **Time trends.** There has been very little change in age-adjusted mortality rates from 1930 to 1981.

3. **Colon and rectum**
   a. **Mortality rate.** Colorectal cancer accounted for 13.6% of all cancer mortality in the United States from 1973 to 1977. The mortality rate for this period was 22.3 individuals per 100,000 population.
   b. **Incidence**
      (1) The age-specific incidence rate of colorectal cancer rises steadily from ages 10–14 to ages 80–84. The rate of increase in incidence is steady until ages 70–75, at which time rectal cancer incidence rates increase more slowly, and then decline after age 85.
      (2) Men and women are affected almost equally, although among whites, the risk for men is somewhat higher than for women; among blacks, the incidence is nearly equal for men and women.
   c. **Time trends.** There has been very little change in mortality rates from 1930 to 1981.

4. **Cervix**
   a. **Mortality rate.** Cervical cancer accounted for 1.3% of all cancer deaths in the United States from 1973 to 1977. The mortality rate for this period was 2.6 individuals per 100,000 population.
   b. **Incidence.** The incidence among whites declined from 38.3 individuals per 100,000 population in 1947 to 11.3 per 100,000 in 1977.
   c. **Time trends.** In the last 2 decades, slight increases in the incidence and mortality rates of cervical cancer have been observed in several Western countries, including the United

Table 5-1. Cancer Incidence and Mortality by Site and Sex

	Incidence*		Deaths*	
	Male	Female	Male	Female
Lung	22%	11%	35%	19%
Breast	. . .	26%	. . .	18%
Colon and rectum	14%	16%	11%	14%
Cervix	. . .	3.5%	. . .	3%
Prostate	19%	. . .	10%	. . .

*Percent of all cancers.

States. These increases are believed to be due in part to changes in sexual practices and increased use of oral contraceptives rather than barrier contraceptives, perhaps leading to more promiscuous behavior and resulting in more venereally transmitted diseases.

5. Prostate

a. Mortality rate. Prostate cancer accounted for 5.3% of all cancer deaths in the United States from 1973 to 1977. The mortality rate for this period was 8.7 individuals per 100,000 population.

b. Incidence

(1) Prostate cancer primarily affects elderly men. The incidence increases with age more rapidly than for any other cancer.

(2) American blacks have the highest prostate cancer incidence rate in the world.

c. Time trends. There has been very little change in mortality rates from 1930 to 1981.

B. Costs. The costs for the first year of treatment for all cancers was estimated to be $4.13 billion in 1975, compared to $1.39 billion for heart disease, $2.86 billion for motor vehicle injuries, and $1.53 billion for stroke.

C. Causal and risk factors

1. Lung

a. Smoking. Case-control and prospective studies have consistently demonstrated that cigarette smoking is a causal factor in lung cancer.

(1) Several cohort studies have shown a relative risk of 9.2 for men who smoke and 2.2 for women who smoke, as compared to a relative risk of 1.0 for nonsmokers of both sexes. The higher risk for men is attributed to the fact that women:

(a) Began smoking later in this century than men.

(b) Start to smoke at older ages than men.

(c) Inhale less deeply than men.

(2) The relative risk for men ranges from 4.6 for those smoking 1–9 cigarettes daily to 18.8 for those smoking over 40 cigarettes daily. The relative risk for women ranges from 1.3 for those smoking 1–9 cigarettes daily to 7.5 for those smoking over 40 cigarettes daily.

(3) The risk of lung cancer also depends on the age at which an individual begins to smoke. Delaying the onset of smoking to the late teens or early adulthood can reduce the risk of developing lung cancer at age 60 or 70 by as much as 20%.

b. Occupational exposure. Industrial carcinogens such as asbestos, radon, nickel, chromium, mustard gas, and other industrial agents, especially in combination with cigarette smoking, can lead to an increased likelihood of developing lung cancer, depending on the length and type of exposure.

c. Air pollution. Air pollution is suspected in the etiology of lung cancer, but evaluation is difficult because the measurement of air pollution is inexact. Lung cancer in urban areas is still overwhelmingly attributed to cigarette smoking. Perhaps 10 cases per 100,000 average smokers may be caused by air pollution.

d. Radiation. High radiation exposure (100+ rads) increases the risk of lung cancer.

e. Family history. Old studies (before 1970) demonstrate an increased tendency for lung cancer to aggregate in families.

2. Breast

a. Pregnancy. Women who have a first pregnancy after the age of 30 have an increased chance of developing breast cancer. For example, women with a first full-term pregnancy before age 20 have a relative risk of breast cancer one-third that of women whose first full-term pregnancy occurs after age 35. The protective effect is confirmed only for full-term pregnancies—that is, pregnancies ending in abortion or miscarriage do not appear to reduce subsequent risk of breast cancer.

b. Family history. The risk to women whose mothers *or* sisters have had breast cancer is twofold, and the risk to those whose mothers *and* sisters have had breast cancer is threefold.

c. Diet. Some studies have shown an association between consumption of fats and oils and breast cancer. Other studies have shown associations of breast cancer rates with total fat and animal protein consumption. Increased intake of fat and animal protein could influence endocrine metabolism and increase the risk of developing breast cancer by:

(1) Promoting growth and sexual development and an early onset of menarche.

(2) Increasing adiposity, leading to greater conversion of androstenedione to estrone.

(3) Increasing prolactin release from the pituitary.

(4) Increasing bile salt production in the gut, leading to altered bacterial flora and the production of carcinogenic substances.

- **d. Radiation.** Exposure to ionizing radiation increases the incidence of breast cancer. Studies from Hiroshima and Nagasaki indicate a marked increase among women exposed to 10 rads or more, following a latent period of 10 years or more. The greatest risks were found at exposures of approximately 100 rads. The risk is significantly greater in women who were irradiated during adolescence.
- **e. Other factors.** The development of breast cancer also is associated with:
  - **(1)** High socioeconomic status.
  - **(2)** Age over 40 years.
  - **(3)** An early menarche.

3. Colon and rectum

- **a. Diet.** Fiber deficiency and high dietary fat consumption appear to be related to colorectal cancer; however, no specific carcinogens associated with the production, preservation, and manufacture of food have been clearly identified.
- **b. Physiologic factors.** Bacteria, which acts upon cholesterol and bile acids in the intestines, produces carcinogens that either act locally or diffuse elsewhere in the body. This reaction is not totally understood.
- **c. Familial predisposition.** Heredity seems to be involved in the development of cancer of the colon.
- **d. Alcohol consumption.** In one case-control study, per capita beer consumption correlated significantly with the colorectal cancer mortality of men 35 to 54 years of age between 1970 and 1974 in the United States, United Kingdom, Australia, and New Zealand.
- **e. Socioeconomic factors.** High socioeconomic groups and whites are more likely to develop colorectal cancer than low socioeconomic groups and blacks.

4. Cervix

- **a. Sexual promiscuity.** Multiple sexual partners, leading to infections and other sexually transmitted diseases, such as herpes, syphilis, and gonorrhea, increase a woman's risk of cervical cancer.
- **b. Oral contraceptive use.** Use of oral contraceptives appears to be a risk factor, although it is not clear whether they in fact increase the risk or whether barrier methods decrease the risk. It could be that users of oral contraceptives are more promiscuous, which increases a woman's risk as a result of infections and other sexually transmitted diseases.
- **c. Coital history.** Age at first coital experience correlates highly with the risk for cervical cancer. Women who had first coitus before 20 years of age have a two- to threefold increase in risk for invasive cervical cancer compared to women whose sexual activity began later. There appears to be a progressive increase in risk the earlier the age at first coitus.
- **d. Smoking.** Women who smoke have a relative risk of 3.0 for developing cervical cancer. The association is strongest in young age groups (i.e., women 20 to 29 years of age) with a relative risk of 17, and is weaker in older women. The risk for black women smokers is similar to that of white women smokers.
- **e. Racial factors.** In general, blacks and Hispanics are at an increased risk for cervical cancer.
- **f. Socioeconomic factors.** Cervical cancer appears to be associated with the socioeconomic class of the patient's husband as indicated by his occupation. Studies suggest that men are a factor in cervical cancer, primarily due to penile hygiene and whether or not they have been circumcised.
- **g. Menarche and menopause.** Age at menarche, age at menopause, and the character of the menses do not appear to be risk factors for cervical cancer, but the interval between menarche and first coitus may be a better predictor of risk than age at first coitus.

5. Prostate. Although the cause of prostate cancer is unknown, it has been associated with the hormone dependence of the prostate and sexual activity. Geographic, occupational, and racial differences in incidence also have been reported.

- **a. Diet.** Dietary fat appears to be related to prostate cancer in the same way it is related to breast cancer and colorectal cancer.
- **b. Occupational exposure.** Workers exposed to industrial carcinogens, such as cadmium oxide dust, reportedly have a higher incidence of prostate cancer than expected.
- **c. Age.** The risk of developing prostate cancer increases with age.
- **d. Religion.** Catholics had 1.5 and Protestants 1.9 times the frequency of prostate cancer deaths as Jewish individuals according to one study.
- **e. Family history.** One study reported that fathers and brothers of 228 prostate cancer patients died from prostate cancer three times more often than the fathers and brothers of controls. Whether there is an environmental or genetic basis for this tendency has not been determined.
- **f. Marriage.** Higher frequencies of prostate cancer have been found in married men than in single men. Rates were particularly high among widowed and divorced men and among married men with children.

D. Prevention and screening

1. **Lung.** Screening for presymptomatic lung cancer is either by pulmonary cytology or chest roentgenography, neither of which is cost-effective for target populations. In addition, screening seems to have no beneficial effect on mortality from lung cancer, although there is a shift to less serious stages at the time of detection.
   a. Preliminary results of a randomized trial of sputum cytology in smokers show no reduction in mortality in those screened.
   b. Individuals with early lung cancer detected by chest x-rays do not have a more favorable prognosis than individuals with lung cancer diagnosed after symptoms appear. In fact, by the time a lung tumor is radiographically visible, it is usually inoperable and incurable.

2. **Breast.** Screening for breast cancer is by mammography and physical examination (palpation) of the breast. Monthly self-examinations are recommended for all women, and the Canadian Task Force recommends annual mammography for women 50 to 59 years of age. There is no concensus on the value of mass screening of women under the age of 50.
   a. Mammography can help to differentiate a benign from a malignant process before it becomes palpable and when it is most curable. Thus, mammography remains the most effective imaging method of detecting nonpalpable cancer. However, 10%–20% of breast cancers cannot be visualized by mammography; in those cases, a woman usually detects the lesion through palpation several months later.
   b. Target populations for screening include women who:
      (1) Are over age 40.
      (2) Are of high socioeconomic status.
      (3) Are white, single, or nulliparous.
      (4) Had their first child after 30 years of age.
      (5) Have a family history of breast cancer.
      (6) Have benign breast disease.
      (7) Have had previous breast cancer.
      (8) Are nuns.

3. **Colon and rectum**
   a. Screening for colorectal cancer is by testing the stool for occult blood. Testing, which is cost-effective for target populations, should be done annually in men and women over 46 years of age.
   b. Target populations for screening include individuals who have a history of:
      (1) Colitis.
      (2) Familial polyposis or villous adenomas.
      (3) Familial cancer of the colon.

4. **Cervix**
   a. Screening for cervical cancer, which is by Pap smear to detect cervical abnormalities, is cost-effective for target populations. Intervals of 1 to 5 years are recommended. The Canadian Task Force recommends testing when a female first becomes sexually active, then every 3 years until the age of 35, and every 5 years thereafter.
   b. Target populations for screening include women who:
      (1) Are between the ages of 25–60.
      (2) Have low socioeconomic status.
      (3) Are prison inmates or prostitutes.
      (4) Have a history of infectious diseases.
      (5) Had first intercourse at an early age.
      (6) Are unmarried mothers.
      (7) Have had induced abortions.
      (8) Have a history of cervical squamous dysplasia.

5. **Prostate**
   a. Screening for prostate cancer is by:
      (1) Digital palpation per rectum.
      (2) Prostatic massage and cytologic examination.
      (3) Determination of serum acid phosphatase concentration.
   b. The target population for screening includes men over age 65.

V. CHRONIC OBSTRUCTIVE PULMONARY DISEASE (COPD)

A. Epidemiology

1. **Mortality rate**
   a. The 1983 death rate for COPD was 16.8 individuals per 100,000 population. Deaths from COPD comprised 2.3% of all deaths in the United States in 1980 and 1981.

b. Approximately 60,000 deaths per year in the United States are due to bronchitis, emphysema, asthma, or COPD; these diseases are also contributory causes of another 60,000 deaths.

2. **Prevalence**
   a. It has been estimated that 16 million Americans have chronic bronchitis, asthma, or emphysema.
   b. Approximately 14% of adult men and 8% of adult women have chronic bronchitis, obstructive airways disease, or both.

3. **Time trends.** Deaths attributed to COPD are increasing; the age-adjusted death rate rose 28% between 1968 and 1978, during which time the death rate from all causes declined by 22%.

B. Costs

1. The estimated cost of COPD to the national economy in 1979 was $6.5 billion. Of this amount, $2.3 billion was for health care, and the remainder was for the indirect costs of morbidity and premature mortality.

2. The National Heart, Lung, and Blood Institute estimates the total cost of respiratory disease in the United States at $25 billion annually—that is, $7 billion for direct costs, $12 billion for the indirect costs of morbidity (e.g., loss of productivity), and $6 billion for the indirect costs of mortality.

C. Causal and risk factors

1. **Smoking.** It has been shown during the past 20 years that smoking, particularly cigarette smoking, is an important cause of respiratory disease.
   a. Risk is related to the number of cigarettes smoked daily and to the duration of the smoking habit.
   b. The lifetime risk of developing lung cancer in a man who is a heavy cigarette smoker may be as high as 25%.

2. **Occupational exposure**, especially among tin, copper, and coal miners; chemical workers; foundry workers; cotton textile workers; and others engaged in heavy industry, increases the risk of COPD.

3. **Air pollution**, including indoor pollutants, may be harmful at high levels; whether or not exposure to low levels of pollutants has a significant effect on health has yet to be determined.

4. **Sex.** Men are at a higher risk than women of developing emphysema and COPD, but not chronic bronchitis; the differences between the sexes increase with age.

5. **Socioeconomic factors.** Morbidity and mortality are generally higher in blue-collar workers than white-collar workers and in those with fewer years of formal education.

6. **Family history.** Offspring of affected parents and brothers and sisters of affected siblings are more likely to develop COPD.

D. Prevention. The only effective approach to COPD appears to be prevention as opposed to early detection or treatment. In fact, there is no method for detection of a precancerous state.

1. **Chest radiographs** have not proven cost-effective as a screening method for identification of individuals with COPD.

2. The most useful screening test is the forced expiratory volume (FEV) measured over 1 second (FEV_1).

3. **Cessation of smoking** *before* symptoms and incapacitation develop reduces the risk of developing COPD. Abstinence from smoking is associated with absence or low frequency of airway obstruction and respiratory disease mortality.

VI. CIRRHOSIS

A. Epidemiology. The 1983 death rate from cirrhosis was 11.1 individuals per 100,000 population. These deaths comprised 1.4% of all deaths in the United States.

B. Causal and risk factors. Excessive daily consumption of alcohol for many years appears to put a drinker at increased risk for developing cirrhosis.

1. **Men** who consume an excess of 40 g of ethanol alcohol per day for many years have a greater chance of developing cirrhosis.

2. **Women** who consume an excess of 20 g of ethanol alcohol per day for many years have a greater chance of developing cirrhosis.

C. Prevention

1. **Primary prevention**
   a. **Health protection measures** include legislative and regulatory controls on:
      (1) Prices of alcoholic beverages.
      (2) Types and locations of liquor outlets.
      (3) Hours and days of liquor sales.
      (4) Drinking age.
      (5) Alcohol content of beverages.
      (6) Differential taxation of various beverages.
      (7) Alcohol distribution systems.
   b. **Health promotion measures** include:
      (1) Public education programs.
      (2) Specifically targeted preventive programs.
      (3) Beverage substitution initiatives.
      (4) Antialcohol promotion and marketing measures.

2. **Secondary prevention**, which is increasingly used by industry, entails the early identification of alcohol abusers through the administration of brief questionnaires to high-risk individuals.

3. **Tertiary prevention** entails intensive treatment to aid the drinker with either moderation or total abstinence from drinking.

VII. SUICIDE

A. Epidemiology. The 1983 death rate was 11.0 individuals per 100,000 population. Deaths from suicide comprised 1.4% of all deaths in the United States in 1983.

B. Causal and risk factors. Risk factors for suicide include:

1. **Mental illness.**

2. **Feelings of helplessness and hopelessness.**

3. **Socioeconomic factors.**

4. **Physical illness or handicap.**

5. **Membership in particular groups** listed below:
   a. Males
   b. Divorced, separated, and widowed individuals (Married individuals have the lowest suicide rates.)
   c. Whites (However, the nonwhite rate is rising faster than the white rate.)
   d. Protestants who commit suicide more often than Catholics or Jews
   e. Unemployed individuals
   f. Individuals who have had contact with a psychiatrist for any reason
   g. Individuals who have already attempted, and failed at, suicide (These people are at the highest risk to complete suicide.)

C. Prevention

1. **Community-based programs** to control suicide through treatment of potential victims, include:
   a. Guidance and referral.
   b. Psychiatric evaluation and consultation.
   c. Provision of psychiatric, medical, legal, and social services.

2. **Education** of the public, of physicians, and of other therapists about the warning signs of suicide may be an effective preventive measure.

3. **Control of the agents used in suicide**, such as guns and drugs, may be an effective preventive measure.

VIII. HOMICIDE

A. Epidemiology

1. **Mortality rate**
   a. The 1980 death rate was 10.5 individuals per 100,000 population in the United States. Deaths from homicide comprised 1.0% of all deaths in the United States in 1983.

b. Homicide is the leading cause of death for black American men between the ages of 15 and 24.

c. Of homicides reported to the Federal Bureau of Investigation in 1980:

(1) 32.9% were committed by friends and acquaintances.

(2) 15.8% were committed by a member of the victim's family.

(3) 12.8% were committed by strangers.

(4) 34.4% were labeled "relationship unknown."

2. Time trends. Homicide rates increased gradually from very low levels in 1900, reaching a peak during the Depression. Rates then declined rapidly to the mid-1940s, remained constant for several years following World War II, then began to rise steadily until 1962. Overall, the rate of homicide declined slightly from 1970 to the early 1980s. However, rates for most age groups of both sexes are as high or higher than any previously recorded in the United States.

B. Causal and risk factors*

1. Age. Individuals 25 to 34 years of age are most likely to be victims of homicide, followed by those 35 to 44 years of age, and then those 15 to 24 years of age.

2. Sex. Men are four times more likely to be victims of homicide than women.

3. Racial factors

a. Nonwhites are 8 to 15 times more likely to be victims of homicide than whites.

b. Hispanic men are two to three times more likely than white men to be victims of homicide.

4. Use of alcohol or other drugs by both the victim and the offender has been documented in at least 45% of all homicides.

5. Socioeconomic factors. Inability to cope with the socioeconomic frustrations of unemployment, underemployment, poverty, inadequate housing, and discrimination is a major risk factor for homicide.

6. Exposure to television violence has been implicated in the likelihood of involvement in homicide.

7. Lack of traditional support systems, such as the family and spiritual institutions, especially among blacks, and a weakening of moral consciousness and sense of identity are associated with an increased risk of homicide.

8. One study that compared 9 juvenile murderers with 91 other juvenile delinquents revealed:

a. Symptoms of psychosis in all of the murderers and in half of the remaining 91 delinquents.

b. Major brain impairment in 90% of the murderers and in 27% of the others.

c. More abuse and violence in the murderers' homes.

d. Psychiatric illness in at least one close relative (parent or sibling) of each murderer.

e. Previously documented violent behavior, including assault, rape, or arson, by each of the murderers.

C. Prevention

1. Education. Individuals under 18 years of age should be considered a "target group" for primary prevention of homicide efforts. Because low academic achievement and high truancy rates are strongly associated with delinquency, educational intervention may be indicated to counteract these patterns.

2. Incarceration of the criminal results in a decrease in homicide rates, mainly because the criminal is removed from society; however, it is not clear whether or not the threat of incarceration or execution deters criminals from murdering.

IX. DIABETES

A. Epidemiology

1. Mortality rate

a. The 1983 death rate for diabetes was 13.4 individuals per 100,000 population. These deaths comprised 1.8% of all deaths in the United States during this time.

b. Of those diagnosed with diabetes before the age of 30, median survival is 10–15 years less

---

*The causal and risk factors listed, which are due to socioeconomic, psychosocial, or racial circumstances, are generally accepted as true but are based on weak evidence. Similarly, the preventive measures recommended have not been rigorously established.

than that of the general population; in 40% of these patients, end stage renal disease develops, and in the remainder, death results from coronary heart disease.

2. **Prevalence**
   a. There are approximately 8.5 million diabetics in the United States between the ages of 20 and 74. Prevalence in the United States population is estimated at 6.7%.
   b. Secondary problems associated with diabetes include:
      (1) Blindness (approximately 5000 new cases every year) due to retinopathy.
      (2) Coronary heart disease.
      (3) Nephropathy.

B. **Costs.** The cost of diabetes is estimated to be $10 billion per year.

C. **Causal and risk factors**

1. **Deficiency in the action of the hormone insulin**, which may result from a quantitative deficiency of insulin, an abnormal insulin resistance to its action, or a combination of deficits, is believed to be the cause of diabetes.

2. **Obesity.** Although the etiology of both insulin-dependent diabetes mellitus (IDDM) and non–insulin-dependent diabetes mellitus (NIDDM) is poorly understood, studies have shown that approximately 80% of people with NIDDM are obese.

3. **Family history** appears to predispose individuals to diabetes. This predisposition is related to HLA DR3/DR4.

4. **Sex.** Men and women have about the same risk for developing IDDM.

5. **Racial factors**
   a. Whites have about 1.5 times the incidence rate of blacks for IDDM.
   b. The incidence of NIDDM is very high among American Indians, Micronesians, Polynesians, black women, and Mexican Americans.

6. **Socioeconomic factors.** Changes in socioeconomic status have been shown to lead to a marked and rapid increase in the incidence and prevalence of NIDDM. This may happen because:
   a. When food sources become more plentiful, a very rapid rise in body weight may occur, with a corresponding increase in the rates of NIDDM.
   b. As socioeconomic status rises, there is generally a decline in the overall level of physical activity, especially that related to work.

D. **Prevention**

1. **Routine screening** for diabetes, by use of urine tests for glucose and fasting and postprandial blood glucose tests, can lead to early treatment, which may help to reduce secondary complications. Testing is recommended for those who:
   a. Have a family history of diabetes.
   b. Have glucose abnormalities associated with pregnancy.
   c. Have physical abnormalities, such as circulatory dysfunction and frank vascular impairment.

2. **Treatment of asymptomatic individuals** has not been shown to be effective in controlling complications. Diabetes itself is not preventable, but secondary complications frequently can be prevented.

3. **Modification of cardiovascular risk factors** such as weight, blood pressure, cholesterol, and smoking are probably the best preventive approaches at the present time.

4. **Home health aides** to assist patients with diet, medication assistance and instruction, urine testing, and monitoring of vital signs have been reported to lead to modest improvements in blood sugar levels for low-income patients.

X. RENAL DISEASE

A. **Epidemiology**

1. **Mortality rate.** The 1983 death rate for renal disease was 6.7 individuals per 100,000 population. These deaths accounted for 0.9% of all deaths in the United States in 1983.

2. **Incidence.** Annual incidence rates for end stage renal disease ranging from 50 to 95 individuals per million population have been reported. In a study of 20 Eastern states from 1973 to

1979, the annual incidence rate increased from 35 individuals per million population in 1973 to 59 individuals per million population in 1979.

3. **Time trends**
   a. Black men had the largest increase in the incidence of end stage renal disease between 1973 and 1979, from 66 to 125 individuals per million, while the incidence for black women increased from 59 to 99 individuals per million from 1973 to 1979.
   b. White men showed an increased incidence from 1973 to 1977, and then stabilized at 60 individuals per million, while white women peaked at around 40 individuals per million in 1977. Incidence rates have stabilized for white women.
   c. Individuals 65 years of age and over experienced the greatest increase in incidence, from 15 individuals per million in 1973 to 125 individuals per million in 1979, with no indication of stabilization or decline.

B. Costs. The costs of end stage renal disease, including dialysis programs and transplantations, were estimated to be $1.6 billion in 1981. In 1982, the cost to Medicare alone, which pays most costs of end stage renal disease programs, was estimated to be $1.6 billion.

C. Causal and risk factors

1. **Immune injury** is the most likely cause of glomerulonephritis, a term used to describe a variety of renal diseases.
2. **Occupational exposure.** Exposure to industrial solvents and gasoline by certain occupational groups, such as painters, is another cause of renal disease.
3. **Racial factors.** Blacks, of all ages except the 0–13-year-old group, are more likely to develop renal diseases, in particular hypertensive nephropathy.
4. **Sex.** Men are slightly more likely than women to develop renal disease.
5. **Age.** Individuals 45–64 years of age are more likely to develop renal disease than those in younger age groups.
6. **Diabetes.** Diabetic nephropathy and hypertensive nephropathy are major causes of morbidity and mortality among diabetics.

D. Prevention

1. **Avoidance of improper exposure to hydrocarbons, industrial solvents, paints, and gasoline** can help to prevent renal disease.
2. **Understanding the immune process and methods to arrest the progression of glomerulonephritis** is currently the focus of most research.
3. **Dialysis and transplantation** are the only ways to prevent imminent death once end stage renal disease develops.
4. **Drug treatment of hypertension in diabetic patients** may reduce the progression of renal failure, according to recent reports. It is unclear whether vigorous control of blood sugar in diabetics also reduces the probability of developing renal failure.
5. **Routine screening for bacteriuria.** Pyelonephritis (bacterial infection of the kidney), bacteriuria (bacteria in the urine), and other urinary tract infections, can lead to chronic pyelonephritis, although this is rare in the absence of structural or neurologic abnormalities or states, such as diabetes or pregnancy. However, high morbidity due to recurring infection, may result. Therefore, diabetic or pregnant women should be screened routinely for bacteriuria.
6. **Control of hypertension.** Antihypertensive drugs, supplemented by general hygienic measures have been shown by clinical trials to be effective in reducing morbidity and mortality due to renal failure.

XI. PEPTIC ULCER DISEASE

A. Epidemiology

1. **Mortality rate.** The 1979 death rate for peptic ulcer disease was 2.0 individuals per 100,000 population (i.e., 1.1 for gastric ulcer and 0.9 for duodenal ulcer). Approximately 6000 deaths per year are due to peptic ulcer disease (i.e., 3000 gastric ulcers and 3000 duodenal ulcers) in the United States.

2. Incidence and prevalence

a. An annual incidence rate of 0.29% was reported in 1975 in the United States, leading to approximately 350,000 new cases per year.

b. The lifetime prevalence of peptic ulcer disease is roughly 5%–10%. The 1-year prevalence of self-reported peptic ulcer disease in the United States was about 1.7%–1.9% between 1961 and 1981. About 4 million Americans suffer from active peptic ulcers during any given year.

c. Overall prevalence has remained fairly stable, although rates for men and women show opposite patterns: Rates for men have decreased from 2.3% to 1.8%, while rates for women have increased from 1.1% to 1.7%. The reasons for these changes are not known.

3. Time trends. The death rate for peptic ulcer disease has decreased by 30% since 1950. Mortality may be influenced by factors such as life-style changes.

B. Costs. It has been estimated that in 1975, the cost of ulcer disease in the United States was between $1.3 and $2.6 billion.

C. Causal and risk factors. Factors such as cigarette smoking, regular use of aspirin, and prolonged use of large steroid doses have been associated with ulcer disease. Less conclusive associations have been reported for alcohol, caffeine, diet, and psychologic stress.

1. Smoking. Men who smoke cigarettes have higher peptic ulcer mortality rates than nonsmokers; strong conclusions cannot be made for women smokers.

a. Prospective studies show that smokers of cigarettes, pipes, or cigars are at a one-third increased risk of developing an ulcer later in life when compared with nonsmokers in their class.

b. Retrospective studies show that cigarette smokers are about twice as likely to have ulcers as nonsmokers. Men who smoke have a 2.1 times greater percentage of peptic ulcer disease, and the prevalence in women who smoke is 1.6 times greater than in nonsmokers. The percentage of people with ulcers increased significantly with the number of cigarettes smoked per day.

2. Aspirin or acetaminophen use is associated with a three to six times higher prevalance of gastric ulcer disease.

3. Family history

a. Family studies have shown that peptic ulcer occurs 2 to 2.5 times more frequently among first-degree relatives of patients with ulcer disease as compared to relatives of those without ulcer disease. The increased risk is only for the same kind of ulcer.

b. Individuals with blood type O are about 37% more likely to develop duodenal ulcer than people with other blood types.

D. Prevention

1. Primary prevention. Avoidance of the agents known to increase the risk of ulcer disease is the basis for prevention.

a. Initial occurrence. A nutritious diet, avoidance of nicotine, and temperance in the use of caffeine and alcohol will decrease the risk of developing duodenal ulcer disease.

b. Recurrence of gastric ulcer may be prevented through avoidance of mucosal-disrupting substances, such as salicylates, nonsteroidal anti-inflammatory drugs, and oral corticosteroids, and by the cessation of smoking.

2. Secondary prevention. Tests for determining a pre-ulcerous condition in asymptomatic individuals do not exist.

3. Tertiary prevention

a. Treatment entails:

(1) Neutralization of gastric acid.

(2) Reduction of gastric acid output.

(3) Increasing the integrity of the gastric and duodenal mucosa.

b. Intense antacid therapy and parenteral cimetidine given intravenously or intramuscularly have been shown to be effective in preventing *recurrence* of stress ulcerations. Cimetidine may also be effective in preventing *recurrences* of duodenal ulcer when given in a dose of 300 to 400 mg at bedtime for 3 months.

XII. ANEMIA

A. Epidemiology

1. Mortality rate. Anemias were the thirteenth leading cause of death of children under the age of 15 in the United States in 1983, accounting for 0.8% of all deaths, with a mortality rate of 0.3 per 100,000 population 1–14 years of age. Anemia accounts for less than 0.05% of deaths overall with a morality rate of 0.1 per 100,000 population.

2. **Incidence and prevalence**
   a. The prevalence of anemia from 1976 to 1980 ranged from 2.3% to 5.9% in a study conducted by the Second National Health and Nutrition Examination Survey.
   b. Prevalence rates in children ranged from 5.7% in infants 1 to 2 years of age to 2.8% in children 9 to 11 years of age, including girls and boys of all races. Children 6 to 8 years of age and boys and men 12 to 44 years of age had the lowest prevalence rates (2.3% and 2.9%, respectively).
   c. The highest prevalence rates, aside from infants, were experienced by girls 15 to 17 years of age (5.9%), young women (4.5%), and elderly men (4.8%).

B. Causal and risk factors

1. **Familial predisposition**
   a. **Sickle-cell anemia** is caused by a lack of Hb A; a deprivation of oxygen results in crescent-shaped cells. This disorder is almost entirely confined to blacks.
   b. **Thalassemia** is caused by partial or complete interference in synthesis of one of the normal hemoglobin peptide chains. Characteristics include unusually thin red corpuscles. This anemia occurs primarily in individuals of Italian, Greek, Syrian, or Armenian heritage, although there is also a high incidence in Thailand and the rest of the Far East.
2. **Iron deficiency**
   a. Children may experience iron deficiency anemia at a time when increased iron is required for rapid growth.
   b. Women are susceptible to iron deficiency due to menstrual blood loss and the iron losses associated with pregnancy.
   c. Individuals of low socioeconomic status are more likely to develop anemia, due to the absence of an iron-rich diet because of poverty or ignorance.
3. **Vitamin B_{12} deficiency.** Pernicious anemia is caused by insufficient intestinal absorption of vitamin B_{12}. It primarily affects individuals over the age of 30, and incidence increases with age. Individuals of northern European extraction are more likely to develop pernicious anemia; it is less common among Orientals and blacks.
4. **Sex and age.** In elderly men, anemia may be linked to a decrease in the androgen stimulation of erythropoiesis that began during puberty; in otherwise healthy subjects, anemia may indicate an overall reduction in hematopoietic reserve.

C. Prevention

1. **Screening** by hematocrit is considered cost-effective for target populations and thus is recommended for the following high-risk groups:
   a. Premature infants
   b. Infants born of a multiple pregnancy or an iron-deficient woman
   c. Individuals in low socioeconomic circumstances
2. **Iron supplements** in foods, primarily cereal products, have been shown to decrease the prevalence of anemia among women in Sweden from 30% in 1965 to 7% in 1975.
3. **Consumption of red meats, organ meats (especially liver), and leafy, green vegetables** that are high in B vitamins is recommended for those at high risk and those previously diagnosed with anemia.

BIBLIOGRAPHY

Akbar N: Causal factors. *Public Health Rep* 95:554–555, 1980

Bennett PH, Knowler WC: Early detection and intervention in diabetes mellitus: is it effective? *J Chron Dis* 37:653–666, 1984

Berg RL, Ornt DB: End stage renal disease: how many, how much? *Am J Public Health* 74:4–5, 1984

Canadian Task Force on the Periodic Health Examination: The periodic health examination. *Can Med Assoc J* 121:3–45, 1979

Cancer statistics, 1986. *CA* 36:9–25, 1986

Cramer DW: Uterine cervix. In *Cancer Epidemiology and Prevention*. Edited by Schottenfeld D, Fraumeni JF Jr. Philadelphia, Saunders, 1982

Dallman PR, Yip R, Johnson C: Prevalence and causes of anemia in the United States, 1976 to 1980. *Am J Clin Nutr* 39:437–445, 1984

Doll R: Prospects for the prevention of cancer. *Clin Radiol* 34:609–623, 1983

Doll R, Peto R: *The Causes of Cancer*. Oxford, Oxford University Press, 1981

Ebert RV, McNabb ME: Cessation of smoking in prevention and treatment of cardiac and pulmonary disease. *Arch Intern Med* 144:1558–1559, 1984

Fielding JE: Smoking: health effects and control. In *Maxcy-Rosenau Public Health and Preventive Medicine*, 12th ed. Edited by Last JM. Norwalk, Conn, Appleton-Century-Crofts, 1986

Fraumeni JF Jr, Blot WJ: Lung and pleura. In *Cancer Epidemiology and Prevention*. Edited by Schottenfeld D, Fraumeni JF Jr. Philadelphia, Saunders, 1982

Garland C, Garland F: Digestive diseases. In *Maxcy-Rosenau Public Health and Preventive Medicine*, 12th ed. Edited by Last JM. Norwalk, Conn, Appleton-Century-Crofts, 1986

Gary LE: Role of alcohol and drug abuse in homicide. *Public Health Rep* 95:553–554, 1980

Greenwald P: Prostate. In *Cancer Epidemiology and Prevention*. Edited by Schottenfeld D, Fraumeni JF Jr. Philadelphia, Saunders, 1982

Haut A, Wintrobe MM: The hemoglobinopathies and thalassemias. In *Harrison's Principles of Internal Medicine*, 6th ed. Edited by Wintrobe MM et al. New York, McGraw-Hill, 1970

Higgins I: Respiratory disease. In *Maxcy-Rosenau Public Health and Preventive Medicine*, 12th ed. Edited by Last JM. Norwalk, Conn, Appleton-Century-Crofts, 1986

Higgins M: Epidemiology of COPD: state of the art. *Chest* 85 (Suppl): 3S–8S, 1984

Hingson R, Merrigan D, Heeren T: Effects of Massachusetts raising its legal drinking age from 18 to 20 on deaths from teenage homicide, suicide, and nontraffic accidents. *Pediatr Clin North Am* 32:221–232, 1985

Hoffer W: Public health strategies eyed to curb homicides. *Am Med News* Oct 25:21–22, 1985

Hopper SV, Miller JP, Birge C, et al: A randomized study of the impact of home health aides on diabetic control and utilization patterns. *Am J Public Health* 74:600–602, 1984

Kannel WB, Doyle JT, Ostfeld AM, et al: Optimal resources for primary prevention of atherosclerotic diseases: atherosclerosis study group. *Circulation* 70:155A–205A, 1984

Kleck G: Capital punishment, gun ownership, and homicide. *Am J Sociol* 84:882–910, 1979

Klein BE: Secondary prevention in diabetes mellitus. *J Chron Dis* 37:671–673, 1984

Kuller LH, LaPorte RE, Orchard TJ: Diabetes. In *Maxcy-Rosenau Public Health and Preventive Medicine*, 12th ed. Edited by Last JM. Norwalk, Conn, Appleton-Century-Crofts, 1986

Kunin CM: Renal disease. In *Maxcy-Rosenau Public Health and Preventive Medicine*, 12th ed. Edited by Last JM. Norwalk, Conn, Appleton-Century-Crofts, 1986

Kurata JH, Haile BM: Epidemiology of peptic ulcer disease. *Clin Gastroenterol* 13:289–307, 1984

Lenfant C, Roccella EJ: Trends in hypertension control in the United States. *Chest* 86:459–462, 1984

Medley ES: Peptic ulcer disease. *J Fam Pract* 18:443–463, 1984

Monk M: Suicide. In *Maxcy-Rosenau Public Health and Preventive Medicine*, 12th ed. Edited by Last JM. Norwalk, Conn, Appleton-Century-Crofts, 1986

Petrakis NL, Ernster VL, King MC: Breast. In *Cancer Epidemiology and Prevention*. Edited by Schottenfeld D, Fraumeni JF Jr. Philadelphia, Saunders, 1982

Pokanzer DC: Neurological disease. In *Maxcy-Rosenau Public Health and Preventive Medicine*, 12th ed. Edited by Last JM. Norwalk, Conn, Appleton-Century-Crofts, 1986

Rankin JG, Ashley MJ: Alcohol-related health problems and their prevention. In *Maxcy-Rosenau Public Health and Preventive Medicine*, 12th ed. Edited by Last JM. Norwalk, Conn, Appleton-Century-Crofts, 1986

Richman J: *Family Therapy for Suicidal People*. New York, Springer, 1986

Rosenberg ML, Stark E, Zahn MA: Interpersonal violence: homicide and spouse abuse. In *Maxcy-Rosenau Public Health and Preventive Medicine*, 12th ed. Edited by Last JM. Norwalk, Conn, Appleton-Century-Crofts, 1986

Schottenfeld D, Winawer SJ: Large intestine. In *Cancer Epidemiology and Prevention*. Edited by Schottenfeld D, Fraumeni, JF Jr. Philadelphia, Saunders, 1982

Scrimshaw NS: Nutrition and preventive medicine. In *Maxcy-Rosenau Public Health and Preventive Medicine*, 12th ed. Edited by Last JM. Norwalk, Conn, Appleton-Century-Crofts, 1986

Strax P: Mammography. In *Screening for Cancer*. Edited by Miller AB. Orlando, Fl, Academic Press, 1985

Sugimoto T, Rosansky SJ: The incidence of treated end stage renal disease in the Eastern United States: 1973–1979. *Am J Public Health* 74:14–17, 1984

Tardiff K: Patterns and major determinants of homicide in the United States. *Hosp Community Psychiatry* 36:632–639, 1985

Thomas DB: Cancer. In *Maxcy-Rosenau Public Health and Preventive Medicine*, 12th ed. Edited by Last JM. Norwalk, Conn, Appleton-Century-Crofts, 1986

Tyroler H: Hypertension. In *Maxcy-Rosenau Public Health and Preventive Medicine*, 12th ed. Edited by Last JM. Norwalk, Conn, Appleton-Century-Crofts, 1986

Watkins LO: Coronary artery disease and hypertension in the U.S. black populations. *Md State Med J* 33:435–436, 1984

Whitehouse GH: An overview on the value of plain radiography and contrast studies in oncologic practice. In *Comprehensive Textbook of Oncology*. Edited by Moossa AR, Robson MC, Schimpff SC. Baltimore, Williams & Wilkins, 1986

Wintrobe MM, Lee GR: Pernicious anemia and other megaloblastic anemias. In *Harrison's Principles of Internal Medicine*, 6th ed. Edited by Wintrobe MM et al. New York, McGraw-Hill, 1970

Woolner LB, Fontana RS: Pulmonary cytology in lung cancer screening. In *Screening for Cancer*. Edited by Miller AB. Orlando, Fl, Academic Press, 1985

Young JL Jr, Pollack ES: The incidence of cancer in the United States. In *Cancer Epidemiology and Prevention*. Edited by Schottenfeld D, Fraumeni JF Jr. Philadelphia, Saunders, 1982

STUDY QUESTIONS

Directions: Each question below contains five suggested answers. Choose the **one best** response to each question.

1. High levels of serum cholesterol are associated with an increased risk of heart disease. However, decreasing daily cholesterol intake by 5 mg results in a decline in the risk of coronary heart disease by

(A) 5%
(B) 10%
(C) 15%
(D) 20%
(E) 25%

2. All of the following trends have been observed in the incidence of lung cancer since 1950 EXCEPT

(A) The incidence of lung cancer in America is increasing faster among women than men
(B) Between 1950 and 1978, the age-adjusted lung cancer rate increased 192% for men and 263% for women
(C) Between 1950 and 1957, the age-adjusted rate for women increased an average of 1% per year, and the age-adjusted rate for men climbed to an average of 6.7% per year
(D) Between 1968 and 1977, the age-adjusted rate for women increased almost 7% per year, but the rate for men fell to 4% per year
(E) Lung cancer accounts for 40% of all cancer mortality and 20% of all deaths in the United States

Directions: Each question below contains four suggested answers of which **one or more** is correct. Choose the answer

A if **1, 2, and 3** are correct
B if **1 and 3** are correct
C if **2 and 4** are correct
D if **4** is correct
E if **1, 2, 3, and 4** are correct

3. Uncontrolled hypertension increases the risk of developing

(1) cerebrovascular disease
(2) coronary heart disease
(3) renal disease
(4) diabetes

4. The risk factors for peptic ulcer disease include

(1) familial predisposition
(2) regular use of aspirin, acetaminophen, or steroids
(3) tobacco smoking
(4) dietary habits

5. Population subgroups that are at increased risk of developing anemias include

(1) children
(2) women
(3) elderly men
(4) blacks

Directions: The group of questions below consists of lettered choices followed by several numbered items. For each numbered item select the **one** lettered choice with which it is **most** closely associated. Each lettered choice may be used once, more than once, or not at all.

Questions 6–9

For each disease listed below, select the description of the screening program that is most likely to be associated with it.

(A) Screening programs are cost-effective for selected populations
(B) Screening programs do not exist for this condition
(C) Screening programs are not cost-effective for this condition
(D) Screening programs are only cost-effective for children under 2 years of age
(E) Screening programs are only cost-effective for women after menopause

6. Coronary heart disease
7. Childhood anemia
8. Cervical cancer
9. Lung cancer

ANSWERS AND EXPLANATIONS

1. The answer is A. (*II C 2; D 2 b*) Studies of blood lipids in healthy adults show consistent and linear increases in individual risk of coronary heart disease, according to levels of total serum cholesterol and low density lipoprotein. Studies have shown that a daily decrease of 5 mg of cholesterol in a population will result in an estimated 5% decline in the population's risk of developing coronary heart disease. Individually, lower cholesterol levels can usually be achieved by decreasing the consumption of milk, butter, eggs, and animal fat.

2. The answer is E. [*IV A 1 b (1)–(3)*] The incidence of lung cancer is now increasing faster among American women than among American men. Between 1950 and 1978, the age-adjusted lung cancer rate increased 192% for men and 263% for women. Between 1950 and 1957, the age-adjusted rate for women increased an average of 1% per year, but between 1968 and 1977, the rate increased almost 7% per year. Between 1950 and 1957, the age-adjusted lung cancer rate for men climbed to an average of 6.7% per year, but between 1968 and 1977, the rate fell to a 4% annual increase. Lung cancer accounts for 25% of all cancer mortality, and 5% of all deaths in the United States.

3. The answer is A (1, 2, 3). (*II C 1; III C 1; X D 4*) Hypertension is a strong and independent risk factor for coronary heart disease and is well established by descriptive studies. Hypertension increases the risk of stroke, and epidemiologic evidence is strong that hypertension is one of the causes of atherosclerosis, particularly in combination with hyperlipidemia. Hypertensive nephropathy is a major cause of morbidity and mortality among diabetics. However, hypertension itself does not increase the risk of developing diabetes.

4. The answer is E (all). (*XI C 1–3*) Factors such as cigarette smoking, regular use of aspirin, and prolonged use of steroids in large doses have been closely associated with ulcer disease. Less conclusive associations have been reported for alcohol, caffeine, diet, and psychologic stress. Family studies have shown that peptic ulcer disease occurs 2 to 2.5 times more frequently among first-degree relatives of patients with ulcer disease as compared to relatives of those without ulcer disease. The increased risk is only for the same kind of ulcer.

5. The answer is E (all). (*XII A 2 c, B 1 a, 2–4*) Children are at an increased risk for anemia because increased iron is required for rapid growth. In women, menstrual blood loss and the iron losses associated with pregnancy can result in anemia. In elderly men, anemia may be linked to a decrease in androgen stimulation of erythropoiesis that began during puberty; in otherwise healthy subjects, anemia may indicate an overall reduction in hematopoietic reserve. In blacks, genetic, socioeconomic, and dietary factors are associated with anemia.

6–9. The answers are: 6-C, 7-A, 8-A, 9-C. (*II D 1; IV D 1 a, b, 4 a–b; XII C 1*) Measurement of blood pressure, which is recommended every 5 years for men and women 16 to 64 years of age and every 2 years after age 65, is the primary screening method for coronary heart disease. Measurement of serum cholesterol levels is also used for screening target populations. However, neither of these screening methods is cost-effective for screening target populations.

Screening for anemia is by hematocrit. Target populations include: premature infants, infants born of a multiple pregnancy or an iron-deficient woman, and individuals of low socioeconomic status. Hematocrit is considered a cost-effective method of screening for anemia for target populations.

Screening for cervical cancer is by Pap smear to detect cervical abnormalities; intervals of 1 to 5 years are recommened. Target populations include individuals who: are between the ages of 25–60, are of low socioeconomic status, are prison inmates, are prostitutes, had first intercourse at an early age, have a history of infectious diseases, are unmarried mothers, have had induced abortions, or have a history of cervical squamous dysplasia. A Pap smear is considered a cost-effective method of screening for cervical cancer.

Screening for presymptomatic lung cancer is by either pulmonary cytology or chest roentgenography, neither of which is considered cost-effective for screening target populations. In addition, screening has no beneficial effect on mortality from lung cancer, although there is a shift to less serious stages at the time of detection.

6
Maternal Health Issues

Sally Faith Dorfman

I. DEFINITIONS

A. **Maternal mortality** consists of deaths attributed to complications of pregnancy, childbirth, and the puerperium, often within a fixed time (42 days, 6 months, or 1 year) of the pregnancy's termination.

1. **Direct maternal mortality** consists of deaths resulting from obstetric complications, omissions, interventions, and their sequelae.
2. **Indirect maternal mortality** consists of deaths resulting from preexisting conditions or conditions aggravated by the pregnancy.
3. **The maternal mortality rate** is the ratio of pregnancy-related deaths to live births over a specified time for a particular geographic area, usually per 100,000 live births.

B. **Preterm terminations of pregnancy**

1. **Abortion.** The **abortion rate** is the number of abortions per 1000 women who are 15 to 44 years of age. The **abortion ratio** is the number of abortions per 1000 live births.
   a. **Induced abortion** is a procedure that terminates a pregnancy, producing a nonviable fetus.
   b. **Spontaneous abortion** includes failure of embryonic development, fetal death in utero, and expulsion of all (complete) or any part (incomplete) of the products of conception before the twentieth week of gestation or expulsion of a fetus weighing less than 500 g.
2. **Ectopic pregnancy** is a pregnancy located outside the normal implantation area in the body of a normally shaped uterus. Continued growth may result in hemorrhagic rupture. In the United States during recent years, approximately one of every 100 reported pregnancies has been ectopic in location, and one of every 1000 ectopic pregnancies resulted in the woman's death. Many factors have been *associated* with increased risk, but *causation* has not been established. Putative risk factors include:
   a. A history of ectopic pregnancy.
   b. Tubal surgery.
   c. Pelvic inflammatory disease.
   d. Progestin exposure.
   e. Infertility.
3. **Stillbirth** is fetal death occurring after the twentieth week of gestation or spontaneous death of a fetus weighing more than 500 g.

C. **Fetal and infant mortality**

1. **Perinatal mortality** consists of fetal and infant deaths occurring between 28 weeks gestation and 1 week postnatal, with fetal or infant weight $\geq$ 500 g.
2. **Neonatal mortality** consists of deaths of live-born infants within 28 days of age.
3. **Infant mortality** consists of deaths of children less than 1 year of age.

II. MATERNAL MORTALITY

A. Maternal mortality overall has decreased in the United States, particularly after the legalization of induced abortion in the early 1970s (Fig. 6-1).

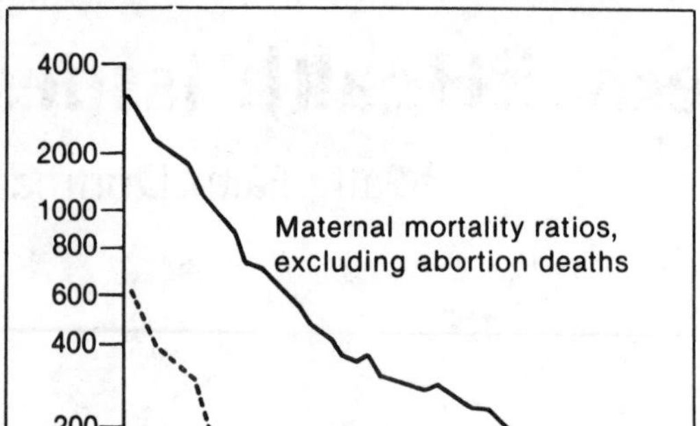

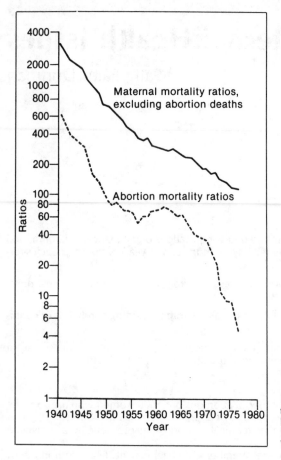

Figure 6-1. Maternal mortality ratios (excluding abortion deaths) and abortion mortality ratios per 1 million live births in the United States, 1940–1977. (Courtesy of Dr. Roger Rochat, National Center for Health Statistics, Washington, D.C.)

B. Analysis of United States maternal mortality rates by race reveals consistently lower rates for white women than for black women and women of other races (Table 6-1).

C. Analysis of international rates by age reveals a "J-shaped curve," with somewhat higher maternal mortality rates for younger and older women; United States rates are higher primarily for older women (see Table 6-1).

D. Embolism, hypertensive diseases of pregnancy, hemorrhage, and infection are the major causes of maternal mortality. Ectopic pregnancy has emerged as another leading cause, despite declining death-to-case rates (Figs. 6-2 and 6-3).

III. PREVENTION OF PREGNANCY

A. **Contraceptive methods.** Criteria for a good contraceptive include efficacy, safety, accessibility, acceptability, and reversibility. Risk/benefit analysis may be done for each method using these criteria and including absence of a method and the resultant unwanted pregnancy.

1. **Abstinence from sex**
   a. **Advantages**
      (1) Accessible, safe, and reversible
      (2) Acceptable to most religious groups
   b. **Disadvantage.** Abstinence is not always an acceptable means of contraception.

2. **Natural family planning** includes calendar, temperature, and cervical mucus analyses.
   a. **Advantages**
      (1) Safe and accessible
      (2) Acceptable to most religious groups
   b. **Disadvantages**
      (1) Requires extensive education

Table 6-1. Death-to-Case Rates for Legal Abortions and Corresponding Childbearing Mortality Rates by Year, Age, and Race (1972–1978)

	Abortion Rate*		Childbearing Rate†		
	Crude	Standardized	Crude	Standardized	Relative Risk‡
Year					
1972	4.1	4.1	15.2	16.8	4.1
1973	3.4	3.2	12.6	13.9	4.3
1974	2.8	2.6	12.1	13.9	5.3
1975	2.8	2.6	10.4	12.0	4.6
1976	0.9	0.8	10.5	11.7	14.6
1977	1.3	1.2	9.3	10.4	8.7
1978	0.5	0.4	8.0	9.1	22.8
Age					
≤ 19	1.3	1.3	8.5	7.7	5.9
20–24	2.1	2.1	7.4	7.9	3.8
25–29	2.0	2.0	9.4	11.6	5.8
30–34	2.5	2.3	17.1	20.1	8.7
≥ 35	3.4	3.2	43.7	46.3	14.5
Race					
White	1.3	1.3	8.3	8.2	6.3
Black and other	3.3	3.5	23.1	23.1	6.6
Overall	1.9	1.8	11.1	12.5	6.9

Reprinted from Centers for Disease Control: *Abortion Surveillance, 1970–1980*. May, 1983.
*Deaths per 100,000 abortions.
†Deaths per 100,000 live births.
‡Ratio of standardized childbearing rate to standardized abortion rate.

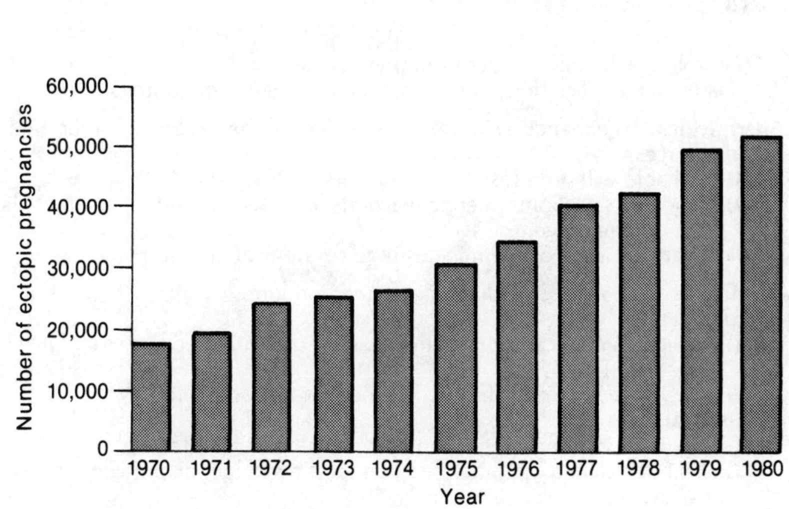

Figure 6-2. Number of ectopic pregnancies in the United States (1970–1980). (National Hospital Discharge Survey; reprinted with permission from Dorfman SF: Deaths from ectopic pregnancy, United States, 1979– 1980. *Obstet Gynecol* 62:334, 1983.)

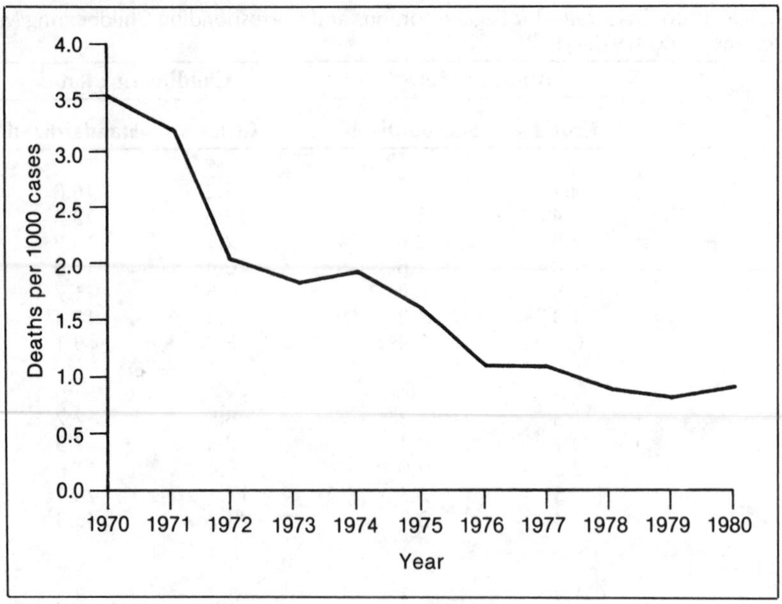

Figure 6-3. Death-to-case rates for women with ectopic pregnancies in the United States (1970–1980). (National Center for Health Statistics; reprinted with permission from Dorfman SF: Deaths from ectopic pregnancy, United States, 1979–1980. *Obstet Gynecol* 62:334, 1983.)

- **(2)** Requires strong motivation
- **(3)** Variable efficacy according to individual motivation and physiologic and pathologic variables

3. Coitus interruptus. The efficacy and acceptability of coitus interruptus may be marginal.

- **a. Advantage.** Coitus interruptus is available to everyone.
- **b. Disadvantages**
  - **(1)** Ineffective from pre-ejaculate sperm
  - **(2)** Requires great motivation and control, which may not be attainable

4. Lactation. The efficacy of lactation is significant on a worldwide basis, but it is unreliable for individual couples.

- **a. Advantages**
  - **(1)** Enhances infant nutrition and health and maternal-infant bonding
  - **(2)** Prolongs the interval between pregnancies
- **b. Disadvantage.** Lactation is an undependable means of contraception.

5. Spermicides. To enhance efficacy, spermicides can be used with other methods.

- **a. Advantages**
  - **(1)** Available without prescriptions or office visits
  - **(2)** Generally safe (Some allergic reactions have been reported, and there is some concern regarding teratogenesis.)
- **b. Disadvantage.** Use of spermicides requires motivation and planning.

6. Barriers (e.g., sponge, cap, diaphragm, and condom)

- **a. Advantages**
  - **(1)** Provide some protection against sexually transmitted diseases and pelvic inflammatory disease (PID)
  - **(2)** May be combined with other methods to enhance efficacy
- **b. Disadvantages**
  - **(1)** Require consistent motivation and planning to be effective
  - **(2)** Minimal risk of toxic shock syndrome from sponge, diaphragm, or cap, especially during menses

7. Intrauterine device (IUD)

- **a. Advantage.** The single insertion of an IUD gives protection for a year or more.
- **b. Disadvantages**
  - **(1)** Significant risks, especially if coupling is not mutually monogamous, including:
    - **(a)** PID

(b) Ectopic pregnancy
(c) Infertility
(2) Heavy menstrual flow and cramping
(3) Limited access and availablity

8. Pills (fixed combinations and phasics)

a. Advantages

(1) Highly effective
(2) Not coitally related
(3) Generally safe and reversible
(4) Thought to be protective against such conditions as anemia, dysmenorrhea, ovarian cysts, and endometrial cancer
(5) Possibly protective against breast and ovarian cancers

b. Disadvantages

(1) Increased risk oı cardiovascular and thromboembolic diseases among:
(a) Women over 35 years of age who smoke (Fig. 6-4).
(b) Women over 35 years of age who do not smoke.
(c) Women taking high-dose pills.
(2) Requires a prescription and regular office visits
(3) Major and minor side effects (e.g., hypertension, migraines, breakthrough bleeding, bloating, and emotional lability)

9. Progestin-only minipills, injectables, and implants

a. Advantages

(1) Effective
(2) Can be used when estrogens are contraindicated

b. Disadvantages

(1) Progestin-only minipills are less effective than combination pills; they are also associated with irregular bleeding.
(2) Injectables and implants are not currently approved for use in the United States.
(3) Depo-provera has been associated with breast tumors in beagle dogs (a species prone to this).

B. Abortion. Table 6-2 and Figures 6-5 and 6-6 illustrate the secular trends and characteristics of women obtaining abortions in the United States (see section II A).

1. Access to safe, legal abortion has had a considerable impact on the decline of maternal mortality and morbidity in the United States. In other countries where induced abortion is not legal, hospital wards are filled with women who have undergone self-induced or illegal abortions.

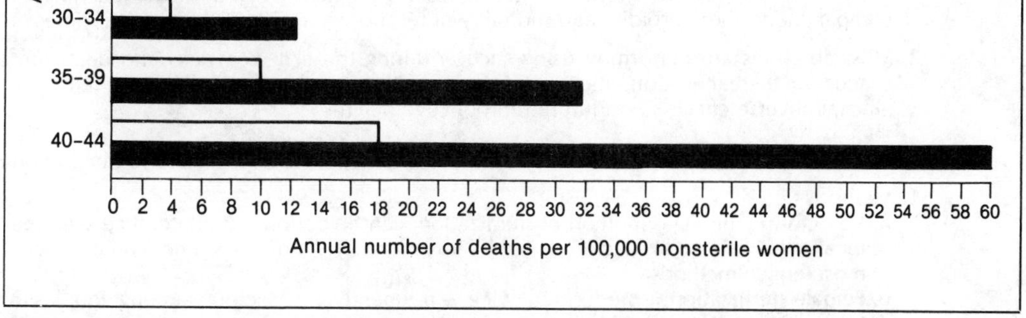

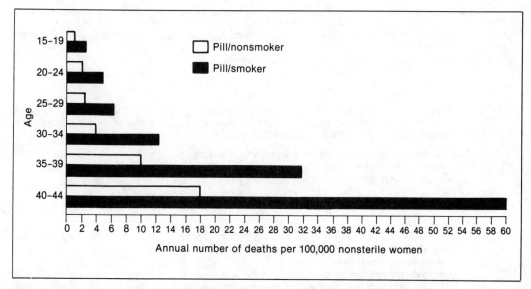

Figure 6-4. Smoking and the pill. (Reprinted with permission from *Contraceptive Technology Update*. Atlanta, GA, November, 1980.)

Table 6-2. Characteristics of Women Obtaining Abortions in the United States (1972–1980)

	Percentage Distribution*								
Characteristics	**1972**	**1973**	**1974**	**1975**	**1976**	**1977**	**1978**	**1979**	**1980**
Residence									
Abortion in-state	56.2	74.8	86.6	89.2	90.0	90.0	89.3	90.0	92.6
Abortion out-of-state	43.8	25.2	13.4	10.8	10.0	10.0	10.7	10.0	7.4
Age									
≤ 19	32.6	32.7	32.7	33.1	32.1	30.8	30.0	30.0	29.2
20–24	32.5	32.0	31.8	31.9	33.3	34.5	35.0	35.4	35.5
≥ 25	34.9	35.3	35.6	35.0	34.6	34.7	34.9	34.6	35.3
Race									
White	77.0	72.5	69.7	67.8	66.6	66.4	67.0	68.9	69.9
Black and other	23.0	27.5	30.3	32.2	33.4	33.6	33.0	31.1	30.1
Marital status									
Married	29.7	27.4	27.4	26.1	24.6	24.3	26.4	24.7	23.1
Unmarried	70.3	72.6	72.6	73.9	75.4	75.7	73.6	75.3	76.9
Number of live births†									
0	49.4	48.6	47.8	47.1	47.7	53.4	56.6	58.1	58.4
1	18.2	18.8	19.6	20.2	20.7	19.1	19.2	19.1	19.5
2	13.3	14.2	14.8	15.5	15.4	14.4	14.1	13.8	13.7
3	8.7	8.7	8.7	8.7	8.3	7.0	5.9	5.5	5.3
≥ 4	10.4	9.7	9.0	8.6	7.9	6.2	4.2	3.5	3.2
Type of procedure									
Curettage	88.6	88.4	89.7	90.9	92.8	93.8	94.6	95.0	95.5
Intrauterine instillation	10.4	10.4	7.8	6.2	6.0	5.4	3.9	3.3	3.1
Hysterotomy/hysterectomy	0.6	0.7	0.6	0.4	0.2	0.2	0.1	0.1	0.1
Other	0.5	0.6	1.9	2.4	0.9	0.7	1.4	1.6	1.3
Weeks of gestation									
≤ 8	34.0	36.1	42.6	44.6	47.0	51.2	52.2	52.1	51.7
9–10	30.7	29.4	28.7	28.4	28.0	27.2	26.9	27.0	26.2
11–12	17.5	17.9	15.4	14.9	14.4	13.1	12.3	12.5	12.2
13–15	8.4	6.9	5.5	5.0	4.5	3.4	4.0	4.2	5.2
16–20	8.2	8.0	6.5	6.1	5.1	4.3	3.7	3.4	3.9
≥ 21	1.3	1.7	1.2	1.0	0.9	0.9	0.9	0.9	0.9

Reprinted from Centers for Disease Control: *Abortion Surveillance, 1970–1980*. May, 1983.

*Excludes unknowns. Since the number of states reporting each characteristic varies from year to year, temporal comparisons should be made with caution.

†For years 1972–1977, data indicate number of living children.

2. In the United States, about 95% of legal abortions are performed during the first 12 weeks of gestation. Morbidity and mortality rates increase with each week of delay, reaching a level comparable to the morbidity and mortality of term pregnancies in the second trimester.

3. Most abortions are performed using suction during the first 12 weeks and dilatation and evacuation thereafter. Contemporary methods of induced abortion do not appear to have significant adverse effects upon future reproductive health.

C. **Sterilization** has become a leading form of contraception, both nationally and internationally.

1. **Methods**
   a. **Vasectomy**, the male method of sterilization, can be performed in an office setting using local anesthesia and is accompanied by less morbidity, mortality, time, and expense than most female methods.
   b. **Female sterilization**, is performed twice as frequently as vasectomy among couples in the United States. It usually involves entering the abdominal cavity to ligate, cauterize, clip, or otherwise interrupt the fallopian tubes, and it often requires extensive anesthesia.
      (1) Advantages. Sterilization is very effective and usually permanent.

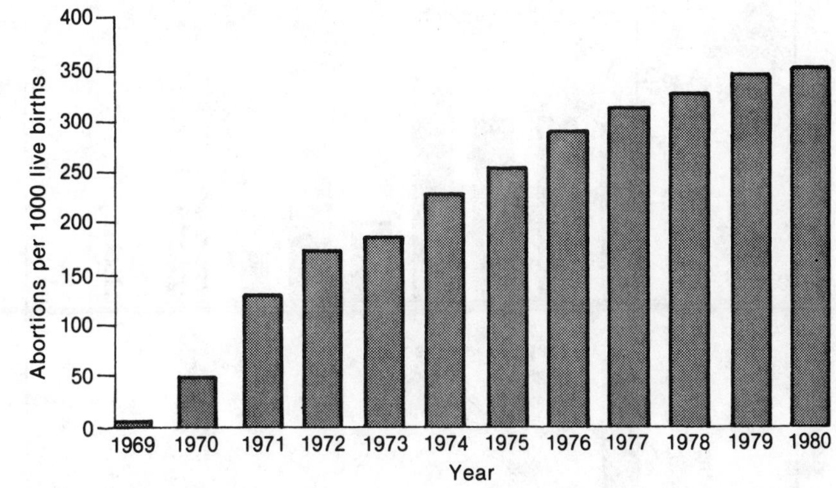

Figure 6-5. Legal abortion ratios in the United States (1969–1980). (Reprinted from Centers for Disease Control, *Abortion Surveillance: 1979–1980*, May, 1983.)

(2) Disadvantages.

(a) As with any surgical procedure, there are always risks, including:

(i) Hemorrhage.

(ii) Infection.

(iii) Anesthetic complications.

(iv) Visceral injury (for females).

(b) Sterilization may fail from spontaneous recanalization of the blocked ducts, or fistula formation, but voluntary reversibility cannot be assumed.

(c) Partial blockage of a fallopian tube may result in an ectopic pregnancy.

(d) Costs may be considerable.

(e) Local or national policies may impede access and availability by mandatory age and consent requirements and waiting periods.

2. Psychosocial and legal issues

a. Counseling and voluntarism are critical issues because of the permanent nature of sterilization surgery. Clients should carefully consider all alternatives in assessing their current and future reproductive possibilities. Most states require a delay between the consent for sterilization and the actual procedure.

b. Reversibility can never be assured, and attempts to reverse female methods may result in ectopic pregnancy. Every effort should be made to identify and discourage clients who are considering future reversal.

IV. PRENATAL CARE AND SCREENING

A. Preconceptional risks to sperm and ova include environmental and occupational hazards, such as pollutants, additives, pesticides, and radiation, that may be present in the home or workplace, resulting in germ cell mutation or expiration.

B. Routine well-woman care during pregnancy

1. Perform a Pap smear and breast and pelvic examinations at the first visit and as indicated thereafter.

2. Give special attention to nutrition, particularly those areas most likely to be marginal, including calcium, folate, and iron. An overall weight gain of 20–30 pounds should be the goal.

3. Check hematocrit and hemoglobin levels to screen for anemia.

4. Stress the importance of good hygiene.

5. Advise sensible exercise levels.

6. Screen and treat sexually transmitted diseases as indicated, including syphilis, gonorrhea, and herpes.

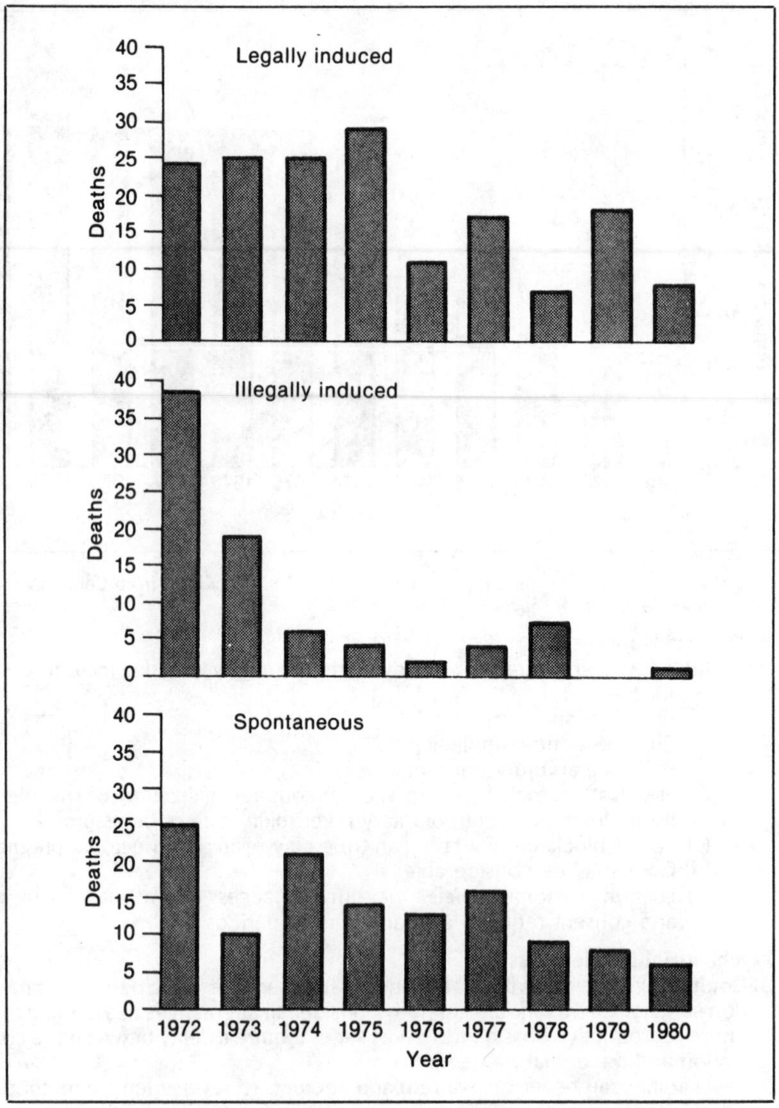

Figure 6-6. Abortion-related deaths by category (excluding unknown category) and year in the United States (1972–1980). (Reprinted from Centers for Disease Control, *Abortion Surveillance: 1979–1980*, May, 1983.)

7. Advise abstinence from hazardous substances, such as cigarettes, drugs, and alcohol.
8. Routinely check weight, blood pressure, reflexes, extremities, and urine. Other screening (e.g., tine testing for tuberculosis) should be performed as indicated.

C. Special pregnancy screening

1. **Infections**
   a. Screen for "TORCH" diseases that may affect the fetus or neonate: toxoplasmosis, rubella, cytomegalovirus, herpes, hepatitis, and others.
   b. Give rubella vaccine to susceptible individuals postpartum.
2. **Rh testing.** Follow special screening protocols for Rh-negative individuals.
3. **Sonography.** Screen for structural abnormalities, multiple gestation, and placental location as indicated.
4. **Amniocentesis and chorionic villus biopsy.** Test for congenital defects by direct sampling of the products of conception as indicated.

5. **Alpha-fetoprotein.** Detect some neural tube defects and other conditions by sampling maternal serum and amniotic fluid as indicated.

D. **Continuous monitoring of maternal well-being.** Check at a minimum blood pressure, weight, extremities, reflexes, and urine at each visit to identify:

1. **Hypertensive diseases of pregnancy** [i.e., preeclampsia/eclampsia ("toxemia") indicated by hypertension, edema, weight gain, hyperreflexia, and proteinuria]
2. **Gestational diabetes.** Many physicians advise routine midpregnancy screening, using a measured glucose load and timed serum sampling in addition to routine urine testing.

E. **Continuous monitoring of fetal development** is accomplished by comparing maternal weight and uterine size at each visit relative to the estimated date of conception in conjunction with other tests, such as, sonography and monitoring of fetal heart rate.

F. **Avoidance of potentially hazardous substances**, including possible teratogens* that are otherwise relatively innocuous (e.g., tetracycline antibiotics and alcohol).

1. **Substance abuse**
   a. **Tobacco** is associated with low birth weight and premature delivery.
   b. **Alcohol** is associated with teratogenic effects.
   c. **Illegal or "recreational" drugs** may result in teratogenic or withdrawal symptoms in neonates.
2. **DES and legal drugs*** (e.g., tetracycline or sulfonamides) may result in assorted teratogenic, structural, functional, or carcinogenic effects on offspring.
3. **Maternal malnutrition, anemia, and diabetes** can result in fetal malnutrition. Low birth weight from multiple causes is a major factor in infant mortality.
4. **Radiation**—either diagnostic, occupational, or environmental—may cause spontaneous abortion, birth defects, or childhood leukemia.*
5. **Occupational and environmental hazards**, including chemicals, pollutants, and radioactive substances that workers may carry home on skin or clothing to their pregnant partners, may cause reproductive problems.*
6. **Infectious agents** [e.g., syphilis, human immunodeficiency virus (HIV), toxoplasmosis, rubella, cytomegalovirus] are associated with assorted negative effects on the fetus.

G. **Cervical testing later in pregnancy** is somewhat controversial regarding frequency and cost/benefit (see below).

V. OBSTETRIC CONCERNS AT THE TIME OF DELIVERY

A. **Infectious diseases of the birth canal**

1. Herpes may be an indication for cesarean section as herpes simplex of the genital tract may lead to encephalitis or disseminated herpes simplex in the infant. Either may be fatal.
2. Gonorrhea, if untreated, may cause blindness in infants.
3. *Chlamydia* may result in ophthalmologic and other damage.
4. *Candida* can cause oral thrush.
5. *Streptococcus* may infect the infant.
6. Hepatitis may be transmitted during or prior to birth.
7. There is good evidence for vertical transmission of human immunodeficiency virus (HIV), the causative agent for acquired immune deficiency syndrome, but details remain sketchy.

B. **Type of delivery** (i.e., spontaneous vaginal delivery, forceps, vacuum extraction, cesarean section, or vaginal birth after cesarean) sometimes is a source of controversy among public health professionals and consumers, as well as obstetricians, midwives, and pediatricians.

---

*For details see *Catalog of Teratogenic Agents* (Baltimore, Johns Hopkins Press, 1980), *Reproductive Hazards of Industrial Chemicals* (New York, Academic Press, 1982), *Work and the Health of Women* (Boca Raton, FL, CRC Press, 1979).

C. **Prenatal health care providers, alternate birthing centers, and home births.** Aspects of contemporary hospital-based care, such as the use of electronic fetal monitoring and ultrasound and the credentials of obstetric attendants, have polarized physicians, certified nurse midwives, public health professionals, lay midwives, and consumer groups.

1. Throughout most of the world, and until recently in the United States and other developed countries, most births occurred at home, with laboring women assisted by lay midwives. Around the time of World War I, care of pregnant women in the United States shifted to physicians, and home births gradually were replaced by hospital deliveries. In the 1960s, a counterculture trend toward family-centered midwife-assisted deliveries increased in popularity. Most births in the United States currently occur in hospitals attended by physicians. Many of these physicians are obstetric specialists, and others are family practitioners who have had training in obstetrics.
2. Certified nurse midwives, working in conjunction with physicians, have provided an increasing amount of prenatal and obstetric care in the United States over the past 2 decades. They often work in hospital-affiliated "home-like" birthing rooms, or in freestanding family-oriented birthing centers.
3. Lay midwives continue to function outside the realm of the regulatory agencies, providing care of variable quality for those unable or unwilling to use established services.

D. **Access to care.** Regionalization efforts have been designed to improve access to comprehensive, quality care for patients at all levels of medical risk by defined geographic areas.

VI. POSTPARTUM PREVENTIVE MEDICINE AND PUBLIC HEALTH CONCERNS

A. Breast-feeding usually enhances infant nutrition, immune defenses, bonding, and contraception, but it is contraindicated in HIV-positive women.

B. Parenting and bonding help to ensure optimal development.

C. Rh immune globulin and rubella vaccines should be administered when indicated for the safety of future pregnancies. Live vaccines should not be given to immunocompromised women.

D. Contraception allows women to recuperate physiologically from pregnancy, adjust to the demands imposed by the new infant, and exercise some control over the timing of any future pregnancy.

BIBLIOGRAPHY

Centers for Disease Control: *Abortion Surveillance, 1970–1980*. May 1983

Centers for Disease Control: *Ectopic Pregnancy Surveillance, 1970–1978*. July 1982

Cherry SH, Berkowitz RL, Kase NG (eds): *Rovinsky and Guttmacher's Medical, Surgical, and Gynecologic Complications of Pregnancy*, 3rd ed. Baltimore, Williams and Wilkins, 1985

Hatcher RA, Guest F, Stewart F, et al: *Contraceptive Technology 1986–1987*, 13th ed. New York, Irvington, 1986

Hern WM: *Abortion Practice*. Philadelphia, Lippincott, 1984

Hodgson JE: *Abortion and Sterilization: Medical and Social Aspects*. New York, Grune and Stratton, 1981

Last JM: *A Dictionary of Epidemiology*. New York, Oxford University Press, 1983

Ory HW, Forrest JD, Lincoln R: *Making Choices: Evaluating the Health Risks and Benefits of Birth Control Methods*. New York, Allan Guttmacher Institute, 1983

Pritchard JA, MacDonald PC: *Williams Obstetrics*, 16th ed. New York, Appleton-Century-Crofts, 1980

STUDY QUESTIONS

Directions: Each question below contains four suggested answers of which **one or more** is correct. Choose the answer

A if **1, 2, and 3** are correct
B if **1 and 3** are correct
C if **2 and 4** are correct
D if **4** is correct
E if **1, 2, 3, and 4** are correct

1. Contraceptives not currently available (1986) in the United States include

(1) triphasic birth control pills
(2) hormonal IUDs
(3) cervicothermal analyses
(4) implantation methods

Directions: The group of questions below consists of lettered choices followed by several numbered items. For each numbered item, select the one lettered choice with which it is most closely associated. Each lettered choice may be used once, more than once, or not at all. Choose the answer

A if the item is associated with **(A) only**
B if the item is associated with **(B) only**
C if the item is associated with **both (A) and (B)**
D if the item is associated with **neither (A) nor (B)**

Questions 2–4

For each case history listed below, select the classification that it most closely represents.

(A) Direct maternal mortality
(B) Perinatal mortality
(C) Both
(D) Neither

2. A woman with a ruptured ectopic pregnancy at 18 weeks gestation hemorrhaged internally and went into shock. She eventually died.

3. A woman with congenital heart disease and labile diabetes had a stillbirth 5 days after her due date. During labor, she developed ketoacidosis and cardiac arrest, which precipitated her death.

4. A woman died of septic shock 4 days after an unsuccessful self-induced abortion attempt at 30 weeks gestation. A male infant was born alive but died 2 days later in a neonatal intensive care unit.

Directions: The group of questions below consists of lettered choices followed by several numbered items. For each numbered item select the **one** lettered choice with which it is **most** closely associated. Each lettered choice may be used once, more than once, or not at all.

Questions 5–8

For each description that follows, select the method of contraception that it best describes.

(A) Estrogen-progestin pills
(B) IUDs
(C) Injectables
(D) Barriers
(E) Lactation

5. Risks are increased for older women and smokers.

6. Septic abortion, pelvic inflammatory disease, ectopic pregnancy, and infertility may be sequelae.

7. A variety of sexually transmitted conditions may be prevented with its use.

8. It carries a very slight increased risk of toxic shock syndrome.

ANSWERS AND EXPLANATIONS

1. The answer is D (4). (*III A 2, 6–8*) Various intrauterine devices (IUDs)—inert, copper, and hormonal—have been available in this country until recently. However, because of the risks of pelvic inflammatory disease, ectopic pregnancy, and infertility among IUD users, some IUDs are being withdrawn from the market. A hormonal IUD is still being marketed (1986); others are approved for use but may be difficult to obtain. Injectables and implants, while used overseas, are not currently approved for use in this country. Birth control pills, both fixed combinations and phasics, are readily available in the United States. Natural family planning involves analysis of the cervical mucus and daily temperature, which is available to anyone.

2–4. The answers are: 2-A, 3-B, 4-C. (*I A 1, 2, C 1–3*) The death of the woman with a ruptured ectopic pregnancy at 18 weeks gestation is classified as direct maternal mortality. Her death was a direct result of the complications of an ectopic implantation; it did not result from a preexisting illness. Although the ectopic pregnancy itself may be categorized as a spontaneous abortion, the question refers to the death of the woman and not the product of conception.

The death of the woman who delivered a stillborn child is classifed as indirect maternal mortality. Her death resulted from preexisting conditions—heart disease and diabetes—that were aggravated by the pregnancy. Although optimal medical and obstetric management may have altered both maternal and fetal outcome, the major factors contributing to her death preceded the pregnancy. The stillborn child is classified as perinatal mortality—that is, death of a fetus or infant between 28 weeks gestation and 1 week postnatal with a fetal weight $\geq$ 500 g.

The death of the woman who died of septic shock is classified as direct maternal mortality. There is no evidence of illness preceding the pregnancy, and her death seems to be the result of the self-induced abortion. The death of the infant can be classified as a neonatal mortality—that is, death of a live-born infant within 28 days of age—or perinatal mortality.

5–8. The answers are: 5-A, 6-B, 7-D, 8-D. (*III A 5–8*) Although birth control pills are highly effective, they carry significant risks of cardiovascular and embolic diseases for older women, especially those who also smoke. They are also thought to be protective against certain conditions such as anemia, dysmenorrhea, ovarian cysts, and endometrial cancer.

The Dalkon Shield is the intrauterine device (IUD) that has been implicated the most as the cause of septic abortion. The association of ectopic pregnancies with IUDs has been attributed, in part, to the method's prevention of intrauterine pregnancy. IUDs are associated with an increased risk of pelvic inflammatory disease, which, along with ectopic pregnancy, may contribute to infertility.

Barrier methods of contraception may prevent the transmission of a variety of sexually transmitted infections. Although protection is not absolute for every infection and every individual episode, the results are significant when large numbers of cases are reviewed. There is a slight increased risk of toxic shock syndrome from the barrier methods (e.g., sponge, cap, and diaphragm), especially during the menses.

7
Health Care of the Young

Marie C. McCormick
Florence B. Schwartz

I. HEALTH OF THE NEWBORN

A. Mortality rates. Several different rates are used to indicate health problems in infancy.

1. **Definition of terms**
   a. **Infant mortality rate (IMR)** is defined as the number of deaths among infants less than 1 year of age per 1000 live births in a given time period, usually 1 year. The IMR traditionally is divided into two segments: the **neonatal mortality rate (NMR)** and the **postneonatal mortality rate (PNMR)**.
      (1) The NMR is calculated as the number of deaths among infants less than 28 days old per 1000 live births.
      (2) The PNMR is calculated as the number of deaths among infants aged 28 days to 11 months per 1000 live births.
   b. **Fetal mortality rate (FMR)** refers to fetal loss in the third trimester of pregnancy, which results in a stillbirth. This rate is defined as the number of stillbirths per 1000 births of gestational age greater than 28 weeks. The gestational age cutoff is meant to indicate that the fetuses are potentially viable. Some fetuses of lower gestational ages currently are surviving; a 20-week cutoff sometimes is used in calculating the FMR.
   c. **Perinatal mortality rate.** Since it may be difficult to determine what constitutes viability, especially in very tiny infants, the perinatal mortality rate is used to indicate infant loss around the time of the birth event. This rate is calculated as the number of deaths of fetuses of gestational age greater than 28 weeks (sometimes 20 weeks) plus the number of deaths of infants less than 7 days old per 1000 total births.

2. **Use of terms.** These mortality rates and the changes in them can be used to assess the type and volume of health problems in infancy because the causes of infant death also result in morbidity among surviving infants.
   a. **Neonatal mortality and perinatal mortality generally reflect causes of death related to maternal health** prior to pregnancy as well as events during pregnancy, delivery, and the early neonatal period. These could include congenital anomalies, asphyxia, birth trauma, and immaturity.
   b. **Postneonatal mortality is more closely linked to environmental factors**, especially socioeconomic disadvantage. The major causes are infection especially respiratory and gastrointestinal, sudden infant death syndrome, injury, and congenital anomalies.

B. Current trends

1. In 1981, the IMR in the United States was 11.9 deaths per 1000 live births, which is a high figure for a developed country. The United States ranks eighteenth among developed countries in infant mortality.
   a. Mortality in infants is higher than that in any group of individuals under the age of 55 and accounts for the majority of deaths among individuals less than 18 years old.
   b. The 1981 IMR represents a major decline in infant mortality since the turn of the century, when the IMR was about 100 in 1000 live births. The decrease has resulted from decreases in both neonatal and postneonatal mortality.
      (1) Most of the decline in the PNMR occurred prior to 1950.
         (a) This decrease is attributed largely to changes in the environment, including improved sanitation and nutrition.
         (b) Little of this change is thought to have resulted from changes in medical care, including the introduction of immunization and antibiotics.
      (2) Although the NMR also decreased early in the twentieth century, a dramatic change has been seen over the past 20 years, when the NMR has been halved.

(a) In contrast to the decrease in PNMR, much of the decrease in the NMR is attributed to medical techniques aimed at increasing the survival of high-risk infants.
(b) Despite this decrease, deaths in the neonatal period account for two-thirds of infant deaths.

2. Trends in infant, neonatal, and postneonatal mortality are summarized in Figure 7-1.

C. Causes of neonatal mortality

1. **The major cause of neonatal mortality reflects failure of intrauterine growth.** This failure can occur in two ways: the infant may be born too soon (**prematurity**), or the infant may not gain weight appropriate to the duration of gestation (**intrauterine growth retardation**).
   a. Prematurity is defined as a gestation of less than 37 weeks since the last menstrual period.
   b. Because gestational age sometimes is difficult to define, birth weight is used to designate the high-risk infant. A birth weight of 2500 g (5.5 lb) or less is believed to increase the risk of neonatal mortality, even if the infant is full-term or of gestational age of 37 weeks or greater.
      (1) Infants with a birth weight of 2500 g or less account for 6%–7% of births but more than 66% of neonatal deaths.
      (2) As birth weight decreases, the NMR increases sharply, such that one-third to one-half of infants with a birth weight of 1500 g or less die in the neonatal period.

2. **Other major causes of neonatal mortality are congenital anomalies and birth injury.** While low-birth-weight infants also may die from these causes, congenital anomalies and birth injury are the primary reasons for death among full-term and normal-birth-weight infants.
   a. **Birth injury and asphyxia** have declined as causes of death in the past 15 years. This is particularly true for infants weighing 4.0 kg or more at birth.
   b. In contrast, the NMR due to **congenital anomalies** has remained relatively constant. While prenatal screening may detect some types of anomalies and genetic disorders, two-thirds of these conditions cannot be anticipated or prevented with current techniques.

D. Causes of postneonatal mortality. The effect of **congenital anomalies** is also reflected in postneonatal deaths, of which about 2 in 1000 can be attributed to congenital anomalies. PNMRs above this level are considered to be directly related to **socioeconomic disadvantage** and **lack of access to medical care**.

1. **The major causes of postneonatal death are lower respiratory tract infection** (e.g., bronchitis and pneumonia) **and gastrointestinal and diarrheal disease.** Most cases are manageable with current medical techniques, and many are preventable with good nutrition and hygiene.

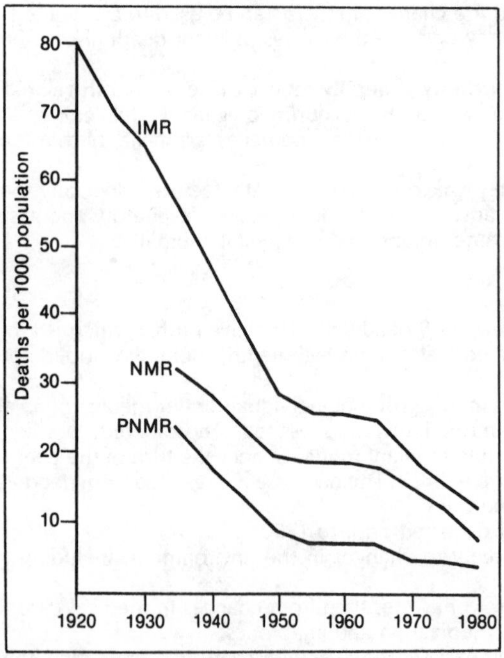

Figure 7-1. Infant mortality rate (*IMR*), neonatal mortality rate (*NMR*), and postneonatal mortality rate (*PNMR*) per 1000 population in the United States between 1920 and 1980.

2. **Sudden infant death syndrome (SIDS) also is a major cause of mortality** and may include a heterogeneous set of conditions. While some of these deaths are not preventable, the link of SIDS to poor environments and the reduction of SIDS-related deaths with services to disadvantaged mothers suggest that some are preventable.

3. **A third cause of postneonatal death is injury.** In particular, infants are at much greater risk of dying in motor vehicle accidents than older children and adults because of their relatively large heads.

E. **Risk factors associated with infant mortality and morbidity** can be divided into those reflecting socioeconomic disadvantage and those reflecting biologic vulnerability of the mother.

1. **Socioeconomic disadvantage** can increase infant mortality in two ways: by increasing the risk of low birth weight and by increasing the risk of postneonatal death regardless of birth weight (e.g., due to infectious causes). The effects of **socioeconomic disadvantage** are believed to account for the increased risk of mortality among black infants, infants born to teenage mothers, and infants born to mothers of low educational attainment.

2. **Biologic vulnerabilities** are reflected primarily in neonatal loss, with an increased risk of low birth weight as well as neonatal mortality regardless of birth weight (e.g., due to conditions secondary to immaturity and congenital anomalies). Biologic vulnerabilities may account for the increased risk of mortality among infants born to mothers aged 35 years and older and mothers with previous obstetric problems.

F. **Management and prevention of infant health problems**

1. **Identification of high-risk parents**
   a. **Maternal age**
      (1) Mothers younger than 18 have an increased risk of delivering a low-birth-weight infant.
      (2) Mothers older than 34 in the past presented an increased risk of delivering low-birth-weight infants but currently account for an insignificant percentage of such births.
   b. **Intrauterine infections.** Several organisms can produce congenital anomalies as well as increase the risk of low-birth-weight infants.
      (1) Two of these infections—rubella and syphilis—are preventable.
      (2) Other infections (e.g., toxoplasmosis, herpes, and cytomegalovirus) can be detected by routine antibody screening of pregnant women.
   c. **Preexisting maternal illnesses.** Such conditions include heart, kidney, and thyroid disease; diabetes mellitus; hypertension; and substance abuse. Early detection and aggressive management of maternal illnesses can reduce the toll of infant loss.
   d. **Maternal history of reproductive problems.** Women who have experienced adverse conditions during prior pregnancies (e.g., premature labor, vaginal bleeding, hypertension, miscarriage, and delivery of a low-birth-weight or stillborn infant) have an increased risk of adverse outcomes in subsequent pregnancies.
   e. **Family history of hereditary disease.** The presence of such a disease may suggest the need for screening and special management.

2. **Prevention of unwanted pregnancies among high-risk parents** may involve genetic counseling, sex education, and family planning.

3. **Management of high-risk pregnancies** includes:
   a. Early antenatal care (within the first trimester).
   b. Regular screening and monitoring throughout pregnancy.
   c. Provision of medical, nutritional, and social services appropriate to the level of risk.
   d. Delivery in a hospital equipped to manage potential problems related to obstetric risk factors.
   e. Monitoring and treatment of the newborn for problems related to obstetric risk factors.

4. **Management of high-risk newborns** includes:
   a. Immediate access to an intensive care nursery.
   b. Continued medical, social, and nutritional monitoring following discharge from the intensive care nursery.

II. HEALTH OF PRESCHOOLERS AND SCHOOLCHILDREN

A. **Mortality**

1. **Mortality rates**
   a. Mortality rates for children aged 1–14 years continue to decline.

(1) Rates have declined from 870 per 100,000 children in 1900 to about 40 per 100,000 currently.
(2) The declining mortality rates are attributed to improvements in sanitation, nutrition, and housing and to the availability of immunization and antibiotics.

b. Despite the declining trend, childhood mortality remains a cause for concern.
(1) Mortality among black children is twice that among white children.
(2) Mortality rates for children in the United States are higher than those for children in other Western nations.
(3) Over the past 10 years, childhood mortality rates have decreased very little.

2. Causes of mortality include:
a. Injuries (e.g., accidents and homicide), which account for 50% of all deaths.
b. Congenital anomalies.
c. Malignant diseases.
d. Infectious conditions (e.g., influenza and pneumonia).
e. Gastroenteritis.

B. Morbidity

1. Morbidity rates
a. Morbidity rates are higher among children than adults. Children average 10 days of restricted activity and 5 days in bed per year, whereas adults 17–64 years of age average 9 days of restricted activity and 3–4 days in bed.
b. Morbidity rates generally are higher among children less than 6 years old and among those in lower income families. Acute conditions that are more common among poor individuals include *Haemophilus influenzae* meningitis, gastroenteritis, and parasitic disease.

2. Acute physical conditions. Most acute conditions in children are attributable to three types of problems.
a. Respiratory illnesses
b. Infections and parasitic conditions
c. Injuries

3. Chronic physical conditions. Although most childhood illnesses are self-limited, serious chronic illnesses affect 5%–10% of children.
a. Congenital anomalies are the most frequently reported conditions among infants. Asthma is the most common chronic illness among older children, affecting 5% of schoolchildren.
b. The current prevalence of serious chronic illness in children is directly related to the successful management of medical problems that previously resulted in early death.

4. "The new morbidity." There is recent concern for conditions that impede a child's achieving his or her full developmental potential. These conditions, referred to as "the new morbidity," include behavior disorders, emotional problems, and specific learning disorders. Up to 15%–20% of children may experience one or more of these conditions.

C. Management and prevention of childhood mortality and morbidity

1. Immunization. Routine immunization of children has been shown repeatedly to be one of the most cost-effective means of preventing mortality and morbidity.
a. Recommended immunization schedules are detailed in Tables 7-1 and 7-2.
b. Immunization services require further attention as those individuals most vulnerable to morbidity are least likely to be protected.

2. Screening for occult treatable conditions
a. Criteria for screening
(1) The condition must represent an important health problem and have a recognizable latent or early symptomatic stage.
(2) Suitable screening tests and accepted treatment for the condition must exist, and diagnostic and treatment facilities must be available.
(3) The natural history of the condition should be understood.
(4) Case finding should be a continuing process, the cost of which should be balanced against the potential expenditures for treatment of symptomatic disease.
(5) There must be a policy dictating who should be treated.

b. Conditions for which screening has proven cost-effective are listed below, with the appropriate timing of the screening noted in parentheses.
(1) Phenylketonuria (in the neonatal period)
(2) Congenital hypothyroidism (in the neonatal period)
(3) Iron deficiency anemia (at 9 months old in high-risk populations)

Table 7-1. Recommended Schedule for Active Immunization of Normal Infants and Children

Recommended Age	Immunization(s)	Comments
2 months	DTP and OPV	Can be initiated as early as 2 weeks of age in areas of high endemicity or during epidemics
4 months	DTP and OPV	2-month interval desired for OPV to avoid interference from previous dose
6 months	DTP (OPV)	OPV is optional (may be given in areas with increased risk of poliovirus exposure)
15 months	MMR	MMR preferred to individual vaccines; tuberculin testing may be done
18 months	DTD* and OPV†	
24 months	Hib	
4–6 years‡	DTP and OPV	At or before school entry
14–16 years	Td	Repeat every 10 years throughout life

Note.—DTP = diphtheria and tetanus toxoids with pertussis vaccine; OPV = oral poliovirus vaccine, containing attenuated poliovirus types 1, 2, and 3; MMR = live measles, mumps, and rubella viruses in a combined vaccine; Hib = *Hemophilus influenzae* type b polysaccharide vaccine; Td = adult tetanus toxoid (full dose) and diphtheria toxoid (reduced dose) in combination. [Reprinted with permission from *Redbook (1986): Report of the Committee on Infectious Diseases*, 20th ed. Elk Grove Village, IL, American Academy of Pediatrics, 1986, p. 9.]

*Should be given 6–12 months after the third dose.

†May be given simultaneously with MMR at 15 months of age.

‡Up to seventh birthday.

Table 7-2. Recommended Immunization Schedules for Children Not Immunized in the First Year of Life

Recommended Time	Immunization(s)	Comments
	Less than 7 Years Old	
First visit	DTP, OPV, MMR	MMR is given if child is ≥ 15 months old; tuberculin testing may be done
Interval after first visit		
1 month	Hib	For children 2–5 years
2 months	DTP and OPV	
4 months	DTP (OPV)	OPV is optional (may be given in areas with increased risk of poliovirus exposure)
10–16 months	DTP and OPV	OPV is not given if third dose was given earlier
4–6 years	DTP and OPV	DTP is not necessary if the fourth dose was given after the fourth birthday; OPV is not necessary if recommended OPV dose 10–16 months following first visit was given after the fourth birthday.
14–16 years	Td	Repeat every 10 years throughout life
	7 Years Old and Older	
First visit	Td, OPV, MMR	
Interval after first visit		
2 months	Td, OPV	
8–14 months	Td, OPV	
14–16 years	Td	Repeat every 10 years throughout life

Note.—DTP = diphtheria and tetanus toxoids with pertussis vaccine; OPV = oral poliovirus vaccine, containing attenuated poliovirus types 1, 2, and 3; MMR = live measles, mumps, and rubella viruses in a combined vaccine; Hib = *Hemophilus influenzae* type b polysaccharide vaccine; Td = adult tetanus toxoid (full dose) and diphtheria toxoid (reduced dose) in combination. Hib can be given, if necessary, simultaneously with DTP (at separate sites). The initial three doses of DTP can be given at 1- to 2-month intervals; for the child in whom immunization is initiated at age 24 months or older one visit could be eliminated by giving DTP, OPV, and MMR at the first visit; DTP and Hib at the second visit (1 month later); and DTP and OPV at the third visit (2 months after the first visit). Subsequent DTP and OPV given at 10–16 months after the first visit are still indicated. [Reprinted with permission from *Redbook (1986): Report of the Committee on Infectious Diseases*, 20th ed. Elk Grove Village IL, American Academy of Pediatrics, 1986, p. 11.]

(4) Lead poisoning (in preschoolers in areas where the positive yield is greater than 6% of those screened)
(5) Tuberculosis (regularly during childhood in high-risk populations)
(6) Vision impairment (in children 3–4 years of age)

c. Additional screening procedures that should be considered include:
(1) Assessment of physical growth and developmental status.
(2) Measurement of blood pressure (in children 3 years of age and older).
(3) Hearing assessment.
(4) Identification of sickle cell disease (in the neonatal period).

3. Prevention of specific health problems

a. Injuries are the major cause of death in this age-group. Two major approaches to prevention have been identified.
(1) Modification of hazards to reduce their potential to cause injury, such as:
(a) Use of products with child-proof caps.
(b) Lowering the temperature of hot water heaters.
(c) Installation of window guards.
(2) Modification of behavior to reduce exposure to hazards, including the use of:
(a) Motorcycle helmets.
(b) Infant car seats.

b. Psychosocial problems are more prevalent among children from socioeconomically disadvantaged families. Early intervention may prevent these problems in targeted groups of children.
(1) The **high-risk groups** include:
(a) Children with an increased risk of morbidity and mortality by virtue of the circumstances of their birth.
(b) Disadvantaged children whose development is hampered by lack of environmental stimulation.
(c) Children with established problems known to result in severe developmental delay.
(2) Preventive strategies include:
(a) Screening and monitoring to detect the emergence of problems, which generally can be conducted as part of well-child care for immunizations and annual checkups using such instruments as the Denver Developmental Screening Test.
(b) Provision of preventive or remedial educational and psychotherapeutic services.

c. Dental caries remain a source of morbidity. Preventive techniques include:
(1) Reduction of sugar in food, drink, and medicines.
(2) Community fluoridation.
(3) Topical fluoride applications.

III. HEALTH OF THE ADOLESCENT

A. Adolescence is the period of life between puberty and full maturity, which is roughly from 12 to 17 years of age. This period is characterized by rapid growth and change in anatomy and physiology as well as shifting values and allegiances. Approximately 11% of the population of the United States falls within this age-group.

B. General health status of adolescents

1. Using traditional morbidity and mortality measures, the health status of the adolescent in the United States is good. Most adolescents fall within a health category bounded by the categories of acute illnesses of childhood and the chronic conditions of later life.

2. Although mortality rates are relatively low (i.e., 35.1 per 100,000 adolescents 10–14 years of age and 101.6 per 100,000 adolescents 15–19 years of age), they may be increasing—the only age-group for which this is true.

C. Causes of adolescent mortality

1. Injuries represent the leading cause of death among adolescents; 36% of adolescent deaths are motor-vehicle related.

2. Other traumatic causes of death include homicide, suicide, and drowning.

3. Cancer is the only major cause of adolescent death that is not related to injury.

4. Use of alcohol and drugs and emotional problems account for a substantial portion of adolescent deaths.

D. Morbidity

1. Physical and mental problems

a. One of five adolescents has some form of **chronic illness, deformity,** or **physical handicap.**

b. Dental problems affect two-thirds of the adolescent population, and vision problems affect one-third.

c. Skin pathology affects more than one-third of the adolescent population.

d. Mental health problems are the fourth leading reason for short-term hospitalization, accounting for 11% of all adolescent hospital stays.

2. Behavior-related problems

a. Alcohol use is increasing among adolescents, with over 90% of the population reporting some alcohol use.

b. Cigarette smoking is reported by more than 10% of the population. Teenage females smoke more than their male counterparts.

c. Drug abuse, including the use of marijuana, inhalants, hallucinogens, and cocaine, is increasing among this population.

d. Pregnancy and sexually transmitted diseases become important concerns as the teenager becomes familiar with his or her sexuality. By age 19, 55.5% of the adolescent population has had sexual intercourse, which leads the way for the serious problem of adolescent pregnancy.

(1) There is a higher incidence of infant mortality among infants born to adolescent mothers.

(2) Adolescent mothers usually are unprepared psychologically, economically, and educationally for parenthood.

(3) Adolescent parents are at increased risk for failure to complete their education and to find employment, thereby limiting their future economic well-being.

E. Management and prevention of adolescent health problems

1. Sex-related problems

a. By providing sex education, the use of contraceptives by adolescents increases and the risk of unwanted pregnancy probably decreases. The same is true for the provision of free contraceptive services.

b. Intensive management of adolescent pregnancies may reduce the increased risk of low-birth-weight infants and, with follow-up, the increased risk of postneonatal death.

2. Smoking and substance abuse

a. Educational campaigns meet with limited success, but intensive school-based efforts may limit cigarette smoking among adolescents.

b. Potentional methods for prevention of substance abuse include:

(1) Enforcement of drinking age laws.

(2) Parental monitoring.

3. Injuries

a. Regulatory activities have proven more effective than educational campaigns. Such activities include the establishment of:

(1) Drinking age laws.

(2) Motorcycle helmet laws.

(3) Requirements for protective gear at athletic events.

(4) Regulations concerning access to firearms.

b. Management of injuries is an essential component of an adolescent health program, which should also include prompt access to emergency services and careful assessment of psychological status.

IV. ORGANIZATION AND FINANCING OF CHILDREN'S HEALTH SERVICES

A. Health care providers

1. Pediatricians

a. Visits to pediatricians account for only 35% of physician visits by children who are 19 years of age or younger. Remaining visits are primarily to family and general practitioners.

b. Visits to pediatricians account for the majority of physician visits by children who are less than 10 years of age and by children in urban areas.

2. Specialists. Children with chronic problems (e.g., diabetes, seizure disorders, and arthritis) may have to rely on **adult specialists** because pediatric specialists are not available.

3. **Nurse practitioners** and **child health associates** may constitute the major health care providers in certain settings, such as:
   a. Schools.
   b. Jails.
   c. Specific populations, such as disadvantaged high-risk groups.

4. **Dentists and dental hygienists** are widely available to children of middle-class families but, because of cost barriers, are less frequently visited by children of low-income families.

B. Sources of care

1. Most (65%) children receive their care from private practitioners in office-based practices.

2. Other sources of care include emergency rooms and outpatient departments (12%), school health services (13%), public health clinics (5%), special government programs (3%), and special volunteer agencies (2%).

3. Minority and disadvantaged children are more likely to rely on hospital and public health clinics. Children relying on hospital clinics have more health problems.

C. Financing care

1. Even with insurance, the payment for most child health care is provided out of pocket by the parents.
   a. Over 80% of children of families with annual incomes exceeding $5000 have some type of private health insurance.
   b. Most children's health services occur in the ambulatory setting and are not covered by insurance.
   c. Few insurance packages cover catastrophic illness (e.g., neonatal intensive care and treatment of cancer).

2. Several mechanisms for health care financing are available to disadvantaged children and children with special health problems.
   a. **Federal services**
      (1) **Medicaid**, which is both state and federally funded, pays for the health care of adults (and their children) who are on welfare (**Aid to Dependent Children**).
      (2) **Social Security Act**
         (a) **Title V** of this act provides services for maternal and child health, crippled children's services, child welfare, and aid to dependent children.
         (b) **Title XX** provides payment for social services related to child neglect and abuse.
      (3) Other child services financed through the federal government include:
         (a) Special Supplemental Food Program for Women, Infants, and Children (WIC).
         (b) PL–142, which provides for the education of all handicapped children.
         (c) Centers for Disease Control programs (e.g., immunization services and screening for lead poisoning).
         (d) Office of Adolescent Pregnancy Program.
         (e) Sudden Infant Death Program.
   b. **State and local services.** State and local governments also have major funding responsibilities, including matching funds for federal programs as well as direct funding of health services. For example, routine pregnancy and well-child care and screening and therapy for lead poisoning and tuberculosis are provided by city and county health departments.

STUDY QUESTIONS

Directions: Each question below contains five suggested answers. Choose the **one best** response to each question.

1. All of the following statements concerning the infant mortality rate (IMR) in the United States are true EXCEPT

(A) the IMR in the United States is considered high for a developed country
(B) the United States ranks about eighteenth among developed countries in infant mortality
(C) the decline in the IMR over the past century has resulted from decreases in only the neonatal mortality rates
(D) the IMR accounts for the majority of deaths among individuals less than 18 years of age
(E) the decline in the IMR is closely linked to both advances in medical care and changes in the environment

2. Postneonatal mortality has been most closely linked to

(A) maternal health prior to pregnancy
(B) events during delivery
(C) environmental factors
(D) maternal health during pregnancy
(E) events during the early neonatal period

3. The leading cause of death among schoolchildren is

(A) congenital anomalies
(B) injuries
(C) malignant diseases
(D) communicable diseases
(E) respiratory illnesses

4. All of the following are criteria for screening EXCEPT

(A) the natural history of the condition should be understood
(B) the condition must represent an important health problem
(C) suitable screening tests for the condition must exist
(D) screening should be available to and used by the entire population
(E) accepted treatment for the condition must be available

5. Screening has been proven cost-effective for all of the following conditions EXCEPT

(A) tuberculosis
(B) iron deficiency anemia
(C) hypertension
(D) vision impairment
(E) phenylketonuria

6. What percentage of the adolescent population reports some alcohol use?

(A) Less than 50%
(B) 60%
(C) 75%
(D) 80%
(E) More than 90%

7. Most physician visits by children 19 years of age or younger are to

(A) pediatricians
(B) family and general practitioners
(C) subspecialty physicians
(D) internists
(E) emergency room physicians

Directions: Each question below contains four suggested answers of which **one or more** is correct. Choose the answer

A if **1, 2, and 3** are correct
B if **1 and 3** are correct
C if **2 and 4** are correct
D if **4** is correct
E if **1, 2, 3, and 4** are correct

8. Measures taken in the management and prevention of infant health problems include

(1) managing high-risk pregnancies
(2) managing high-risk newborns
(3) preventing unwanted pregnancies among high-risk parents
(4) providing neonatal intensive care units at all hospitals offering obstetric services

9. Mortality rates in the United States are increasing for

(1) infants
(2) preschoolers
(3) schoolchildren
(4) adolescents

10. The recommended immunization schedule for children includes vaccination against

(1) polio
(2) pertussis
(3) tetanus
(4) smallpox

ANSWERS AND EXPLANATIONS

1. The answer is C. (*I B 1 a–b*) The infant mortality rate (IMR) is based on both neonatal and postneonatal mortality. Thus, the decline in the infant mortality rate has resulted from decreases in both neonatal and postneonatal mortality. Most of the decline in postneonatal mortality occurred prior to 1950. The more dramatic change in neonatal mortality rates has occurred over the last 20 years. Despite this decrease, the United States has a high IMR for a developed country, ranking about eighteenth.

2. The answer is C. (*I A 2 b; I E*) Postneonatal mortality has been closely linked to environmental factors, especially economic disadvantage. Maternal health prior to pregnancy as well as events during pregnancy, delivery, and the early neonatal period are more closely linked to neonatal and perinatal mortality.

3. The answer is B. (*II A 2*) Injuries are the major cause of death among schoolchildren, accounting for 50% of all deaths. Other causes of death in this age-group include congenital anomalies, malignant diseases, infectious conditions (e.g., influenza and pneumonia), and gastroenteritis. Two approaches to prevention of injury-related childhood mortality have been identified: modification of hazards to reduce their potential to cause injury (e.g., use of products with child-proof caps) and modification of behavior to reduce exposure to hazards (e.g., use of infant car seats).

4. The answer is D. (*II C 2 a*) Screening procedures have been found to be most effective when there are policies dictating who should be treated. In general, all screening tests may not be warranted or cost-effective for the entire population. Screening should be used only when: the natural history of the condition is understood, the condition represents an important health problem, suitable screening tests exist, and an accepted treatment for the condition is available.

5. The answer is C. (*II C 2 b, c*) Targeted screening among children has been proven cost-effective for tuberculosis, iron deficiency anemia, vision impairment, and phenylketonuria. Although screening for hypertension (i.e., blood pressure measurement in children 3 years of age and older) should be considered, this technique may not be cost-effective because the natural history of hypertension in this age-group is not well understood and blood pressure measurement is difficult.

6. The answer is E. (*III D 2 a*) Alcohol use is increasing among adolescents. More than 90% of the high school students report some alcohol use; about 73% of these students report use within the last month. In contrast, use of marijuana and tobacco among high school students is decreasing.

7. The answer is B. (*IV A 1 a–b*) Most physician visits by children 19 years of age or younger are to family and general practitioners. Visits to pediatricians account for only 35% of physician visits by children in this age-group. However, visits to pediatricians account for the majority of physician visits by children who are younger than 10 and by children in urban areas.

8. The answer is A (1, 2, 3). (*I F*) It is not necessary to have neonatal intensive care units at all hospitals offering obstetric services. Rather, these services should be effectively regionalized, guaranteeing accessibility to those in need of the services. Management of high-risk pregnancies, identification of high-risk parents, management of high-risk newborns, and prevention of unwanted pregnancies all contribute to the management and prevention of infant health problems.

9. The answer is D (4). (*I B 1 a–b; II A 1 a–b; III B 2*) Although mortality rates for adolescents are relatively low, they are increasing. This is the only age-group in the United States exhibiting increasing mortality rates. Conversely, the mortality rates for infants in this country is quite high but is decreasing. Mortality among infants is higher than that among any other group of individuals under the age of 55 years. Mortality rates for children 1–14 years of age continue to decline in the United States but remain a cause for concern. Childhood mortality rates in this country are higher than those in other Western nations and, over the last 10 years, have decreased very little.

10. The answer is A (1, 2, 3). (*II C 1 a; Table 7-1*) Polio, diphtheria, pertussis, tetanus, measles, mumps, *Hemophilus*, and rubella vaccines all are recommended, and a schedule for their administration is well established. Smallpox vaccine is no longer recommended for the general population. Routine immunization of children has been shown repeatedly to be one of the most cost-effective means of preventing childhood mortality and morbidity.

8 Injuries

Lawrence D. Budnick

I. INTRODUCTION

A. Definition

1. The term injury is derived from the Latin term *in juris* meaning "not right."
2. An injury is the physical damage to a person that occurs as a result of exposure to physical or chemical agents at rates greater than the body can tolerate. An injury is generally considered to occur acutely after exposure.
3. Injuries are often considered separately from diseases, although they are part of the spectrum of diseases. The difference between an injury and a disease may be only one of the dose of the causal factor, the time course during which the causal factor operates, or the body's adaptation and response to the causal factor.
   - **a.** Injuries and diseases are often caused by the same factors, although the amount or the rate of exposure may differ; for example:
     - **(1)** Radiation can cause a burn (injury) and cancer (disease).
     - **(2)** Carbon monoxide can cause brain damage and encephalopathy (injury) and secondary polycythemia (disease).
     - **(3)** Kinetic energy can cause a fracture (injury) and arthritis (disease).
   - **b.** Although the symptoms of an injury are usually immediately obvious as compared to the symptoms of disease, the duration of latency periods for injuries and diseases overlap; for example:
     - **(1)** Whiplash, an acceleration extension injury of the cervical spine, may not cause symptoms until days after the injury occurred.
     - **(2)** Lead poisoning damage may not be evident until long after the exposure, but once evident, may progress rapidly.
     - **(3)** Foodborne *Bacillus cereus* disease has an incubation period as short as 1 hour.
     - **(4)** Altitude decompression sickness, or caisson disease, which is due to nitrogen bubbles forming in the blood and tissues, occurs immediately after a too rapid decompression from a high pressure environment.

B. Accidents

1. Injuries, especially unintentional injuries (see section IV A 2) have often been referred to as "accidents." The term "accident," however, inappropriately implies chance misfortune and lack of predictability, which inaccurately describe the epidemiology of injuries (see section II A).
2. Although the term "accident" is imprecise and unscientific, it continues to be used in some classification and surveillance systems (see Tables 8-1 and 8-2); for example:
   - **a.** The United States National Center for Health Statistics classifies unintentional injuries as "accidents and adverse effects."
   - **b.** Statistics Canada classifies all injuries as "accidents, poisonings, and violence."
3. The convention of describing the injury and the injury-causing event should be followed rather than using the term "accident."

II. EPIDEMIOLOGIC CONSTRUCTS

A. Basic concepts

1. An injury is a problem of medical ecology—that is, it is a problem in the relationship between one or more individuals and the surrounding environment, related to time.

2. As with infectious and chronic diseases, an epidemiologic web consisting of factors relating to the host or individual, the physical and social environments, the agent, and the vector can be delineated for injuries (see Chapter 1, section III A).

B. Host

1. The host, or the **individual affected**, has been the principal focus of research related to injuries and preventive measures aimed at decreasing injury rates.

2. An injury may result when the demands of a task being performed exceed an individual's performance capacity, which varies with the individual's physical, psychological, and cognitive abilities.

3. Host factors that affect the risk of injuries differ according to the type of injury, as do some risk indicators.*
   a. **Age.** Young children and the elderly have less control over their environments, and young adults often take great risks, particularly in situations with which they are inexperienced.
   b. **Sex.** Males appear to be more prone to violent behavior than females.
   c. **Race.** Blacks have a decreased risk of suicide and an increased risk of homicide, which is the leading cause of death for adolescent and young adult blacks. Native Americans have an increased risk of all injuries.
   d. **Alcohol and other drug use.** The use of alcohol and other drugs increases the risk of injuries. About one-half of all drivers who die in motor vehicle crashes have blood alcohol concentrations above the legal limit.
   e. **Chronic medical conditions.** Some chronic medical conditions, such as poor vision and uncontrolled epilepsy, increase the risk of injuries.
   f. **Physiologic status.** Osteoporosis, which is often related to endocrine status, increases the risk of fall-related injuries.

C. Environment

1. **The physical environment** is the location at which the injury occurs. Examples of alterations made in the physical environment that can increase or reduce the risk of injuries follow.
   a. Road design can decrease or increase the risk of injuries. A road barrier can assist an automobile to come to a safe stop or can become a hazard by functioning as a spear and piercing an occupant of an automobile.
   b. Homes can be built or equipped with safety features, such as smoke detectors and automatic sprinkler systems, in which cases they are less likely to result in fire and flame-related injuries than are homes without such devices.
   c. Swimming pools with fences are safer than pools without fences.

2. **The social environment** is comprised of societal attitudes, laws, and regulations that control or tolerate the occurrence of events that can lead to injuries. Examples of social environmental factors that increase the risk of injuries follow.
   a. Tolerance of violent behavior
   b. Acceptance of the use of alcohol and other drugs
   c. Economic deprivation
   d. Racism
   e. Sexism

D. Agent. The injury-causing agent is **energy**. As noted above, a large amount of energy quickly transmitted may result in injury, while a small amount of energy transmitted over a long period of time may result in disease (see section I A 3). The five types of energy that cause injuries follow.

1. **Kinetic energy**, or mechanical energy, is the most common cause of injuries; for example:
   a. In an automobile crash, the energy transferred by the motor vehicle that injures a person is kinetic energy. The energy imparted is proportional to the square of the speed of the vehicle. Thus, if the speed doubles, the amount of energy transmitted to the occupant quadruples.
   b. The energy resulting from a fall that injures a person is also kinetic energy.

2. **Thermal energy**, when excessive, is the most common cause of burns. A marked lack of thermal energy results in hypothermia and frostbite.

3. **Electrical energy** causes electrocutions and burns.

---

*According to Dr. Duncan W. Clark, characteristics that are associated with a condition but are neither causal nor controllable, such as age, sex, and race, are more appropriately called risk indicators, not risk factors.

4. **Radiation energy** causes burns.

5. **Chemical energy**, by interfering with the body's energy metabolism, can cause injuries; for example:
   a. Inhaled water interferes with pulmonary function, which can result in drowning.
   b. Carbon monoxide interferes with the oxygen-carrying capacity of blood, which can result in acute brain injury.

E. Vector. The vectors, or vehicles of injury, are the carriers of the energy. The design of the vector markedly alters the amount of energy available to cause an injury. Examples of vector factors that alter the occurrence of injuries follow.

1. Weapons are vectors of kinetic energy. Firearm design can decrease or increase the risk of injuries.
   a. Firearms with safety locks discharge unintentionally less frequently than firearms without safety locks.
   b. Small, easily concealed firearms can increase the risk of aggravated assault.

2. Automobiles are vectors of kinetic energy. Automobile design can decrease or increase the risk of injuries.
   a. Automobiles with air bags and automatic seat belts can protect occupants from many potentially fatal or injury-causing crashes.
   b. Small automobiles are associated with an increased risk of fatal injuries.

3. Electric wires are vectors of electrical energy. Insulated electric wire is safer than noninsulated wire.

III. MEASURES OF IMPACT IN THE UNITED STATES

A. Morbidity

1. Incidence
   a. About 70 million people are injured yearly in the United States for an annual incidence rate of about 31 people injured per 100 people.
   b. The incidence rate of injuries among males is about 40% greater than among females.
   c. Overall, the incidence rate of injuries decreases with increasing age.
   d. Injuries account for about 16% of all acute conditions, ranking second after respiratory conditions.

2. Disability prevalence
   a. Restricted activity
      (1) Injuries and impairments due to injuries account for about 804 million days of restricted activity for an annual rate of about 357 days of restricted activity per 100 people.
      (2) Acute injuries are associated with about 23% of all days of restricted activity due to acute conditions, ranking second after respiratory conditions.
   b. Bed disability
      (1) Injuries and impairments due to injuries account for about 195 million days of bed disability for an annual rate of about 87 days of bed disability per 100 people.
      (2) Acute injuries are associated with about 15% of all days of bed disability due to acute conditions, ranking second after respiratory conditions.

3. Productive activity loss
   a. Days lost from school
      (1) Acute injuries account for about 14 million days lost from school for an annual rate of about 37 days lost from school per 100 schoolchildren (6–16 years of age).
      (2) Acute injuries are associated with about 8% of all lost school days due to acute conditions, ranking third after respiratory conditions and infective and parasitic diseases.
   b. Days lost from work
      (1) Acute injuries account for about 97 million days lost from work for an annual rate of about 97 days lost from work per 100 currently employed people.
      (2) Acute injuries are associated with about 29% of all lost workdays due to acute conditions, ranking second after respiratory conditions.

B. Mortality

1. Mortality rates
   a. Injuries accounted for over 140,000 deaths (7.0% of all deaths) for a rate of 61 deaths from injuries per 100,000 people in 1984.

b. For all ages, injuries are the fourth leading cause of death after diseases of the heart (750,000 deaths), malignant neoplasms (430,000 deaths), and cerebrovascular diseases (150,000 deaths).
c. For people 1–34 years of age, injuries cause over one-half of all deaths. For people 1–44 years of age, injuries are the leading cause of death.
d. Injury mortality rates are greatest among the elderly, although injuries are ranked behind other causes of death.
e. For all injuries, except homicide and suicide, injury mortality rates are higher in rural areas.

2. Years of potential life lost (YPLL). Injuries are the leading cause of YPLL, accounting for about 3.5 million YPLL (to age 65) annually. In comparison, malignant neoplasms, the next leading cause of YPLL, account for about 1.8 million YPLL (to age 65) annually.
a. YPLL is a measure of premature death; it is the difference between the age at death and an arbitrary cutoff of potential or productive age, generally taken as either 65 or 70 years.
b. The impact of mortality is based on the age at death with the YPLL varying inversely with the age at death. Comparisons among causes of death based on YPLL emphasize the causes that have a greater impact on young people than on elderly people. For example, three individuals, 20, 35, and 50 years of age, die. If the arbitrary cutoff for potential life is 65 years, then the YPLLs for the three are 45, 30, and 15 years, respectively. Note that the YPLL for the 20-year-old individual is three times the YPLL for the individual who is 50 years old. The total YPLL is the sum of the individual YPLLs, or 90 YPLL.

C. Medical care utilization

1. Physician office visits
a. Injuries and poisonings are the principal diagnoses recorded for over 45 million (8%) of the physician office visits annually.
b. Injuries are the fourth leading cause of physician office visits after respiratory, circulatory, and neurologic diseases.

2. Emergency department visits
a. Over 25 million people are treated for injuries in emergency departments annually.
b. Injuries account for over 25% of emergency department visits.

3. Hospitalizations
a. Injuries and poisonings are the first listed diagnoses for about 3.5 million (9%) of the patients discharged from short-stay hospitals.
b. Injuries are the fourth leading cause of hospitalization after circulatory and digestive diseases and obstetric care.
c. The average hospital stay for all injuries (6.8 days) is similar to that for all conditions (6.6 days).

D. Direct and indirect costs

1. Economic costs include medical and related expenses, wage losses, insurance administration costs, indirect work losses, and associated property damage. Economic costs for all injuries are estimated to be over $90 billion annually. The societal cost for motor vehicle-related injuries alone is estimated to be over $40 billion annually.

2. Pain and emotional sequelae of individuals injured and their families are incalculable.

IV. CLASSIFICATIONS

A. **Intent.** Injuries are classified by the intent or purposefulness of occurrence.

1. Intentional injuries—that is, injuries that are purposely inflicted and often are associated with violence—cause about 50,000 deaths and represent about 1.2 million YPLL (to age 65) annually in the United States. The injuries can be inflicted by one person on another or can be self-directed. Examples include:
a. Child abuse.
b. Domestic violence.
c. Sexual assault.
d. Aggravated assault.
e. Homicide (the eleventh leading cause of death).*
f. Suicide (the ninth leading cause of death).*
g. Parasuicide.

*Suicide and homicide together represent the fifth leading cause of death in the United States.

2. **Unintentional injuries**—that is, injuries that are not purposely inflicted—cause about 91,000 deaths and represent about 2.3 million YPLL (to age 65) annually in the United States. They are the leading cause of death in people 1–44 years of age and the fourth leading cause of death for all people in the United States after cardiovascular diseases, malignant neoplasms, and cerebrovascular diseases. Examples include:
   a. Motor vehicle-related injuries.
   b. Fall-related injuries.
   c. Fire and burn-related injuries.
   d. Drownings.
3. **Distinction between intentional and unintentional injuries.** It is often difficult to define the intent of an injury; thus, the distinction between intentional and unintentional injuries can be tenuous and artificial. For example:
   a. Although motor vehicle-related injuries are generally classified as unintentional, vehicular assault is not uncommon.
   b. Automobiles intentionally built without certain safety features (i.e., without air bags) could result in injury to the occupants during a crash, and while the crash may be unintentional, the resultant injuries could be considered preventable, and, conceivably, intentional.
   c. The decrease in carbon monoxide levels in domestic gas has been accompanied by decreases in both unintentional poisonings and suicides due to domestic gas.

B. **Place of occurrence.** Injuries are classified by the place of occurrence. There are four principal locations at which injuries occur.

1. **Motor vehicles.** Motor vehicle-related injuries involve all transport vehicles in motion. The most common cause of motor vehicle-related injuries and deaths are automobile collisions. Some risk factors for motor vehicle-related injuries include alcohol use, decreased vehicle size, increased vehicle speed, and night driving.
   a. **Morbidity.** About 5 million people sustain motor vehicle-related injuries annually in the United States. Of these injuries, about 1.7 million are disabling, of which about 150,000 result in permanent impairment.
   b. **Mortality.** Motor vehicle-related injuries cause about 46,000 deaths and represent about 1.7 million YPLL (to age 65) annually in the United States. Motor vehicle-related injury mortality rates are greatest for individuals 15–24 years of age.
2. **Workplace.** Occupational injuries occur at the work site or result from incidents in the work environment. The most commonly occurring occupational injury is injury to the trunk.
   a. **Morbidity.** About 11 million people sustain occupational injuries annually in the United States. Of these injuries about 1.9 million are disabling, of which about 70,000 result in permanent impairment.
   b. **Mortality.** Occupational injuries cause about 11,000 deaths and represent about 300,000 YPLL (to age 65) annually in the United States. Approximately one-third of all fatal occupational injuries are motor vehicle-related. Falls result in 10% of fatal occupational injuries.
3. **Home.** Home injuries occur in the home and the surrounding premises.
   a. **Morbidity.** About 25 million people sustain injuries at home annually in the United States. Of these injuries, about 3.2 million are disabling, of which about 80,000 result in permanent impairment.
   b. **Mortality.** Home injuries cause about 22,000 deaths annually in the United States. Falls are the most common cause of home injury deaths.
4. **Public places.** These injuries occur in places used by the public and include recreational injuries and injuries resulting from natural events, such as lightening or floods.
   a. **Morbidity.** About 29 million people sustain injuries in public places annually in the United States. Of these injuries, about 24 million are disabling, of which about 60,000 result in permanent impairment.
   b. **Mortality.** About 19,000 deaths occur annually in public places in the United States. The most common cause of death from injury in a public place is drowning in a natural body of water.

C. **Nature of injury**

1. The International Classification of Diseases (ICD), the principal classification scheme that defines the nature of injuries (**N codes**):
   a. Is the *primary* coding mechanism for diseases and conditions.
   b. Is a *secondary* coding mechanism for injuries after classification by external cause (see section IV D).

c. Provides information concerning necessary health care resources and services.
d. Is most useful when accompanied by the classifications by external cause and by severity of injury. Examples of severity classifications include the:
(1) Abbreviated Injury Scale.
(2) Injury Severity Score.
(3) Consumer Product Safety Commission Hazard Index.

2. Injuries classified by the nature of the injury are classified by the part of the body that was injured and the type of damage that occurred, including injuries resulting from infectious or parasitic agents. For example, the ICD code for fractures of the neck of the femur includes fractures from all causes, including fractures resulting from falls and automobile crashes, whether intentionally or unintentionally inflicted.

D. External cause of injury

1. The ICD Supplementary Classification of External Causes of Injuries and Poisonings (**E codes**) is the principal classification scheme that:
a. Defines the external cause of injuries.
b. Classifies the injuries by apparent intent.
c. Provides information concerning etiology.
d. Is used in conjunction with the nature of injury codes.

2. Injuries classified by external cause, regardless of the resultant body damage, are classified by the etiologic environmental events and circumstances.

3. The most important external causes of injury are listed in Table 8-1.
a. Injuries by motor vehicle are the leading cause of injury mortality.
b. Falls are the leading cause of injury morbidity for all age groups and of injury mortality among people at least 75 years of age.
c. Mechanical suffocation or asphyxiation is the leading cause of injury mortality among children less than 1 year old.
d. Firearms cause two-thirds of all homicides and one-half of all suicides.

E. Other classifications are dependent upon the purposes for which the injury data are being used.

1. Product. The United States Consumer Product Safety Commission classifies and studies injuries by the type of consumer product associated with the injury (see Table 8-2).

2. Criminality. Police departments often classify injuries by the criminal nature of the event that caused the injury (see section V B 3).

V. SURVEILLANCE SYSTEMS for injuries, the quality of which varies greatly, measure the extent of

Table 8-1. International Classification of Diseases: Supplementary Classification of External Causes of Injury and Poisoning (The E Code Classification)

Transport accidents*
Accidental poisonings†
Surgical and medical procedures‡
Accidental falls
Accidents caused by fire and flames
Accidents due to natural and environmental factors
Accidents caused by submersion, suffocation, and foreign bodies
Other accidents
Late effects of accidental injury
Drugs, medicinal and biologic substances causing adverse effects in therapeutic use
Suicide and self-inflicted injury
Homicide and injury purposely inflicted by other individuals
Legal intervention
Injury undetermined whether accidentally or purposely inflicted
Injury resulting from operations of war

*Include railway, motor vehicle traffic, motor vehicle nontraffic, other road vehicle, water transport, air and space transport, and vehicle accidents not classifiable elsewhere.

†Include by drugs, medicinal substances, and biologicals, and by other solid and liquid substances, gases, and vapors.

‡As the cause of abnormal reaction of a patient or later complication, with or without mention of misadventure at the time of the procedure.

various injuries, describe the risk factors and indicators involved, and measure the effectiveness of interventions (see Chapter 1, section III D).

A. **Federal agencies.** Table 8-2 lists some of the federal agencies that conduct national injury surveillance and study injuries.

1. The Centers for Disease Control conduct and support studies on the epidemiology and prevention of injuries and violence.
2. The Health Resources Services Administration; the Alcohol, Drug Abuse, and Mental Health Administration; and the National Institutes of Health study injury epidemiology and prevention.
3. The Federal Aviation Administration, the Federal Railroad Administration, the Occupational Safety and Health Administration, the Bureau of Labor Statistics, the Coast Guard, the Veterans Administration, and the Federal Highway Administration study injuries.

B. **State and local agencies**

1. Departments of health conduct surveillance of fatal injuries as part of their vital statistics function (see Chapter 3, section I A 1 b). Some health departments also conduct surveillance of nonfatal injuries (e.g., the Massachusetts Department of Public Health as part of its Statewide Childhood Injury Prevention Program).
2. Transportation departments conduct surveillance of motor vehicle crashes and injuries.
3. Police departments conduct surveillance of violent and intentional injuries and motor vehicle crashes and injuries.
4. Departments of labor conduct surveillance of occupational injuries.
5. Fire departments conduct surveillance of fire and flame-related injuries.

C. **Other organizations**

1. The National Safety Council, a nongovernmental, nonprofit, public service organization chartered by an Act of Congress, annually compiles data from many sources on injury morbidity, mortality, and costs and conducts injury prevention programs.
2. The Insurance Institute for Highway Safety, sponsored by the insurance industry, conducts and supports research into injury epidemiology and prevention. For example, it supported the Northeastern Ohio Trauma Study, a major population-based study of injury incidence.
3. Researchers in public health and medical schools, universities, hospitals, and corporations conduct studies on injury epidemiology and prevention.
4. Many organizations, such as the American Academy of Pediatrics, the American Association for Automotive Medicine, the American College of Preventive Medicine, the American Medi-

Table 8-2. Selected Federal Agencies That Conduct National Injury Surveillance

Agency	Surveillance System
Federal Bureau of Investigation	Uniform Crime Reports
Federal Emergency Management Agency	National Fire Incident Reporting System
National Center for Health Statistics	Vital Statistics Surveillance
	National Ambulatory Care Survey
	National Health and Nutrition Examination Survey
	National Health Interview Survey
	National Hospital Discharge Survey
National Highway Traffic Safety Administration	Fatal Accident Reporting System
	National Accident Sampling System
National Institute of Justice	National Crime Survey
National Transportation Safety Board	Transportation Safety Reports
Consumer Product Safety Commission	Medical Examiners and Coroners Alert Program
	National Electronic Injury Surveillance System
	Product-related Death Certificate File
	Product-related Incidents File
Food and Drug Administration	Poison Control Case Reports

cal Association, the American Public Health Association, and the American Red Cross, provide support for the study and prevention of injuries.

VI. MODELS OF PREVENTION.

The practical approach to prevent and control injuries should involve strategies chosen on the basis of their actual effectiveness in reducing injuries, not on the relative importance or the time of occurrence of the causal or contributing factors they influence. Usually a combination of strategies and interventions are most effective. For example, the safest automobile restraint system incorporates both air bags and seat belts.

A. Passive and active strategies

1. **Passive strategies** are automatic, require no individual or repetitive action to be protective, and are generally the most effective. For example, the installation of air bags in motor vehicles is a passive strategy because the occupants of the automobile will be protected in a crash regardless of their individual actions.

2. **Active strategies** are voluntary, require repetitive, individual action to be protective, and are generally less effective than passive strategies. For example, seat belts in most motor vehicles must be buckled by the occupant every time the vehicle is used in order to be effective.

B. The four E's of intervention

1. **Engineering interventions** are aimed at the vectors and physical environments that promote or support the occurrence of injuries. These interventions, which are often passive, are among the most effective in decreasing the occurrence of injuries. For example, medicine containers were redesigned to be childproof.

2. **Economic interventions** are aimed at influencing behavior based on monetary incentives and rewards or penalties. For example, many insurance companies have low rates for residences equipped with smoke detectors and sprinkler systems.

3. **Enforcement interventions** are aimed at influencing behavior by laws and regulations. These interventions are only effective when the laws and regulations are applied. For example, a number of states have made the use of automobile seat belts and of special car seats for children mandatory. The enforcement of these two requirements, however, is variable.

4. **Educational interventions** are aimed at influencing behavior through reasoning and knowledge. These interventions are usually the least effective, especially when used alone without other interventions. Educational interventions could be more effective if they were directed toward societal leaders and decision-makers. For example, because high school driver education programs are often accompanied by licensure at young ages and by an increase in the proportion of young people who drive, populations with these programs have relatively *more* motor vehicle crashes among young people than populations that do not have such programs.

C. The Haddon Models are useful for determining possible interventions and prevention measures for particular injuries.

1. **The Haddon Matrix**, formulated by Dr. William H. Haddon, Jr., arranges intervention and prevention strategies by agent, vector, host, and physical and social environmental factors, according to the time at which the strategy would be effective in relation to the occurrence of the injury event. Table 8-3 depicts the Haddon Matrix and provides examples of each factor- and phase-specific strategy.

Table 8-3. The Haddon Matrix

			Environment	
	Agent and Vector	**Host**	**Physical**	**Social**
Pre-event strategy	Use self-extinguishing cigarettes	Insure anticonvulsant therapy for epileptics	Use nonslip surfaces in bathtubs	Revoke driver licenses of intoxicated drivers
Event strategy	Use air bags	Use motorcycle helmets	Use roadside poles that break away	Assist others being assaulted
Post-event strategy	Have emergency safety releases for machines	Obtain emergency medical care	Implement a rapid emergency transportation system	Support medical and rehabilitative services

a. **Pre-event strategies** are designed to prevent the agent from reaching the susceptible host and, therefore, prevent the occurrence of the injury-producing event.
b. **Event strategies** are effective at the time the injury could occur and are designed to minimize the interaction between the agent and the host to prevent or minimize the damage.
c. **Post-event strategies** are designed to limit or repair the damage already incurred.

2. **The Ten Countermeasure Strategies**, also known as the Tiger Strategies (they were introduced in a paper entitled, "On the Escape of Tigers: An Ecologic Note"), were also formulated by Dr. Haddon (Table 8-4). They evolved from the Haddon Matrix and were based on the energy exchanges that result in injuries and the need to minimize injuries that have occurred.

Table 8-4. The Ten Countermeasure Strategies

Countermeasure Strategy	Example
1. Prevent the marshalling of potentially injurious agents.	1. Eliminate nuclear weapons.
2. Reduce the amount of the agent.	2. Reduce the speed capability of motor vehicles.
3. Prevent the inappropriate release of the agent.	3. Make bathtubs slip-resistant.
4. Modify release of the agent.	4. Use seat belts.
5. Separate the host from the agent by time or space.	5. Use traffic lights at hazardous intersections.
6. Separate the host from the agent by physical barriers.	6. Use bulletproof vests.
7. Modify surfaces and basic structures.	7. Use air bags in motor vehicles.
8. Increase resistance to injury.	8. Prevent or treat osteoporosis.
9. Improve emergency responses.	9. Provide good emergency medical services.
10. Improve medical care and rehabilitation.	10. Provide good clinical services.

BIBLIOGRAPHY

Baker SP, O'Neill B, Karpf RS: *The Injury Fact Book*. Lexington, Kentucky, DC Heath, 1984

Barancik JI, Chatterjee BF, Greene YC, et al: Northeastern Ohio Trauma Study. I. Magnitude of the Problem. *Am J Public Health* 73:746–751, 1983

Committee on Trauma Research, Commission on Life Sciences, National Research Council and the Institute of Medicine: *Injury in America: A Continuing Public Health Problem*. Washington DC, National Academy Press, 1985

Haddon W Jr: On the escape of tigers: an ecologic note. *Am J Public Health* 60:2229–2234, 1970

Haddon W Jr, Baker SP: Injury control. In *Preventive and Community Medicine*, 2nd ed. Edited by Clark DW, MacMahon B. Boston, Little Brown, pp 109–140, 1981

National Safety Council: *Accident Facts*. Chicago, National Safety Council, 1985

Waller JA: Prevention of premature death and disability due to injury. In *Public Health and Preventive Medicine*, 12th ed. Edited by Last JM. New York, Appleton-Century-Crofts, pp 1543–1576, 1986

STUDY QUESTIONS

Directions: Each question below contains five suggested answers. Choose the **one best** response to each question.

1. The correct rank order for the five leading causes of years of potential life lost is

(A) injuries, cancer, heart disease, stroke, liver disease
(B) cancer, injuries, heart disease, stroke, liver disease
(C) cancer, heart disease, injuries, stroke, liver disease
(D) heart disease, cancer, stroke, injuries, liver disease
(E) cancer, heart disease, stroke, liver disease, injuries

2. Agents of injury include all of the following EXCEPT

(A) kinetic energy
(B) thermal energy
(C) potential energy
(D) electrical energy
(E) radiation energy

3. The most common cause of occupational injury deaths is related to

(A) manufacturing equipment
(B) agricultural equipment
(C) motor vehicles
(D) electrocutions
(E) falls

4. The National Electronic Injury Surveillance System

(A) is based on data from hospital pathology departments
(B) is run by the Consumer Product Safety Commission
(C) provides information on motor vehicle-related injuries
(D) is useful in defining "accident-prone" individuals
(E) None of the above

Directions: Each question below contains four suggested answers of which **one or more** is correct. Choose the answer

A if **1, 2, and 3** are correct
B if **1 and 3** are correct
C if **2 and 4** are correct
D if **4** is correct
E if **1, 2, 3, and 4** are correct

5. Vectors that are associated with injuries include

(1) electric wires
(2) electricity
(3) bullets
(4) carbon monoxide

6. Measures of injury morbidity include

(1) incidence rates
(2) disability prevalence
(3) productive activity loss
(4) physician office visits

7. The Haddon Matrix is based on the

(1) surveillance of injuries
(2) factors associated with injuries
(3) International Classification of Diseases
(4) time course of the injury event

8. The Ten Countermeasure Strategies are

(1) based on the transfer of energy
(2) host factor specific
(3) used to define interventions for many injuries
(4) used to enforce interventions for many injuries

9. Characteristics of fatal intentional injuries include which of the following?

(1) They are caused by handguns in over 50% of cases
(2) They number about 50,000 deaths per year
(3) They are associated with the acceptance of violence as an appropriate behavior
(4) They are the leading cause of death for blacks 20–34 years of age

Directions: The groups of questions below consist of lettered choices followed by several numbered items. For each numbered item select the **one** lettered choice with which it is **most** closely associated. Each lettered choice may be used once, more than once, or not at all.

Questions 10–13

Four medical students are involved in an automobile crash on a rainy Saturday night after a party that followed a national medical examination. The compact car went off the road at 70 miles per hour and hit a tree. Two of the students died, and two were hospitalized. The driver had a blood alcohol concentration of 10 mg per 100 ml. None of the students were wearing seat belts. For each risk factor present in the case history, select the risk factor category that is most appropriate.

(A) Agent factor
(B) Host factor
(C) Vector factor
(D) Social environmental factor
(E) Physical environmental factor

10. Elevated blood alcohol concentration

11. Rainy night

12. Compact car

13. Speed of 70 miles per hour

Questions 14–18

For each injury category listed below, select the type of injury that is most likely to be responsible for it.

(A) Motor vehicle-related injuries
(B) Fall-related injuries
(C) Suffocation-related injuries
(D) Knife-related injuries
(E) Firearm-related injuries

14. Leading cause of injury morbidity

15. Leading cause of injury mortality

16. Leading cause of homicide

17. Leading cause of injury mortality among the elderly

18. Leading cause of injury mortality among infants less than 1 year old

ANSWERS AND EXPLANATIONS

1. The answer is A. (*III B 2 a–c; IV A 1, 2*) Injuries are the leading cause of years of potential life lost (YPLL), with unintentional injuries accounting for about 2.3 million and intentional injuries about 1.2 million YPLL each year. Malignant neoplasms, the second leading cause of YPLL, account for about 1.8 million YPLL. Heart disease, stroke, and liver disease account for 1.6, 0.3, and 0.2 million YPLL each year, respectively.

2. The answer is C. (*II D 1–5*) Energy is an injury-causing agent that may be transmitted quickly, resulting in injury, or over a long period of time, resulting in disease. Kinetic energy, or mechanical energy, is the most common cause of injuries (e.g., automobile collisions). Thermal energy, when excessive, is the most common cause of burns. A marked lack of thermal energy results in hypothermia and frostbite. Electrical energy causes electrocutions and burns, and radiation energy also causes burns. Potential energy describes the energy inherent in an object that has not yet been dissipated. Because it has yet to be transmitted, potential energy does not *cause* injuries.

3. The answer is C. (*IV B 2*) Occupational injuries are injuries that occur as a result of trauma or exposure to toxins or harmful substances in the workplace. The most common cause of fatal occupational injuries is related to motor vehicles, which account for about one-third of all occupational injury deaths. Falls, the next most common cause of occupational injury deaths, account for about 10%.

4. The answer is B. (*V A; Table 8-2*) The National Electronic Injury Surveillance System collects confidential data on the incidence of consumer product-related injuries from 66 representative hospital emergency treatment departments in the United States. It is run by the Consumer Product Safety Commission. Data on motor vehicle-related injuries is available from the Fatal Accident Reporting System, run by the National Highway Traffic Safety Administration.

5. The answer is B (1, 3). (*II E*) Vectors are the carriers of the injury agents, or energy. The design of the vector markedly alters the amount of energy available to cause an injury. Electric wires are vectors of electrical energy (electricity). Bullets are vectors of kinetic energy. Carbon monoxide and electricity are injury-causing agents not vectors.

6. The answer is A (1, 2, 3). (*III A 1–3*) Injury morbidity is measured by incidence rates, disability prevalence, and productive activity loss. About 70 million people are injured annually in the United States for an incidence rate of 31 people injured per 100 people per year. Disability prevalence includes restricted activity and bed disability. Injuries account for about 804 million days of restricted activity for an annual rate of 357 days of restricted activity per 100 people and for 195 million days of bed disability for an annual rate of 87 days of bed disability per 100 people. Productive activity loss includes days lost from school and work. Injuries account for about 14 million days lost from school for an annual rate of 37 days lost from school per 100 schoolchildren and for 97 million days lost from work for an annual rate of 97 days lost from work per 100 employed people. Physician office visits are a measure of medical care utilization.

7. The answer is C (2, 4). (*VI C 1 a–c; Table 8-3*) The Haddon Matrix arranges intervention and prevention strategies by agent, vector, host, and physical and social environmental factors, according to the time course of the injury event. Pre-event strategies are designed to prevent the agent from reaching the susceptible host and thus prevent the injury-producing event. Event strategies are effective at the time the injury could occur; they are designed to minimize the interaction between the agent and the host to prevent or minimize the damage. Post-event strategies are designed to limit or repair the damage already incurred. The Haddon Matrix is not associated with the surveillance of injuries or the International Classification of Diseases.

8. The answer is B (1, 3). (*VI C 2; Table 8-4*) The Ten Countermeasure Strategies are based on the energy exchanges that result in injuries and on the need to minimize injuries. These strategies are useful for defining interventions. The strategies relate to all factors and do not emphasize host factors. Enforcement of the interventions, however, depends on society.

9. The answer is E (all). (*II C 2 a–c; IV A 1*) Intentional injuries are injuries that are purposely inflicted by one person on another or by one person on him- or herself. Fatal intentional injuries, which include homicide (if the injury is caused by another person) and suicide (if the injury is self-inflicted), are responsible for about 50,000 deaths per year. Handguns are the leading vector for fatal intentional injuries. Family members and acquaintances are responsible for about three-fourths of the homicides. The mortality rate for homicides among blacks is more than five times greater than among whites; however, the suicide rate among whites is about double that of blacks.

10–13. The answers are: 10-B, 11-E, 12-C, 13-A. (*II B–E*) Elevated blood alcohol concentration is a host factor, which indicates individual abuse of alcohol. In most states, a blood alcohol concentration of at least 10 mg (or 0.01 g) per 100 ml or 0.10% weight/volume defines legal intoxication. The tolerance of drunk driving, however, is a social environmental factor.

A rainy night is a physical environmental factor that is not controllable. However, the effects of a rainy night can be modified with road lights, improved highway surfaces, and good tires.

The compact car is a vector factor. Small cars are less safe than large cars, particularly in a collision, and are associated with an increased risk of injuries.

The speed of the car is an agent factor. The force of impact is related to the square of the speed. The force for a speed of 70 miles per hour, for example, is four times the force for a speed of 35 miles per hour.

14–18. The answers are: 14-B, 15-A, 16-E, 17-B, 18-C. (*IV D 3*) The leading cause of injury morbidity is falls. In the Northeastern Ohio Trauma Study, falls accounted for one-fourth of all injuries. In one year, 5% of the population received emergency treatment for a fall-related injury.

The leading cause of injury mortality is motor vehicles. Overall, motor vehicles account for about one-half of the unintentional injury deaths that occur each year. Among persons aged 15–24 years, motor vehicles account for about three-fourths of unintentional injury deaths that occur.

The leading cause of homicides is firearms. Firearms are the cause of two-thirds of all homicides and one-half of all suicides. They are the sixth leading cause of fatal unintentional injuries for all ages and the third for people 10–19 years of age.

The leading cause of injury mortality among the elderly is falls. There are about 13,000 fatal falls yearly and over two-thirds occur among the elderly.

The leading cause of injury mortality among infants is mechanical suffocation or asphyxiation due to food or a foreign object. Suffocation is the cause of death for about 40% of the 1000 children less than 1 year old who die yearly from unintentional injuries.

9
Mental Health

Christina L. Herring

I. MENTAL HEALTH VERSUS MENTAL DISORDER

A. Mental health. A comprehensive definition of mental health is that given by Ginsburg, who stresses the relationship of mental health to mastery of the environment as manifested in three crucial areas of living—love, work, and play. He states that mental health is "the ability to hold a job, have a family, keep out of trouble with the law, and enjoy the usual opportunities for pleasure."

B. Mental disorder. The problem in defining mental disorder is that the consensus that exists regarding the undesirability of symptoms of a medical disorder—pain, disability, and death—does not always exist for the symptoms of a mental disorder.

1. The lack of consensus over a definition of mental disorder concerns:
   - **a.** Whether or not a given condition should be regarded as undesirable.
   - **b.** The degree to which the condition should be considered undesirable in order to be designated as an illness.
   - **c.** Whether or not the condition should be regarded as within the domain of psychiatry or some other discipline.
2. Two approaches to defining mental disorder include:
   - **a.** Viewing mental disorder as any significant deviation from an ideal state of positive mental health. This approach, which accepts the basic psychoanalytic principles, is characteristic of the approach taken by most psychiatrists in the United States.
   - **b.** Accepting the notion of a continuum of conditions from highly desirable to highly undesirable but placing the cutoff point for mental disorder close to the highly undesirable end of the continuum; thus, only conditions unequivocally associated with suffering and disability are designated as illness or disorder. This approach is characteristic of European psychiatrists and may explain why epidemiologic studies conducted in the United States report a much higher incidence of mental disorder than European studies.
3. The most comprehensive definition of mental disorder is that proposed by Spitzer who states that:
   - **a.** The manifestations of the condition are primarily psychologic and involve alterations in behavior.
   - **b.** The condition in its full blown state is regularly and intrinsically associated with subjective distress, generalized impairment in social effectiveness or functioning, or voluntary behavior that the subject wishes he could stop because it is regularly associated with physical disability or illness.
   - **c.** The condition is distinct clinically from other conditions and ideally, follow-up studies, family studies, and response to treatment are also distinct.

II. APPLICATION OF EPIDEMIOLOGY TO MENTAL ILLNESS

A. Types of case definitions. To define a case of mental illness, studies have used the following sources:

1. Hospital admissions and discharges
2. Physicians' examinations and diagnoses
3. Register statistics, which entail a central listing of every individual who makes use of either outpatient or inpatient psychiatric services

B. **Problems of case definitions** are greatest in chronic diseases of known etiology—for example, schizophrenia and manic-depressive illness. Since the disease persists over the patient's lifetime, the symptoms usually wax and wane, and not all physicians would agree on a diagnosis every time the patient is examined.

1. **Schizophrenia**
   a. **The incidence** of schizophrenia is approximately 50 to 250 cases per 100,000 population.
   b. **The prevalence** of schizophrenia is a more subjective estimate than that of incidence. Taking a very narrow basis for case definition—that is, hospitalized schizophrenics on any given day in the United States—it was found that there were 160 schizophrenics per 100,000 population in mental hospitals in 1965.
   c. **Admission rates** for schizophrenia for both sexes primarily involve people 20 to 40 years of age, with a peak occurrence at 25 to 34 years of age.
   d. **The differential in rates** of schizophrenia among various population groups was most striking among different socioeconomic groups.
      (1) Faris and Dunham found that the areas of Chicago with high rates of schizophrenia were characterized by high mobility and social disorganization.
      (2) Odegaard compared rates of first hospital admissions among a native-born population of Minnesota and a Norwegian-born population that had migrated there. There was definitely a higher rate of schizophrenia among the Norwegians who had migrated to Minnesota.
      (3) These two studies led to the drift and origin hypotheses of schizophrenia.
         (a) **The drift hypothesis** holds that the schizophrenic is a highly mobile individual who tends to drift into areas of high social mobility and great social disorganization, thus accounting for the high rates of schizophrenia found in these areas.
         (b) **The origin hypothesis** holds that certain etiologic factors create a higher rate of schizophrenia among the inhabitants of these mobile and disorganized areas and that these etiologic factors are not present in stable areas. The high rate of schizophrenia among the lower socioeconomic groups is supported by hospitalization statistics.

2. **Manic-depressive illness**
   a. **The incidence** of manic-depressive reactions has decreased markedly in the last 50 years.
      (1) In 1900, 17% of all admissions to the Boston State Hospital and 37% of admissions to the McLean Hospital were diagnosed as manic-depressive.
      (2) In 1950, the figures were 8% and 16%, respectively.
   b. **Admission rates**
      (1) In all classes of hospitals, women outnumber men, and, in sharp contrast to schizophrenia, the upper classes are more likely to be represented than the lower classes.
      (2) In Kraepelin's series, 58% of first attacks occurred between 20 and 35 years of age, and 35% occurred between 35 and 60 years of age. The manic form of the reaction occurs primarily in the younger individuals and the depressed reaction in the older group.
      (3) A large percentage of manic-depressive individuals are married—particularly as compared to the number of married schizophrenics; however, unlike in schizophrenia, marital status is not related to prognosis.

III. EXTENT AND COST OF MENTAL ILLNESS

A. **Extent of mental illness.** At least 10% of the population of the United States (about 30 million Americans) have some form of mental disorder that could benefit from professional help. The extent of mental illness is often related to the number of hospitalized patients.

1. There are more patients in hospitals with mental disorders at any one time than all other diseases combined, including cancer and heart disease.

2. Recent figures indicate that approximately 360,000 individuals are receiving psychiatric care in public and private mental hospitals, psychiatric services of general hospitals, and Veterans Administration psychiatric facilities on any given day of the year and that 1.75 million individuals receive treatment at these institutions annually.

3. Readmissions to mental hospitals are common: Of the 972,000 individuals admitted to mental hospitals and psychiatric services of general hospitals annually, nearly 360,000 (or more than one-third) are readmissions.

B. **Professional services** for mental disorders are carried out by a number of different practitioners.

1. There are 27,000 practicing psychiatrists in the United States (1300 are psychoanalysts), but the distribution is very uneven: Five states (i.e., New York, New Jersey, Pennsylvania, Massa-

chusetts, and California) have more than one-half of all psychiatrists, while two-thirds of all counties in the United States have none at all.

2. There are 20,000 psychologists, 19,000 psychiatric social workers, and 30,000 psychiatric nurses, resulting in a ratio of 35 mental health workers for every 100,000 people in the United States.

C. The cost of mental illness is quite high.

1. About $4 billion are spent annually for the treatment of mental illness in federal, state, county, and private mental hospitals and psychiatric units of community hospitals.

2. Tax monies pay approximately two-thirds of this bill with the other third coming from the private sector.

D. The burden of mental illness on industry is impressive.

1. The National Association for Mental Health estimates that individuals hospitalized for mental illness lose nearly $2 billion per year in purchasing power.

2. Mental disorders account for at least 50% of all absenteeism, which costs industry $5 billion annually.

3. Mental disorders are important factors in the etiology of 75% of all accidents, which cost industry $3 billion annually in injury to workers and damage to their machines.

IV. CARE OF THE MENTALLY ILL. The history of care of the mentally ill in the United States is not a record to be viewed with pride. It was once widely believed that individuals suffering from mental illness were possessed by demons and should be put away in jails, poorhouses, or kennels or punished in stocks or at whipping posts.

A. Early reformers

1. In 1756, Benjamin Franklin was instrumental in opening Pennsylvania Hospital in Philadelphia to the mentally disturbed.

2. In 1773, the first hospital in the United States devoted exclusively to mental patients was opened in Williamsburg, Virginia.

3. Dr. Benjamin Rush began a scientific study of mental illness at Pennsylvania Hospital in 1800.

4. Dorothea Lynde Dix, the greatest early reformer in the nineteenth century, is best known for:
   a. Crusading for intelligent and humane treatment of the mentally ill.
   b. Founding Saint Elizabeth's Hospital in Washington, D.C.
   c. Awakening the public conscience.
   d. Stimulating the movement toward the creation of the state mental hospital system.

B. State-supported mental hospitals were established in most states by the end of the nineteenth century.

1. There are presently 327 state and county mental hospitals in the United States.

2. The number of patients in these mental hospitals increased steadily until around 1955 after which the population of the institutions dropped continually as a result of:
   a. The use of psychotropic drugs.
   b. Advanced methods of intensive therapy, including group therapy and milieu therapy.
   c. The development of community mental health centers in the 1960s.

C. Private psychiatric hospitals

1. Although there are about 200 private psychiatric hospitals in the United States, 18 states have no private facilities, and 11 states have only one.

2. Private hospitals account for approximately 15,000 beds as compared to 500,000 beds in public institutions.

3. Private psychiatric hospitals offer many obvious advantages to mental patients who can afford to pay since these patients are more likely to receive individual psychotherapy; they are, however, unevenly distributed: 40% of the hospitals and 25% of the beds are found in California and New York.

D. Community hospitals. Approximately 800 community hospitals, or 1 out of every 7, have separate units for treating psychiatric patients.

1. Approximately 19,000 beds are reserved for treating the mentally ill in these institutions, but the average stay is only 3 weeks.
2. The admissions to psychiatric services in community hospitals are approximately equal to those of state mental institutions.

V. CHANGING CONCEPTS AND ATTITUDES

A. The development of psychotropic agents, one of the most outstanding changes in the field of mental health, has had the following effects:

1. It has allowed mental patients to return to the community and in some cases to their families and their jobs.
2. It has had a profound impact upon public acceptance of mental illness. As a result of increased public and private awareness, federal grants from the Hospital Improvement Program and the Hospital Staff Development Program have helped to provide better facilities and better trained personnel than ever before.
3. Prior to the availability of these drugs, there was small chance for a short hospital stay or rapid recovery. The period of hospitalization has been reduced from years to months and even weeks for some patients; for example, the average stay for the first psychiatric admission is 3 weeks.

B. Insurance coverage of mental illness

1. **Inpatient coverage**
   a. Although coverage of mental disorders is now a basic feature of most hospital insurance written for groups, the current practice of health insurance agencies is to provide only those benefits specified by service contracts.
   b. With improved treatment methods, resulting in shorter hospital stays, and the increased use of general hospitals to treat psychiatric patients, insurance restrictions are more liberal with respect to inpatient services.
   c. Medicare and Medicaid provide some benefits, but there are significant limitations both in duration of coverage and financial allowance.
2. **Outpatient coverage.** Insurance coverage for outpatient services and partial hospitalization services is dismal.
   a. Outpatient coverage is often only available under an extended benefit or major medical certificate.
   b. In addition, the initial deductible and co-insurance features discourage early referral and treatment.
   c. In most of these policies, there is almost no coverage for day care or for the services of psychologists, social workers, and other professionals who have become increasingly important in the treatment of mental disorders.

C. Community mental health centers have had a lasting effect on the care of the mentally ill in this country.

1. The Joint Commission on Mental Illness and Health established by Congress in 1955 issued a report in 1961 entitled "Action for Mental Health." This report revealed the deficiencies that existed in the public mental hospital system and called for a number of significant changes, including:
   a. A need for more community clinics for outpatient treatment.
   b. A recommendation to increase the use of general hospitals for the inpatient treatment of psychiatric illness.
   c. A need for a change in the nature of the public mental hospital.
2. President John F. Kennedy presented his now historic special message, "Mental Illness and Mental Retardation," in which he proposed a new approach to the care of the mentally ill.
   a. This new approach was designed and implemented in an attempt to:
      (1) Use federal resources to stimulate state, local, and private action to create, at the community level, a significant number and range of mental health services.
      (2) Reduce patient populations in state mental hospitals.
   b. Although the establishment of community mental health centers has provided needed services, disastrous consequences have resulted from reliance on these services.
      (1) Although the population of patients in state mental hospitals has been markedly reduced, the number of readmissions has risen so sharply that the state hospital system

has become a revolving door. Psychiatrists now agree that they have been overly optimistic about the efficacy of psychotherapeutic drugs.

(2) Community resources have proven inadequate to handle the large number of former state hospital patients, resulting in an extraordinary number of homeless mentally ill people.

(3) Federal funding has not provided the impetus to the state, local, or private funding so that when federal funding is curtailed, so are services.

D. ***The Diagnostic and Statistical Manual for the Classification of Mental Disorders (DSM)*** has provided a significant change in the diagnosis of mental disorders.

1. **The *DSM-I*** was the first publication to contain a glossary of descriptions of diagnostic categories. Its use of the term "reaction" throughout the classification reflected the influence of Adolf Meyer's psychobiologic view that mental disorders represented reactions of the personality to psychologic, social, and biologic factors.

2. **The *DSM-II*** (the second edition) based the classification of mental disorders on the eighth edition of the *International Classification of Diseases (ICD-8)*. The *DSM-II* did not use the term "reaction"; it used diagnostic terms that did not imply a particular theoretical framework for understanding nonorganic mental disorders.

3. **The *DSM-III*** (the third edition) provides a classification of mental disorders based on the *ICD-9*, but there is still no satisfactory definition that specifies precise boundaries for the concept "mental disorder." The approach taken in the *DSM-III* is atheoretical with regard to etiology. It attempts to describe disorders comprehensively and to provide specific diagnostic criteria as guides for making each diagnosis, unlike the *DSM-I*, *DSM-II*, and *ICD-9*.
   a. Each of the mental disorders is conceptualized as a clinically significant behavioral or psychologic syndrome that occurs in an individual and is typically associated with either a painful symptom (distress) or impairment in one or more important areas of functioning (disability).
   b. There is no assumption that each mental disorder is a discrete entity with sharp boundaries between it and other mental disorders or between it and no mental disorder.

VI. PREVENTION OF MENTAL DISORDER

A. **Primary prevention** is both the promotion of general mental health and the protection against the occurrence of specific diseases.

1. Promoting mental health is a perplexing problem.
   a. There must be a definition of mental health.
   b. It must be assumed that mental health can be affected by measures undertaken during the lifetime of the individual who is the target of the measures.

2. Specific diseases are the aim of primary prevention.
   a. Organic brain syndrome, resulting from diseases such as syphilis and vitamin deficiencies, was the leading cause of mental hospital admissions 50 to 75 years ago, although it is unusual to find cases in the United States today.
   b. Crisis or situational reaction is a condition that is currently receiving much attention in terms of preventive efforts.
   (1) Caplan developed a theory and techniques for preparing individuals in advance to deal with crises in the hope of avoiding the distress that usually results.
   (2) There are two aspects to crisis preparation:
   (a) Anticipatory guidance—the cognitive aspect—consists of a group discussion of the crisis situation that the indiviudal will potentially face, of techniques others have found effective, and the individual's own experiences in mastering previous crises.
   (b) Emotional innoculation—the emotional aspect—involves putting an individual through a series of increasingly stressful experiences to the point at which he or she is almost overwhelmed.
   c. Schizophrenia is a disease for which preventive efforts have received considerable attention.
   (1) Unfortunately, all evidence suggests that the rate of schizophrenic breakdown has remained stable for many years in spite of preventive efforts.
   (2) There also seems to be an inherited tendency toward schizophrenia but no one knows what is inherited: It is presently one of several theories of etiology.
   d. Senility has become a serious problem in our society as the number of people over 65 years of age increases. There has been a strong trend to classify elderly people with problems of living as psychiatric patients and admit them to mental hospitals.

(1) Effective prevention probably requires a change in life-style and attitudes in society so that elderly people have a respected niche.

(2) Young people can be prepared in advance with the skills, resources, and attitudes necessary to combat the disengagement common to old age.

e. **Personality disorders** result from distorted relationships in childhood. Bowlby has shown that raising infants in institutions leads to disturbed development in childhood. The implication of these findings for preventive efforts is that orphaned or abandoned children should not be raised in institutions or shifted between foster homes.

B. **Secondary prevention** encompasses early diagnosis and prompt and adequate treatment to prevent sequelae and limit disability. The value of secondary prevention is untested with regard to most mental disorders. Current efforts at early diagnosis and treatment of mental disorders are in four major areas.

1. **Screening large population groups** to find mentally ill people who may then be directed into treatment has been done only as part of research projects. Although most studies have methodological problems, it seems safe to say that a minimum of 10% of the general American population report significant psychiatric disability at any one time and therefore are in need of treatment. Schools are an obvious setting in which clinical screening procedures followed by treatment would be logical and effective.

2. **Crisis intervention** offers service immediately. Service is brief and focuses on the presenting problem. There is no attempt to bring about major personality changes but rather to return the individual to his or her previous level of functioning. Because of the vulnerability of the individual in crisis, the mental health worker who intervenes is in a very powerful position.

a. Crisis intervention has its roots in the work of three groups.

(1) **Lindemann** studied survivors of the famous Coconut Grove fire and members of several other bereaved and distressed groups during World War II and found that a normal grief reaction is expected. In fact, if this reaction does not appear, other more disabling manifestations were likely to occur.

(2) **Tyhurst** included grief reactions in a group that he called "transition states—circumstances representing significant change, often sudden or intense, in the life situations of individuals."

(3) **Thomas** saw crisis as "a threat, a challenge, a strain on the attention, a call to new action."

b. Other pioneers in crisis intervention include the following:

(1) **Querido** attempted to reduce the mental hospitalization rate for the city of Amsterdam in the early 1930s. The services he instituted included home visits and a variety of social welfare activities beyond traditional psychotherapy and medication.

(2) **Shneidman** at the Los Angeles Suicide Prevention Center pioneered techniques for intervening with apparent suicide-prone individuals through telephone interviews.

(3) **Bard** trained teams of policemen as family crisis intervention workers.

(4) **Glass**, a United States Army psychiatrist during World War II and the Korean conflict, pioneered techniques for crisis intervention during military conflict.

3. **Educating the public** to recognize mental illness in the early stages and then to seek help early seems to be a useful but yet unproven approach.

a. **Davis** has done an extensive review of the mental health education efforts. He suggests that when mental health education aims only to provide information, it is likely to succeed; when it aims to change behavior, it is likely to fail.

b. **Avnet** found that use of mental health services was surprisingly low even after intensive efforts to educate insured people about the availability of their coverage.

4. **Increasing the availability of services**

a. Major steps to increase the availability of services have been taken through the funding of community mental health centers by the federal and state governments.

b. Mental health centers have increased availability even further by developing satellite clinics and outreach measures.

c. It is unknown whether the increased use is occurring among those groups that can benefit most from services.

C. **Tertiary prevention** encompasses rehabilitation after defect and disability have occurred in an attempt to reduce the disability.

1. Despite major reductions in hospital use, there are over 400,000 patients in state and veterans' psychiatric hospitals, many of whom suffer from the chronic disability of schizophrenia. Although much remains to be discovered about schizophrenia, a great deal is known about its course.

a. Pinel, working in the eighteenth century, found that schizophrenics under the influence of moral treatment, became less disabled mentally.

b. By the middle of the nineteenth century, under the influence of Quaker groups, mental hospitals became completely open, and these institutions were reporting 100% cure rates.

c. At the turn of the twentieth century, mentally ill people were elaborately studied, but hospitals became much larger, conditions in them deteriorated, and cure rates went from 100% to 0%. Deterioration became common, and admission to a hospital became a sentence of life imprisonment.

d. After World War II, British hospitals began to be unlocked, and severely mentally ill individuals in England no longer deteriorated; American hospitals began similar practices after learning of the success rate reported by the British.

e. Pasamanick demonstrated that for most schizophrenics hospitalization was not necessary. They could be handled as well at home with regular visits from public health nurses and with medication.

2. The general objective of psychiatric rehabilitation is to produce behavior in the patient that will enable him or her to function in society. Thus, it is obvious that the institutional setting must permit and even encourage behavior appropriate for life outside.

a. Human behavior:

(1) Can be changed by gradually shaping completely new responses.

(2) Responds to the presence or absence of specific factors in the environment, as well as to the general influence of social pressure.

b. Social pressure:

(1) Can be exerted through involvement in a group and interaction with members of the group. The attitude and social forces with the group are crucial in determining the behavior of group members.

(2) Can be inferred from, modified for, and exerted on the individual through observing, modifying, and exerting the group's expectations of the individual.

3. The aged mentally disabled differ in that they previously had a full range of social skills but have lost these through a combination of lack of use, depression, and apathy in response to change in life circumstances and central nervous system tissue damage. Reality orientation:

a. Resembles remotivation as practiced with the mentally ill.

b. Starts with simple social interaction and progresses to more complicated skills.

BIBLIOGRAPHY

Avnet H: *Psychiatric Insurance: Financing Short-Term Ambulatory Treatment—A Research Project Report*. New York, Group Health Insurance, 1962

Bard M: *Training Police as Specialists in Family Crisis Intervention*. Washington, DC, US Government Printing Office, 1970

Bowlby J: Maternal care and mental health. *WHO*, monograph series no. 2, 1951, p 355

Caplan G: *Principles of Preventive Psychiatry*. New York, Basic Books, 1964

Davis JA: *Education for Positive Mental Health: A Review of Existing Research and Recommendations for Future Studies*. Chicago, Aldine, 1965

Diagnostic and Statistical Manual of Mental Disorders (DSM-I). Washington, DC, American Psychiatric Association, 1952

Diagnostic and Statistical Manual of Mental Disorders (DSM-II). Washington, DC, American Psychiatric Association, 1968

Diagnostic and Statistical Manual of Mental Disorders (DSM-III). Washington, DC, American Psychiatric Association, 1980

Faris RE, Dunham WE: *Mental Disorders in Urban Areas*. Chicago, University of Chicago Press, 1939

Ginsburg SW: The mental health movement and its theoretical assumptions. In *Community Programs for Mental Health*. Edited by Kotinsky R, Witmer H. Cambridge, Harvard University Press, 1955, p 7

Glass AJ: Principles of combat psychiatry. *Milit Med* 117:27, 1958

International Classification of Diseases, 8th ed (ICD-8). Washington, DC, World Health Organization, 1968

Kraepelin E: *Manic-Depressive Insanity and Paranoia*. Edited by Robertson GM. Edinburgh, Livingstone, 1921

Lindemann E: Symptomatology and management of acute grief. *Am J Psychiatry* 101:141, 1944

Odegaard O: Emigration and insanity. *Acta Psychiatr Neurol* 4(Suppl 4): 546, 1932

Pasamanick B, Scarpitte FP, Dinitz S: *Schizophrenics in the Community*. New York, Appleton-Century-Crofts, 1967

Pinel P: *Traite Medico—Philosophique sur 1'Aberration Mentale*. New York, Hafner, 1962

Querido A: The shaping of community mental health care. *Br J Psychiatry* 114:293, 1968

Shneidman EB: The national suicide prevention program. In *Organizing the Community to Prevent Suicide*. Edited by Zusman J, Davidson DL. Springfield, Ill, Charles C Thomas, 1971, p 19

Spitzer RL, Endicott J: Computer diagnosis in an automated record keeping system: a study of clinical acceptability. In *Progress in Psychiatric Information Systems: Computer Application*. Edited by Crawford JL, Morgan DW, Grantinco DT. Cambridge, Ballinger Books, 1973, p 103

Thomas WI: *Source Book for Social Origins*. Boston, Badger, 1909, p 18

Tyhurst JS: The role of transition states—including disasters—in mental illness. In *Symposium on Social and Preventive Psychiatry*. Washington, DC, Walter Reed Army Institute of Research, US Government Printing Office, 1958, pp 149–169

STUDY QUESTIONS

Directions: Each question below contains five suggested answers. Choose the **one best** response to each question.

1. All of the following statements concerning the care of the mentally ill in the United States is true EXCEPT

(A) two-thirds of the counties in the United States have no psychiatrists at all
(B) state-supported mental hospitals are responsible for the care of the mentally ill more often than private and community hospitals combined
(C) the annual admissions to the psychiatric services in community hospitals are approximately equal to those in state institutions
(D) the history of the care of the mentally ill is not a record to be viewed with pride
(E) Dorothea Dix is best known as the first woman psychiatrist who crusaded for humane treatment of the mentally ill

2. Manic-depressive illness occurs more frequently

(A) among lower class individuals than among upper class individuals
(B) as a manic reaction among patients 20–35 years of age than among older patients
(C) among men than women
(D) than it occurred 50 years ago
(E) among unmarried individuals, particularly as compared to married schizophrenics

3. Tertiary prevention of mental disorder involves

(A) early diagnosis and prompt treatment to prevent sequelae and limit disability
(B) hospitalization for mentally disturbed individuals who are unable to function under the stress of everyday life
(C) individual psychotherapy, since groups are not able to shape behavior as well as individual therapists
(D) screening large population groups followed by appropriate treatment
(E) psychiatric rehabilitation designed to produce behavior that will enable the mentally disturbed individual to function in society

4. Insurance coverage of mental illness is best characterized by which of the following statements?

(A) It is liberal in terms of financial allotments for the services of psychologists, social workers, and psychoanalysts
(B) It encourages early referral because of inconsequential deductibles
(C) It encourages return to the community by providing for coverage for day care
(D) It is now a basic feature of most hospital group insurance but only for inpatient status
(E) It is supplemented by liberal Medicare and Medicaid benefits for those who qualify

Directions: Each question below contains four suggested answers of which **one or more** is correct. Choose the answer

A if **1, 2, and 3** are correct
B if **1 and 3** are correct
C if **2 and 4** are correct
D if **4** is correct
E if **1, 2, 3, and 4** are correct

5. Correct statements concerning the definition of mental disorder include which of the following?

(1) There is general consensus regarding the undesirability of the symptoms of a mental disorder
(2) Only conditions unequivocally associated with suffering and disability are characterized as illness by American psychiatrists
(3) The manifestations of mental disorder are both psychologic and physical and, therefore, are measurable
(4) Mental disorder is associated with subjective distress and impairment in social functioning

6. The third edition of *The Diagnostic and Statistical Manual for the Classification of Mental Disorders (DSM-III)* is characterized by

(1) the assumption that each mental disorder is a discrete entity
(2) an atheoretical approach with regard to the etiology of syndromes
(3) the use of the term "reaction" throughout to reflect a psychobiologic view
(4) the conceptualization of each mental disorder as a clinically significant behavioral or psychologic syndrome

Directions: The group of questions below consists of lettered choices followed by several numbered items. For each numbered item select the **one** lettered choice with which it is **most** closely associated. Each lettered choice may be used once, more than once, or not at all.

Questions 7–10

Match the research in crisis intervention with the appropriate researcher.

(A) Tyhurst
(B) Querido
(C) Schneidman
(D) Lindemann
(E) Glass

D 7. Research into the Coconut Grove fire, which showed that a normal grief reaction is expected

C 8. Research in techniques for suicide prevention

B 9. Research into social welfare activities, including home visits to reduce mental hospitalization rates

E 10. Research in crisis intervention during military conflict

ANSWERS AND EXPLANATIONS

1. The answer is E. (*III B 1; IV A 4, B 1, C, D 2*) The care of the mentally ill in the United States is not a record to be viewed with pride; mental patients were often put away in jails or poorhouses.

Dorothea Dix, the greatest early reformer in the nineteenth century, was not a psychiatrist; however, she did crusade tirelessly for intelligent and humane treatment of the mentally ill.

State-supported mental hospitals were established in most states by the end of the nineteenth century. Today they account for about 500,000 beds as compared to private hospitals with 15,000 beds and community hospitals with 19,000 beds. Community hospitals, however, have approximately an equal number of admissions annually as those of state institutions.

Although there are 27,000 practicing psychiatrists in the United States, two-thirds of the counties in this country have no psychiatrist.

2. The answer is B. (*II B 2 a–b*) The incidence of manic-depressive reactions has decreased markedly in the last 50 years. In all classes of hospitals, women outnumber men, and the upper classes are more likely to be represented than the lower classes. Also, a large percentage of manic-depressive individuals are married, particularly as compared to the number of married schizophrenics. The manic form of the reaction occurs primarily among patients 20–35 years of age, and the depressed reaction, among individuals 35–60 years of age. Patients need not have a bipolar disorder to be labeled manic-depressive.

3. The answer is E. [*VI B 1, C 1 e, 2 b (1)*] Tertiary prevention of mental disorder entails rehabilitation *after* defect and disability have occurred. Psychiatric rehabilitation is designed to produce behavior that will enable the patient to function in society. Group therapy, in particular, is important in exerting social pressure, which can modify behavior. Pasamanick demonstrated that hospitalization, particularly for schizophrenics, was not necessary as they could be handled as well at home with medication and regular visits from public health nurses. Early diagnosis and treatment, including the screening of large population groups, characterize secondary prevention efforts.

4. The answer is D. (*V B 1–2*) Inpatient coverage is now a basic feature of most hospital insurance written for groups. With improved treatment methods, resulting in shorter hospital stays, and increased use of general hospitals to treat psychiatric patients, insurance restrictions are more liberal with respect to inpatient services. While Medicare and Medicaid provide some benefits, the financial allotments are limited. Insurance coverage for outpatient services is dismal. Not only do the initial deductible and co-insurance features discourage early referral, but there is almost no coverage for day care or for the services of psychologists, social workers, and psychoanalysts.

5. The answer is D (4). (*I B 1–3*) There is no consensus regarding the undesirability of symptoms of a mental disorder. American psychiatrists view mental disorder as any significant deviation from an ideal state of positive mental health, while European psychiatrists are more likely to consider only conditions associated with suffering and disability as illness or disorder. The manifestations of a mental disorder are psychologic, not usually physical, and, therefore, cannot easily be measured. The most comprehensive definition of mental disorder is a condition that is associated with subjective distress, impairment in social functioning, and voluntary behavior that the patient wishes he or she could stop because it is regularly associated with physical disability or illness.

6. The answer is C (2, 4). (*V D 1–3*) The third edition of *The Diagnostic and Statistical Manual for the Classification of Mental Disorder (DSM-III)* uses an atheoretical approach with regard to etiology. It attempts to describe disorders comprehensively and to provide specific diagnostic criteria as guides for making each diagnosis. Each mental disorder is conceptualized as a clinically significant behavioral or psychologic syndrome. However, there is no assumption that each mental disorder is a discrete entity with sharp boundaries. The term "reaction" was used throughout the *DSM-I*, reflecting the influence of Adolf Meyer's psychobiologic view that mental disorders represented reactions of the personality to psychologic, social, and biologic factors.

7–10. The answers are: 7-D, 8-C, 9-B, 10-E. (*VI B 2*) Crisis intervention offers brief and immediate service, which focuses on the presenting problem. There is no attempt to bring about a major personality change, but rather to return the individual to his or her previous level of functioning.

Lindemann studied the survivors of the famous Coconut Grove fire and found that a normal grief reaction is expected. In fact, if this reaction does not appear, other more disabling manifestations were likely to occur.

Schneidman at the Los Angeles Suicide Prevention Center pioneered techniques for intervening with apparent suicide-prone individuals through telephone interviews.

Querido attempted to reduce the mental hospitalization rate for the city of Amsterdam in the 1930s. He instituted home visits and a variety of social welfare activities beyond traditional psychotherapy and medication.

Glass, a United States Army psychiatrist during World War II and the Korean War, pioneered techniques for crisis intervention during military conflict.

10
Mental Retardation

Christina L. Herring

I. INTRODUCTION

A. Mental retardation is an impairment of the mind characterized by subnormal intellectual development. It is not a single entity but a group of syndromes resulting from many causes; thus, it is not classified as a disease or an illness.

B. According to the American Association on Mental Deficiency (AAMD), mental retardation refers to significantly below average general intellectual functioning that exists concurrently with deficits in nonadaptive behavior and shows up during the developmental period. The AAMD definition:

1. Emphasizes aberrations that interfere with learning ability and social functioning, which occur before the completion of growth and development.
   a. In more than 90% of cases, mental retardation exists at birth or occurs within the first 2 years of life.
   b. In more than 95% of cases, mental retardation occurs before the fifth year.

2. Excludes mental deficiency acquired in adulthood and conditions in which intelligence may be masked by illness or emotional, drug-induced, or epileptic syndromes.

II. EPIDEMIOLOGY

A. **The incidence** of mental retardation is determined by the number of new cases documented each year.

1. **Severe mental retardation** is usually caused by genetic disorders or prenatal conditions; it is usually obvious at birth or in the immediate postnatal period because of particular characteristics recognizable by health professionals.
   a. The incidence of some genetic disorders, such as Down's syndrome, has remained constant for the past 50 years.
   b. The incidence of infectious disorders and their sequelae, such as congenital syphilis, has declined sharply with the widespread use of antibiotics.

2. **Mild mental retardation** often is not recognized until a child enters school.
   a. Estimates of mild mental retardation are accurate only where there is widespread compulsory education.
   b. Since detection of mild mental retardation is based on verbal and numerical skills specific to the schoolchild in industrialized societies, this defect may have very little influence on job performance in later life.

B. **The prevalence** of mental retardation in the United States, which is based on incidence and duration, is about 3% of the population; that is, there are approximately 7 million mentally retarded individuals in the United States.

1. Mental retardation is four times more common than rheumatic heart disease and nine times more common than cerebral palsy in the United States.

2. Of the 4.5 million infants born this year in the United States, slightly more than 100,000 will be classified as mentally retarded.

III. CLASSIFICATIONS. Mental retardation can be classified according to the objectives sought such as intelligence quotient (IQ), etiology, and specific syndromes.

A. **Classification by IQ** is an arbitrary method based on the results of standardized tests. To determine IQ, mental age is divided by chronologic age, and the result is multiplied by 100.

1. **General classifications by IQ** include the following:
   a. Genius: 140 and above
   b. Superior: 110 to 139
   c. Average: 90 to 109
   d. Low normal: 80 to 89
   e. Mentally retarded: 79 and below

2. **Mental retardation classifications by IQ** include the following:
   a. Mild (individuals with IQs of 70 to 79 are considered borderline cases): 53 to 79
   b. Moderate: 36 to 52
   c. Severe: 20 to 35
   d. Profound: below 20

B. **Etiology.** Etiologic classifications often are based on whether the condition is acquired prenatally, at birth, or postnatally. Since it is often difficult to determine prenatal or natal causes, these two etiologic groups are often combined as congenital causes of mental retardation.

1. **Prenatal causes of mental retardation**
   a. Genetic transmission is reported to be the most common cause of mental retardation, accounting for about 50% of all cases.
   b. Conditions acquired in utero include maternal infections (e.g., rubella), maternal metabolic diseases (e.g., diabetes and toxemia of pregnancy), and maternal ingestion of alcohol or other drugs (e.g., fetal alcohol syndrome).
   c. Although more than 200 diseases and conditions can cause mental retardation, the exact cause cannot be determined in over 75% of cases.

2. **Natal causes of mental retardation** primarily are traumatic and anoxic, resulting from abnormal presentations, accidents of delivery, and maternal oversedation. Although fetal monitoring has reduced the incidence of severe neurologic impairment by indicating the need for emergency cesarean section, it is still impossible to predict the need for cesarean section from an antepartum course. Recent studies have reported a combined rate of neonatal death and severe neurologic impairment to be over 2%.

3. **Postnatal causes of mental retardation** include infections, such as encephalitis and meningitis, trauma, such as skull fractures or cerebral hemorrhage, or lead ingestion.
   a. Lead encephalopathy, as a result of ingestion of lead paint, is responsible for 1 in 500 cases of institutionalized retarded individuals.
   b. Measles encephalitis, prior to immunization, was responsible for mental retardation in 50% of survivors who were affected before the age of 2 or 1% of all cases of mental retardation.
   c. There has been a sharp decline in the case-fatality rate of bacterial meningitis since modern treatments were introduced, but cytomegalovirus, mycoplasma, and toxoplasma are still causes of mental retardation after perinatal infection.
   d. Head injuries in children seldom produce serious brain damage and mental retardation.

IV. GENETIC AND NONGENETIC CAUSES OF MENTAL RETARDATION

A. **Genetic conditions**

1. **Disorders of amino acid metabolism**
   a. **Phenylketonuria (PKU)** is a rare defect of amino acid metabolism.
      (1) **The prevalence** is 1/15,000 in an average white population; it is quite rare among blacks.
      (2) **The biochemical defect** involves a deficiency of enzymes essential for the breakdown of phenylalanine.
         (a) The fetus is not affected since the mother has the essential enzyme for the breakdown of phenylalanine; the problem arises when the infant must break down the protein postnatally.
         (b) Since phenylalanine cannot be broken down, it accumulates in the blood, and the resulting hyperphenylalanemia adversely affects the brain of the developing infant.
         (c) After the age of 5, intellectual function is not affected by high levels of phenylalanine.
      (3) **Genetics.** PKU is transmitted by an autosomal recessive gene; both parents are unaffected carriers.
         (a) One in four offspring will be unaffected and not carriers.

(b) Half of the offspring will be unaffected carriers.
(c) One in four offspring will have PKU.

(4) **Prevention of mental retardation** in infants with PKU results from protecting them from high levels of circulating phenylalanine during the first 5 years of life.
(a) **The screening objective** must be to identify every affected newborn as soon as possible. This is done by:
(i) **Identifying a family at risk** after an affected child has become mentally retarded; however, it should be noted that the retardation is not reversible.
(ii) **Identifying parent carriers.** To date, however, no reliable carrier tests are available.
(iii) **Screening all newborns** for the presence of PKU.
(b) **Before screening** was instituted, the prevalence of PKU-related retardation was 1% of all institutionalized mentally retarded individuals.

(5) **Clinical features** of PKU include:
(a) Severe or profound mental retardation.
(b) Epilepsy.
(c) Fair complexion.
(d) Blond hair.
(e) Slight build.

(6) **Successful dietary treatment** has created a new problem: There are now women who are capable of reproduction, but who, as adults, lack the appropriate enzyme to break down phenylalanine. They, therefore, have high levels of phenylalanine in their blood, which may cause decreased intrauterine growth of their offspring and an increased risk of fetal death or mental retardation.

b. Maple syrup urine disease

(1) **The biochemical defect** interferes with decarboxylation of the branched chain amino acids—leucine, isoleucine, and valine—which accumulate in the blood and cause overflow aminoaciduria. The urine has a characteristic odor, from which the condition derives its name, due to derivatives of the ketoacids.
(2) **The genetics** of this disease are unknown.
(3) **Characteristic pathologic changes** include:
(a) A small brain with a thin cortex.
(b) Poorly myelinated fibers.
(4) **Clinical features**, which are obvious in the first week of life, include:
(a) Decerebrate rigidity.
(b) Seizures.
(c) Irregularity of respiration.
(d) Hypoglycemia.

2. Disorders of fat metabolism

a. Cerebromacular degeneration involves a group of disorders in which there is progressive mental deterioration and loss of visual function that are transmitted by an autosomal recessive gene.

(1) **Four types**, which differ as to age of onset, include the following:
(a) **Tay-Sachs disease**, which occurs chiefly among Ashkenazi Jewish infants, begins at 4 to 8 months of age. Infants look normal at birth but become weak and hypotonic. Spasticity, convulsions, and progressive physical and mental deterioration follow, leading to death in 2 to 4 years. Screening is available for the identification of Tay-Sachs carriers.
(b) **Bielschowsky-Jansky disease** has its onset at 2 to 4 years of age. It is characterized by pigmentary degeneration and mental retardation.
(c) **Spielmeyer-Stock-Vogt-Koyanagi disease**, the juvenile form, occurs in children 5 to 6 years of age, but the progress is slow. Impairment of vision, the first symptom, leads to blindness. Ataxia, convulsions, and mental deterioration then occur, leading to death at 10 to 15 years of age.
(d) **Kufs' disease**, the late juvenile form, is rare. It occurs after 15 years of age.

(2) **Characteristic pathologic findings** include the accumulation of lipid substances called gangliosides in the nerve cells throughout the central nervous system. There is no treatment available. Amniocentesis and chorionic villous sampling can determine whether a fetus is affected.

b. Niemann-Pick disease is transmitted by an autosomal recessive gene and occurs predominately in Ashkenazi Jews but does occur in all races. The onset is usually in infancy after initial normal development.

(1) **The biochemical defect**, which involves the storage of sphingomyelins in the neurons, liver, and spleen, can be identified by biopsy of the rectum or brain.

(2) **Characteristic pathologic findings** include:
(a) Developmental arrest and mental regression.
(b) Abdominal enlargement due to hepatosplenomegaly.
(c) Anemia.
(d) General emaciation.
(e) A cherry-red spot in the retina.

c. **Gaucher's disease** is transmitted by an autosomal recessive gene and occurs predominately in Ashkenazi Jews.
(1) **The metabolic defect** consists of a diminution of the enzyme activity of glucocerebrosidase, which leads to the accumulation of cerebrosides in the neurons and the cells of the reticuloendothelial system.
(2) **Types**
(a) **An acute neuronopathic form**, which manifests in infancy
(b) **A chronic non-neuronopathic or adult form**, which is the most common
(c) **A juvenile form**, which may begin at any time in childhood
(3) **Clinical features**
(a) In the acute neuronopathic form the infant has hepatosplenomegaly and strabismus; the head is retroflexed, and the limbs are spastic. It is rapidly fatal—that is, 80% die within the first year.
(b) In the chronic non-neuronopathic form, IQ is normal, but there is hepatosplenomegaly and bone pain; fractures often result from minor trauma. The disease may lead to early death, depending on how extensively the heart and lungs are infiltrated.
(c) In the juvenile form, children usually have neurologic abnormalities, which cause behavior problems, low IQ, seizures, tremors, and dysmetrias.

3. **Down's syndrome** occurs when there is an excess of chromosomal material relating to chromosome 21.
a. **Types**
(1) **Trisomy 21** is the most common. There are three 21 chromosomes; the extra chromosome is acquired because of a failure in chromosomal pairing of one of the parental germ cells.
(2) **Translocation** occurs when the long arm of chromosome 21 becomes attached to another chromosome (13, 18, or another 21). This disorder, unlike trisomy 21, is usually inherited. The translocation chromosome may be found in unaffected parents and siblings; these asymptomatic carriers have only 45 chromosomes.
(3) **Trisomy mosaic 21** is the rarest form; only some of the cells are trisomic while others are normal.

b. **The incidence** of Down's syndrome in the United States is about 1 in 700 births. Women over 35 years of age have a 1 in 100 chance of having a Down's syndrome child (trisomy 21). If a translocation is present, the risk is about 1 in 3 for all women.

c. **Characteristic pathologic findings** include:
(1) Embryonic convolutional patterns of the brain.
(2) A small cerebellum and brain stem.
(3) Abnormalities of the pituitary gland.
(4) Cardiac anomalies, particularly septal defects.

d. **Clinical features** include:
(1) Mental retardation. Most patients are moderately or severely retarded with only a minority having an IQ above 50. Mental development appears to progress normally up to 6 months after which IQ decreases from near normal at 1 year to about 30 at older ages.
(2) Hypotonia.
(3) Oblique palpebral fissures.
(4) Abundant neck skin.
(5) A small flattened skull.
(6) High cheek bones.
(7) Broad, thick hands with a transverse palmar crease.
(8) Short and inwardly curved little fingers.
(9) A fissured and thickened tongue.

e. **Prevention.** Down's syndrome can be prevented by prenatal screening with amniocentesis or chorionic villous sampling. However, these methods have several drawbacks.
(1) There is a risk to the fetus.
(2) They are primarily performed on women over 35 years of age; thus, Down's syndrome births among young women are still possible.
(3) Prevention is possible only by abortion, which raises additional ethical and religious concerns.

4. **Spina bifida** is a neurological defect, which permits leakage of cerebral spinal fluid. Surgery can sometimes correct the spinal cord defect but not always.
   a. **Incidence** is variable among different nationalities, but it occurs most frequently in infants of Irish extraction.
   b. **Occurrence** is not linked to maternal age, but may be as high as 5% if either parent or a sibling has the disorder.
   c. **Characteristic pathologic findings** include:
      (1) Mental retardation.
      (2) Paraplegia.
      (3) Incontinence.
   d. **Prevention.** Amniocentesis at midgestation can be used to detect elevation of alpha-fetoprotein consistent with a neural tube defect. Thus, prevention, as in Down's syndrome, depends on induced abortion.

B. Nongenetic conditions

1. **Infections**
   a. **Syphilis.** While uncommon, this preventable disorder does occur, resulting in congenital syphilis.
      (1) **Clinical features**
         (a) **In early congenital syphilis**, the most severely affected fetuses are stillborn. Of the live-born syphilitic infants, most have no lesions at birth but develop papular skin rashes, osteochrondritis, and jaundice. Invasion of the central nervous system is usually asymptomatic.
         (b) **In late congenital syphilis**, the stigmata represent the end stage of an early lesion and include Hutchinson's teeth, notched or peg-shaped central incisors, interstitial keratitis often leading to blindness, and symmetric synovial effusions of the knees. Involvement of the central nervous system may result in paresis.
      (2) **Treatment**
         (a) Syphilitic infections are responsive to penicillin therapy.
         (b) The fetus may be successfully treated in utero via medication given to the mother.
         (c) The neonate is successfully treated by a dose of 50,000 or 100,000 units of penicillin G per kilogram of body weight.
   b. **Rubella virus** affects the fetus only if it is contracted between the eighth and thirteenth weeks of pregnancy. Congenital rubella syndrome includes:
      (1) Deafness.
      (2) Blindness.
      (3) Heart defects.
      (4) Mental retardation.

2. **Environmental factors**
   a. **Lead and mercury exposure** can cause mental retardation in young children.
   b. **Fetal alcohol syndrome**, associated with maternal alcoholism, may cause mental retardation.
      (1) **Clinical features**
         (a) Low birth weight
         (b) Microcephaly
         (c) Flattened facial features
         (d) Mild to moderate mental retardation
      (2) **An incidence** of at least 0.02% has been suggested.
      (3) **Prevention** involves abstinence or at least strict moderation of alcohol intake during pregnancy.
   c. **Nutritional deficiencies**
      (1) **Maternal iodine deficiency** at conception and during early pregnancy leads to cretinism, which includes mental retardation.
         (a) It typically occurs in noncoastal areas and can be prevented by maternal iodine supplementation.
         (b) Early treatment of infants prevents mental retardation.
         (c) Sporadic cretinism that is not associated with iodine deficiency in the diet is rare.
      (2) **Low birth weight** (less than 2500 g) is associated with mental retardation. The incidence of mental retardation among low-birth-weight infants has declined in the United States in the last 30 years.
         (a) In the United States, maternal smoking, drinking, and drug abuse affect birth weight more than maternal diet.
         (b) In developing countries, malnutrition and maternal infections are more important causes of low birth weight.

(c) In the United States, undernourishment solely during pregnancy does not cause mental retardation.

(d) Premature infants of very low birth weight (less than 1500 g) previously suffered high mortality rates in the perinatal period. Cerebral palsy and mental retardation occurred in survivors. Although mortality rates in the United States have been reduced, rates of cerebral palsy and mental retardation have not fallen correspondingly.

V. PREVENTION OF MENTAL RETARDATION

A. Primary measures

1. Continue research into the causes of mental retardation.
2. Provide genetic counseling, prenatal diagnosis, early detection, and proper treatment to prevent mental retardation of genetic origin.
3. Prevent infections and parasitic diseases as well as monitor the environment to protect against chemical and physical hazards.
4. Improve social and economic conditions, which may lead to secondary phenomena, such as malnutrition, prematurity, obstetric hazards, and understimulation.
5. Provide good obstetric, prenatal, and postnatal care, including treatment of maternal illness; fetal monitoring; recognition of obstetric abnormalities; and prediction, prevention, and treatment of biochemical abnormalities.

B. Secondary measures

1. Provide a stimulating and emotionally stable environment for the infant and growing child.
2. Provide suitable educational programs for infants and children with normal intellectual potential who have isolated motor, sensory, perceptual, behavioral, and intellectual difficulties.
3. In the case of culturally determined retardation, provide more sensory, verbal, and emotional stimulation, and introduce new experiences and useful skills to widen the child's intellectual horizon.

C. Tertiary measures include core and community services.

1. **Behavioral and personality difficulties**
   - a. The chief obstacle to effective therapy is the difficulty in establishing communication with the child. Engaging the child in shared activities is probably the most effective way to establish a relationship.
   - b. Individual and group psychotherapy are effective only if they are integrated into the total milieu of the child.
   - c. Drugs may play an important role in treatment if the child is hyperactive or overstimulated. Phenothiazines are the most commonly prescribed drugs.
2. **Behavior modification** is a commonly used treatment, involving:
   - a. Delineating the behavior that needs to be changed.
   - b. Recording the frequency of that behavior.
   - c. Reinforcing either positively or negatively the target behavior.
3. **Parental counseling**
   - a. Early diagnosis of mental retardation can improve the chances of harmonious parent-child relationships.
   - b. The parents' helplessness is best handled by giving the parents specific tasks to do and stressing their role in helping the child to develop as normally as possible.
   - c. The most difficult decision to be made is whether or not to institutionalize the child. Communication with appropriate community services should be established and maintained for counseling and support in this decision.
4. **Training, education, treatment, and rehabilitation**
   - a. The main obstacle to these goals in most state institutions is their large size and their inclusion of patients with all degrees of mental and physical handicaps.
   - b. Some facilities may serve the needs of mildly retarded persons who cannot be cared for at home but do not require institutionalization.
   - c. At present, there are about 200,000 mentally retarded individuals in institutions, which is between 3% and 4% of the total retarded population in the United States.

5. **Special education.** The present system of special education distinguishes between educable and trainable individuals to prepare the mentally retarded student for future life adjustments.
   a. Other than reading, writing, and basic mathematics, there is less emphasis on academics and more emphasis on vocational training.
   b. There is an attempt to discover precise assets of individuals so that a specific program can use these assets.
   c. Operant conditioning techniques based on the principles of reinforcement of desired behavior, such as rewarding self-dressing with hard candy, has been introduced successfully.
   d. The value of psychiatric guidance and consultation has been recognized.

VI. FUTURE NEEDS IN MENTAL RETARDATION

A. Training medical students is an essential step in the process of physicians' education in mental retardation.

B. Diversity of handicaps associated with mental retardation requires a variety of services; the concept of a comprehensive multipurpose center in the community might be the answer to providing a thorough evaluation and treatment of the problems associated with mental retardation.

C. Future research is essential in mental retardation.

1. There are many areas in biochemical research that may aid in the prevention and treatment of mental retardation, including the inborn errors of metabolism, storage diseases, and structure of chromosomes.
2. Modern research may bring the possibility of the alteration of genetic material.
3. There is a need for a better understanding of fetal metabolism and placental function.
4. Basic and applied research is still required to improve present teaching methods.

STUDY QUESTIONS

Directions: Each question below contains five suggested answers. Choose the **one best** response to each question.

1. Phenylketonuria (PKU), a disorder of amino acid metabolism, has which of the following characteristics?

(A) It occurs in blacks 10 times more frequently than in whites
(B) It is caused by a deficiency in the enzyme that breaks down the protein phenylalanine
(C) It is successfully treated by giving massive doses of the missing enzyme
(D) It is transmitted by a sex-linked recessive gene
(E) It is prevented by identification of affected fetuses in utero by amniocentesis

2. Tay-Sachs disease is characterized by

(A) the accumulation of lipid substances in the nerve cells in the central nervous system
(B) a biochemical defect that involves the storage of sphingomyelins in the neurons, liver, and spleen
(C) transmission by a sex-linked recessive gene
(D) four separate disease entities distinguished by age of onset
(E) profound mental retardation evident at birth

Directions: Each question below contains four suggested answers of which **one or more** is correct. Choose the answer

A if **1, 2, and 3** are correct
B if **1 and 3** are correct
C if **2 and 4** are correct
D if **4** is correct
E if **1, 2, 3, and 4** are correct

3. The treatment of the mentally retarded with core and community services involves

(1) behavior modification
(2) helping parents decide whether or not to institutionalize the mentally retarded child
(3) operant conditioning techniques
(4) providing a stimulating environment for the growing child

4. For the future, there are many needs in special education, including

(1) building modern institutions to house more of the mentally retarded
(2) training medical students to assess and treat the mentally retarded
(3) training psychiatrists in dynamic psychotherapy for the mentally retarded
(4) biochemical research into the inborn errors of metabolism

Directions: The group of questions below consists of lettered choices followed by several numbered items. For each numbered item select the **one** lettered choice with which it is **most** closely associated. Each lettered choice may be used once, more than once, or not at all.

Questions 5–8

For each description of mental functioning listed below, select the intelligence quotient score that is most appropriate.

(A) 79 and below
(B) 20 to 35
(C) 70 to 79
(D) 110 to 139
(E) 90 to 109

5. Severe mental retardation
6. Mental retardation
7. Average intelligence
8. Superior intelligence

ANSWERS AND EXPLANATIONS

1. The answer is B. [*IV A 1 a (1)–(6)*] Phenylketonuria (PKU) is a rare defect in amino acid metabolism, involving a deficiency of enzymes essential for the breakdown of phenylalanine. Since phenylalanine cannot be broken down, it accumulates in the blood, and the resulting hyperphenylalanemia adversely affects the brain of the developing infant. The fetus is not affected, as the mother has the essential enzyme; the problem arises postnatally. However, dietary treatment of infants with PKU has been successful in preventing mental retardation. Since the genetic defect (it is transmitted as an autosomal recessive trait) cannot be detected by amniocentesis, all infants are screened at birth for PKU. The prevalence is 1 in 15,000 in an average white population; it is rare in blacks.

2. The answer is A. [*IV A 2 a (1)–(2)*] Tay-Sachs disease involves the accumulation of lipid substances known as gangliosides in the nerve cells throughout the central nervous system. Niemann-Pick disease involves the storage of sphingomyelins. Tay-Sachs disease, which occurs chiefly among Ashkenazi Jewish infants, is transmitted by an autosomal recessive gene. Tay-Sachs is one of four separate disease entities called cerebromacular degeneration, which are distinguished by age of onset. Infants with Tay-Sachs appear normal at birth, but progressive mental and physical deterioration begins at 4 to 8 months of age.

3. The answer is A (1, 2, 3). (*V B 1, C 2, 3 c, 5 c*) Core and community services are tertiary prevention measures, which include behavior modification, counseling to determine whether institutionalization is a proper choice given that large institutions group patients together regardless of their disabilities, and operant conditioning techniques, which are based on the principles of reinforcement of desired behavior. Provision of a stimulating environment for a growing child is a secondary prevention measure.

4. The answer is C (2, 4). (*VI A–C*) It has been shown that the mentally retarded are better handled in the community if at all possible. Training medical students so that they can assess and treat mentally retarded individuals in the community is an essential step in the process of a physician's education. Future research is essential in mental retardation, including biochemical and genetic research and research in fetomaternal health. Dynamic psychotherapy is reserved for those individuals with normal intellect.

5–8. The answers are: 5-B, 6-A, 7-E, 8-D. (*III A 1–2*) Mental retardation is classified according to the objectives sought, such as intelligence quotient (IQ), etiology, and specific syndromes. Classification by IQ is an arbitrary method based on the results of standardized tests. To determine IQ, mental age is divided by chronologic age, and the result is multiplied by 100. Mental retardation encompasses all IQs below 79; however individuals with IQs of 70 to 79 are considered borderline cases. Severe mental retardation is indicated by an IQ between 20 and 35. Average intelligence is measured as between 90 and 109, and superior intelligence is measured as between 110 and 139.

11
Substance Abuse

Christina L. Herring

I. INTRODUCTION. Historically, there has been confusion concerning the difference between drug addiction and drug dependence.

A. ***The Diagnostic and Statistical Manual for the Classification of Mental Disorders-II (DSM-II)*** used the term drug dependence instead of drug addiction and listed drug and alcohol abuse as distinct entities.

B. **The *DSM-III*** combines drug and alcohol abuse under Substance Abuse Disorders.

1. **Nonpathologic substance use** is distinguished from **substance abuse** by the following three criteria:
   - **a.** A pattern of pathologic use, including:
     - **(1)** Intoxication throughout the day.
     - **(2)** Inability to moderate or stop.
     - **(3)** Continuation of use despite medical contraindications.
     - **(4)** A need for daily use for adequate functioning.
   - **b.** Impairment in social or occupational functioning.
   - **c.** Duration of at least 1 month.

2. **Substance dependence**, a more severe form of substance abuse disorder than substance abuse, is determined by physical dependence as evidenced by either tolerance or withdrawal.
   - **a. Tolerance** means that increased amounts of the substance are required to achieve the desired effect.
   - **b. Withdrawal** means that following cessation or reduction in intake a substance-specific syndrome will result.

II. EPIDEMIOLOGY OF SUBSTANCE ABUSE. Substances associated with both abuse and dependence include alcohol, barbiturates, opioids, amphetamines, and cannabis. Three additional substances—cocaine, phencyclidine (PCP), and hallucinogens—are associated with abuse only; physical dependence has not yet been demonstrated.

A. **Alcohol.** Alcohol abuse constitutes the most serious drug problem in the United States.

1. **Incidence.** Nearly 100 million people in the United States drink alcohol, and although more than 90% do so without harm, an estimated 9 million Americans suffer from alcoholism.

2. **Sex.** Population surveys indicate that between 3% and 5% of adult men and between 0.1% and 1% of adult women are alcoholics.

3. **Injuries.** Alcoholics are associated with an annual toll of 25,000 traffic fatalities, 15,000 homicides and suicides, and 20,000 deaths from alcohol-associated diseases.

4. **Crime.** One-third of the arrests that occur each year are for public intoxication. If arrests for drunken driving, disorderly conduct, vagrancy, and other alcohol-related offenses are included, the proportion rises to 50% of arrests.

5. **Social profile.** One study showed that heavy drinkers tended to be:
   - **a.** Men and women 45–49 years old.
   - **b.** Members of low socioeconomic groups.
   - **c.** Service workers.
   - **d.** Unmarried.

e. City dwellers.
f. Catholic or Protestant.
g. American Indians.

B. Drugs

1. Barbiturates. Barbiturates are legitimately manufactured in immense quantities and are readily available in numerous forms. For example, in 1954, at least 800,000 pounds of barbiturates were produced in the United States, and since 1962, production has increased to over 1 million pounds per year. Production is presently sufficient to supply every individual in the country with 50 doses.

a. Social profile. Individuals with a dependence on barbiturates fall into one of three patterns of use.

(1) Chronic intoxication occurs in 30- to 50-year-old individuals who obtain drugs from their physicians rather than from illegal sources. They are members of the middle or upper classes, and their drug dependence may go unnoticed by family members or close friends for months or years.

(2) Episodic intoxication occurs in teenagers or young adults who ingest barbiturates for the same purpose that they consume alcohol—to produce a "high."

(3) Intravenous barbiturate use occurs in young adults who are involved in the illegal drug culture. They may also use amphetamines and heroin. They use barbiturates because they are less expensive.

b. The incidence and prevalence of barbiturate abuse are impossible to estimate.

2. Opioids. Most addiction rates are calculated according to the Baden formula, which assumes that the number of heroin deaths reported in New York City represents 1% of all addicts.

a. Incidence. The National Institute of Mental Health reported that there were 62,045 active narcotic addicts in 1969. More than half of the known addicts live in New York City. The Federal Bureau of Narcotics and Dangerous Drugs reported that there were 560,000 active narcotic addicts, or 0.3% of the population, in 1973.

b. Sex. Men are primarily affected: the men to women ratio is approximately 5:1.

c. Social profile

(1) In the 1950s, the typical heroin addict was an urban dweller, a member of a minority group, especially black or Spanish-speaking, male, and in his late twenties or early thirties.

(2) In New York City, however, there has been a shift toward younger ages with the average age of patients in drug-free programs just over 17 years. In fact, the Board of Education of New York City estimates that 8% of high school age youngsters use heroin.

(3) In 1966, 98% of the addicts admitted to the Lexington and Fort Worth Public Health Service Hospitals were urban residents.

(4) Among the medical profession, the narcotic addiction rate is estimated to be between 1% and 2% as contrasted with the overall rate of 0.3% for the entire United States population.

3. Amphetamines. Recent surveys among student populations have revealed that in some cities significant amphetamine abuse occurs in children in the fifth and sixth grades and that between 15% and 25% of all high school students are regular speed users. However, cocaine is now replacing amphetamines as the drug most abused so that amphetamine abuse is confined to teenagers who experiment with drugs.

a. The incidence of amphetamine abuse is impossible to determine because most abusers do not come to the attention of the medical profession.

(1) By 1958, the legal production of amphetamines in the United States was 3.5 billion tablets—enough to supply every citizen with about 20 standard (5 mg) doses.

(2) By 1968, the drug industry was producing 8 billion tablets.

(3) By 1970, production exceeded 10 billion tablets.

b. Uses. In the 1950s, amphetamines were popularly prescribed as a safe way to diet since the addiction potential was not known. Today, few physicians prescribe amphetamines as there are few legitimate indications.

4. Marijuana

a. Social profile. The Commission on Marijuana and Drug Abuse conducted the first large scale probability study of individuals over 12 years of age and found that:

(1) Young adults 18 to 25 years of age are the heaviest drug users with about one-fourth currently using marijuana.

(2) Approximately 11% of high school seniors use marijuana daily.

(3) There appears to be a sharp decline in use after the age of 25.

b. The demand for marijuana has not increased substantially over the past 10 years.

III. ETIOLOGY OF ADDICTION TO ALCOHOL

A. Family studies on alcoholism consistently emphasize the high prevalence of alcoholism among relatives of alcoholics. In most studies, at least 25% of male relatives are alcoholic. These studies also show a higher than expected frequency (between 5% and 10%) of alcoholism among female relatives. Identification of hereditary factors in family studies involves:

1. **Twin studies**, which study identical and fraternal twins to determine concordance for alcoholism.
2. **Genetic marker studies**, which examine the relationship between a known inherited biologic trait and a familial disease, suggesting that the latter is genetically transmitted.
3. **Adoption studies**, which involves interviewing children of alcoholics.

B. Twin, adoption, and genetic marker studies

1. Identical twins are more often concordant for alcoholism than are fraternal twins.
2. Identical twins are more concordant for quantity and frequency of drinking but not for the adverse consequences of drinking.
3. Associations between a genetic marker and alcoholism have not been determined unequivocally.
4. Children of alcoholics are particularly vulnerable to alcoholism whether they are raised by their alcoholic parents or by nonalcoholic foster parents. This vulnerability is specific for alcoholism and does not involve risk for other psychopathology.
5. Individuals raised apart from their alcoholic parents were significantly more likely to have a drinking problem if a biologic parent was alcoholic than if a surrogate parent was alcoholic.
6. Although women are less often heavy drinkers than are men, among those who do drink heavily, an unusually high percentage become alcoholic. Also, women from alcoholic families are prone to be depressed, while men in these families are prone to alcoholism. In one study, 30% of daughters raised by alcoholics had been treated by age 32 for depression, compared to about 5% of controls.

C. Familial alcoholism. A useful subcategory of alcoholism, "familial alcoholism," has been proposed, which should include:

1. A family history of alcoholism.
2. Early onset of alcoholism.
3. Severe symptoms, requiring treatment at an early age.
4. Absence of other conspicuous psychopathology.

IV. THEORIES OF ADDICTION

A. Psychoanalytic theories

1. **Freud** believed that addiction was the result of strong oral influences in childhood. Drugs provide an escape from reality.
2. **Menninger** held that a self-destructive drive is the prime component in addiction—that is, addiction was considered the means by which individuals who had a powerful, but unconscious, urge for self-destruction could destroy themselves. This urge was thought to be derived from the guilt that resulted from a child's anger toward his or her parents who frustrated his or her needs for oral gratification.
3. **Adler** attributed the cause of addiction to powerful feelings of inferiority related to a perpetual state of insecurity and a desire to escape responsibility.
4. **Rado** was the first psychoanalyst to suggest that drug use might represent an individual's attempt to cope with difficult emotional states. Rado argued that it was not the drug but rather the individual's impulse to use it that made him or her an addict.
5. **Chein, Gerard, Lee, and Rosenfeld** argued that not only depression but also states of anxiety, panic, and self-rejection fed the impulse to use drugs.

6. **Vaillant** urged practitioners to assess the addict's ego functions and then attempt to:
   a. Find a substitute for each immature defense.
   b. Control self-destructive behavior.
   c. Provide a context for involvement and acceptance.
7. **Wurmser** emphasized the heterogeneity of drug abusers and proposed a hierarchical model of causation for drug dependence.
8. **Khantzian** focused on how specific drug effects—energizing (amphetamines and cocaine), relaxing (sedative-hypnotics), and controlling (opiates)—interact with distinct personality factors and behavior patterns. He suggested that individuals select one drug over another in an attempt to cope with specific problems in their internal and external environments, which would be unmanageable and unbearable without the particular drug effect.

B. Learning theories. Learning theorists are concerned with setting responses into motion.

1. **Rewarded responses.** When response is followed by reward, the relationship between stimulus and response is strengthened. This strengthening of the cue-response connection is the essence of learning.
   a. **Dollard and Miller** pointed out that alcohol results in a temporary reduction of fear and conflict.
   b. **Shoben** held that the release from anxiety arising from the first drinking experience is the method by which reinforcement principles operate in alcoholism.
2. **Unrewarded responses.** Whenever a response is unrewarded by a reaction that lessens the drive to respond, the response tends to disappear, letting others appear. The extinction of successive unrewarded responses produces random behavior.

C. Sociologic theories

1. **Horton** studied the consumption of alcohol, subsistence security, and accessibility of alcohol in 77 cultures. He found a high degree of correlation between subsistence insecurity and excessive drinking.
2. **Bales** relates social organization and cultural practice to alcoholism based on:
   a. The degree to which a culture influences the needs for adjustment or inner tensions in its members.
   b. The attitudes toward drinking, which the culture encourages in its members.
   c. The degree to which the culture provides suitable substitute means of satisfaction.

V. PREVENTION OF SUBSTANCE ABUSE.

Approaches to the prevention of alcohol- and drug-related problems have been derived mainly from three important models.

A. Public health model. Although critics question whether the health field is capable of preventing alcohol and drug problems as they may be more social than medical in nature, the public health model proposes three points of intervention.

1. **Host.** The individual's knowledge about alcohol and drugs and the attitudes that influence abuse patterns must be considered.
2. **Agent.** The content, distribution, and availability of alcohol and drugs are important factors that influence abuse patterns.
3. **Environment.** The setting or context in which substance use occurs and the community mores that influence it must be examined.

B. Distribution of consumption model. A direct relationship appears to exist between per capita consumption and the prevalence of heavy use of alcohol and drugs.

1. **de Lint** reviewed research on control measures and concluded that minor variations in density, location, and type of outlet, hours and days of sales, or other regulations have no measurable effect on the rates of alcohol consumption.
2. **Popham** and associates noted that an increase in opportunities to drink results in increased drinking and drunkenness; however they also found that widespread availability promoted moderate drinking. In addition, they reviewed the effect of the legal restraints on drinking and discovered that:
   a. Highly restrictive controls on accessibility lead to lower consumption levels and fewer alcohol problems.
   b. Controls are unlikely to be implemented in the absence of substantial public support.

c. Controls usually involve a variety of social and political costs that eventually are perceived to outweigh their benefits.

3. **Smart** concluded that lowering age limits for purchase and consumption of alcohol leads to increased alcohol consumption and alcohol problems among young people.

4. Reviews indicate that a rise in alcohol prices generally led to a decrease in alcohol consumption, and a rise in the income of consumers generally led to an increase in alcohol consumption.

C. **Sociocultural model** emphasizes the relationship between alcohol problems and the normal patterns of alcohol use within a society. Alcohol-related problems are likely to occur:

1. In the presence of personal ambivalence and anxiety about alcohol.
2. In situations in which the juxtaposition of drinking events and social situations generate social conflict and problematic consequences.
3. In the presence of norms that encourage excessive and problem drinking.
4. As one set of problems in a cluster of other problems that occur in the individual's relationship to social structures.

VI. TREATMENT AND REHABILITATION OF SUBSTANCE ABUSERS

A. **Alcohol withdrawal.** Studies indicate that recovery rates and improvement rates for alcoholics following treatment depend on a number of factors.

1. Alcoholics of higher socioeconomic status and higher social stability have significantly higher improvement rates than alcoholics of lower socioeconomic status and lower social stability.
2. Recent studies of treatment outcome for socially stable, middle-class alcoholics provide evidence that alcoholism inpatient treatment is effective. However, the length of inpatient stay for primary alcoholism treatment has been reduced for the typical alcoholic patient as continued outpatient treatment services have become available.
3. A multidisciplinary approach was more effective than individual psychotherapy.
4. Patients with few psychologic problems improved in any treatment program, while patients with serious psychologic problems showed virtually no improvement in any program.
5. Abstention remains the ideal treatment goal for alcoholics.

B. **Drug withdrawal**

1. The first step in drug-free and antagonist treatment programs is withdrawal from the drug of abuse. The user is then stabilized or a substitution of methadone is made immediately. After a satisfactory initial suppression of the abstinence syndrome, the methadone is withdrawn over a period of 3 to 7 days at the rate of 5 mg/day.
2. Present treatment approaches appear to stress either nonbiologic or biologic models.
   a. **Nonbiologic models.** Among the nonbiologic models are various psychotherapeutic attempts, including:
      (1) Group psychotherapy.
      (2) Residential treatment centers, such as Synanon and Daytop.
      (3) Religious, political, and social pressures, such as those exerted by Black Muslims and Black Panthers.
      (4) Punitive legal enforcements.
      (5) Therapeutic communities, such as Odyssey House and Phoenix House.
         (a) The idea of the therapeutic community originated with Chuck Dederick, the founder of Synanon, whose rehabilitation efforts rely on harsh group encounters, re-education, and hard work. Synanon's major tenet is that addicts are immature people in flight from reality and responsibility who need to be given a second chance to grow up.
         (b) The therapeutic communities adhere to the concept that the abuse of drugs is symptomatic of underlying antisocial personality problems and behavior patterns.
         (c) The largest therapeutic community, Phoenix House in New York City, consisted of 15 houses and more than 1000 residents in 1970. From 1967 to 1970, during the first 3 years of its existence, only 148 Phoenix House residents completed a 2½ year program and returned to a drug-free life.

b. Biologic models. Five biologic models have been proposed for the treatment of narcotics addiction. Two (i.e., methadone maintenance and narcotic antagonists) are in current use, and three (i.e., biochemical blockade, receptor blockade, and immune therapy) are still experimental.

(1) Methadone maintenance is based on the assumption that heroin addiction is a metabolic disease. It is also assumed that if the addict is supplied with adequate quantities of opiate, he will not find it necessary to resort to criminal activity. The patients return to the clinic six times a week for 3 months. Those who adhere to the program and appear to be showing substantial progress in rehabilitation are placed on a three-times-a-week schedule, receiving one dose at the clinic and a 2-day supply to take at home. In a highly selective original group, 80% of patients remained in the program over a 5-year period.

(2) Narcotic antagonists prevent opiates from acting; they do not exert a narcotic effect nor are they addictive. The extinction of drug-seeking behavior could provide a means to reverse the pathophysiology of addiction. If the relief afforded by narcotics during the period of conditioned abstinence were blocked, the extinction of physical and psychic dependence could occur. The major weakness of the antagonist model is the lack of any mechanism compelling the addict receiving the antagonist to continue.

BIBLIOGRAPHY

Adler A: Individual psychiatry of alcoholic patients. *J Crim Psychopathol* 3:74, 1941

American Psychiatric Association: *Diagnostic and Statistical Manual of Mental Disorders*, 3rd ed. Washington, DC, American Psychiatric Association, 1975

Baden, M: Narcotic abuse: a medical examiner's view. *NY State J Med* 72:834, 1972

Bales RF: Cultural difference in rates of alcoholism. *Q J Stud Alcohol* 6:480, 1946

Bruun K, Edwards G, Lumo M, et al: *Alcohol Control Policies in Public Health Perspective*, vol 25. Finnish Foundation for Alcohol Studies, New Brunswick, NJ, Rutgers Center for Alcohol Studies, 1975

Cahalan D, Cisin, IH, Crossley HM: *American Drinking Practices: A National Survey of Drinking Behavior and Attitudes*. New Brunswick, NJ, Rutgers Center of Alcohol Studies, 1969

Chein I, Gerard DL, Lee RS, et al: *The Road to H: Narcotics, Delinquency and Social Policy*. New York, Basic Books, 1964

de Lint J: Alcohol control policy as a strategy for prevention: a critical examination of the evidence. Presented at the International Conference on Alcoholism and Drug Dependence, Liverpool, England, 1976

Dollard JA, Miller NE: *Personality and Psychotherapy: An Analysis in Terms of Learning, Thinking and Culture*. New York, McGraw-Hill, 1950

Federal Register, vol 38 (90), sect 130 44(8), May 10, 1973

Goodwin DW: Is alcoholism hereditary? A review and critique. *Arch Gen Psychiatry* 25:545–549, 1971

Horton D: Function of alcohol in primitive societies: cross-cultural study. *Q J Stud Alcohol* 4:199, 1943

Jellinek EM, Jolliffe N: Effect of alcohol on the individual: review of the literature of 1939. *Q J Stud Alcohol* 1:110–181, 1940

Kaij L: Studies on the Etiology and Sequels and Abuse of Alcohol. Thesis, University of Lund, Sweden, 1960

Kalant QJ: *The Amphetamines: Toxicity and Addiction*. Toronto, University of Toronto Press, 1966

Khantzian EJ: Self-selection and progression in drug dependence. *Psychiatry Digest* 36:19–22, 1975

McLennan AT, O'Brien CP, Krou R, et al: Matching substance abuse patients to appropriate treatments: a conceptual and methodological approach. *Drug Alcohol Depend* 5:189–195, 1980

Menninger KA: *Man Against Himself.* New York, Harcourt Brace, 1938

National Commission on Marijuana and Drug Abuse: *Marijuana: A Signal of Misunderstanding: First Report of the National Commission on Marijuana and Drug Abuse.* Washington, DC, United States Government Printing Office, 1972

National Institute of Mental Health: *The Mental Health of Urban America*. Washington, DC, United States Public Health Service, 1969

Parlanen J, Bruun K, Markkanen T: *Inheritance of Drinking Behavior: A Study on Intelligence, Personality, and Use of Alcohol of Adult Twins*. Helsinki, Finland, Finnish Foundation for Alcohol Studies, 1966, pp 14–159

Popham RE: A critique of the genetotrophic theory of the etiology of alcoholism. *Q J Stud Alcohol* 14:228, 1953

Rado A: The psychoanalysis of pharmacothymia. *Psychoanalytic Q* 2:1–23, 1933

Schuckit MA, Goodwin DW, Winokur G: A half-sibling study of alcoholism. *Am J Psychiatry* 128: 1132–1136, 1972

Smart RG: The relationship of availability of alcoholic beverages to per capita consumption and alcoholism rates. *Q J Stud Alcohol* 38:891–896, 1976

Swartz J: Barbiturates. *Tex Med* 68:54, 1972

Vaillant GE: A 12 year follow-up of New York narcotic addicts (IV). *Am J Psychiatry* 123:573–584, 1966

Wikler A: Diagnosis and treatment of drug dependence of the barbiturate type. *Am J Psychiatry* 125: 758, 1968

Wurmser L: Psychoanalytic considerations of the etiology of compulsive drug use. *J Am Psychoanal* 22:820–843, 1974

STUDY QUESTIONS

Directions: Each question below contains five suggested answers. Choose the **one best** response to each question.

1. Which of the following substances is associated with both abuse and dependence?

(A) Cocaine
(B) Cannabis
(C) LSD
(D) Phencyclidine (PCP)
(E) "Ecstacy"

2. Studies on the epidemiology of barbiturate use have shown that

(A) together legitimate manufacturing and illegal production of barbiturates produce over 1 million pounds per year
(B) because it is an expensive habit to maintain, users often resort to petty crime to finance their addiction
(C) chronic intoxication may go unnoticed for years, even by family members and close friends.
(D) the incidence is relatively easy to compute since barbiturate prescriptions are controlled by the Food and Drug Administration
(E) most users engage in intravenous administration since that is the most intense high

3. Epidemiologic studies of heroin use show that

(A) addiction rates assume that the number of heroin deaths in New York City represent 1% of all addicts
(B) the men to women ratio is about 2:1
(C) the Board of Education of New York City estimates that 18% of high school students use heroin
(D) within the medical profession, the addiction rate is estimated at between 5% and 6%.
(E) the number of addicts found by the National Institute of Mental Health is much larger than that estimated by the Federal Bureau of Narcotics and Dangerous Drugs

Directions: Each question below contains four suggested answers of which **one or more** is correct. Choose the answer

A if **1, 2, and 3** are correct
B if **1 and 3** are correct
C if **2 and 4** are correct
D if **4** is correct
E if **1, 2, 3, and 4** are correct

4. Treatment for drug use involves which of the following methods?

(1) Methadone maintenance
(2) Group psychotherapy
(3) Withdrawal from the drug of abuse
(4) Residence in a therapeutic community

5. Family studies of alcoholism have shown that

(1) there is a high prevalence of alcoholism among relatives of alcoholics
(2) children of alcoholics are vulnerable to alcoholism even if raised by nonalcoholic foster parents
(3) female relatives of alcoholics are more apt to be depressed, while male relatives are more apt to become alcoholic
(4) identical twins are more concordant for the adverse consequences of drinking than for the quantity and frequency of drinking

ANSWERS AND EXPLANATIONS

1. The answer is B. (*II*) There are five classes of substances that are associated with both abuse and dependence: alcohol, barbiturates, opioids, amphetamines, and cannabis. Three additional substances—cocaine, phencyclidine, and LSD—are associated with abuse only; physical dependence has not yet been demonstrated.

2. The answer is C. (*II B 1*) Barbiturates are legitimately manufactured in immense quantities (over 1 million pounds per year) and are readily available in numerous forms. Barbiturate use is a habit that is relatively inexpensive to maintain since barbiturates are manufactured for a medical use. Chronic intoxication is not easily detected and may go unidentified even by family members for months or years. The incidence and prevalence are impossible to estimate because most abusers are undetected. Intravenous barbiturate use does occur, but it involves a small number of people—usually young adults involved in an illegal drug culture.

3. The answer is A. (*II B 2*) Most addiction rates are calculated according to the Baden formula, which assumes that the number of heroin deaths reported in New York City represent 1% of all addicts. The men to women ratio has been reported to be 5:1. The Board of Education of New York City estimates that 8% of high school students use heroin. Within the medical profession, the narcotic addiction rate is estimated to be between 1% and 2%. The estimate of addiction done by the Federal Bureau of Narcotics and Dangerous Drugs was much larger than that done by the National Institute of Mental Health.

4. The answer is E (all). (*VI B 1–2*) Treatment for substance abuse can be either nonbiologic where former addicts are asked to take responsibility for their addiction or biologic where heroin addiction is assumed to be a metabolic disease and methadone is prescribed. Synanon relies on harsh group therapy encounters—the major tenet being that addicts are immature people in flight from reality and responsibility. The first step in withdrawal is that the user is withdrawn from the drug of abuse. Therapeutic communities, which have shown some success, adhere to the concept that the abuse of drugs is symptomatic of underlying antisocial personality problems and behavior problems.

5. The answer is A (1, 2, 3). (*III A 1–2*) Most studies show a high prevalence of alcoholism among relatives of alcoholics—that is, at least 25% of male relatives and 5% of female relatives are alcoholic. In one study, identical twins were more concordant for quantity and frequency of drinking but not for the adverse consequences of drinking. Other studies have shown that children of alcoholics are vulnerable to alcoholism whether raised by their alcoholic parents or by nonalcoholic foster parents. Family studies have shown that female relatives of alcoholics are prone to depression, while male relatives are prone to alcoholism.

12
Occupational Medicine

Peter Orris
Stephen Michael Hessl
Daniel Oleh Hryhorczuk

I. INTRODUCTION

A. Labor force. In 1984, the labor force in the United States numbered 113,544,000 of a total population of 176,383,000 individuals who were 16 years or older.

1. Approximately 56.2% of the labor force were men and 43% were women in 1984. The percentage of women in the labor force has increased by 2.2% since 1980 and 6.2% since 1975.

2. Approximately 86.7% of the labor force were white and 10.6% were black in 1984.

B. Distribution of the labor force. From 1979–1984, the percentage of the labor force engaged in manufacturing and agriculture declined, while those engaged in service and trade increased. See Table 12-1 for the distribution of the work force in 1979 and 1984.

C. Occupational diseases and injuries

1. Occupational injuries increased from 4.9 million in 1983 to 5.3 million in 1984, the first yearly increase in this decade.

2. The United States Bureau of Labor Statistics reported 124,800 new cases of occupational illnesses in 1984, which represented an increase of 19,000 cases over 1983.

D. Definitions

1. **American Conference of Governmental Industrial Hygienists (ACGIH)** is a voluntary independent association that publishes a set of recommended safe exposure levels for industrial toxins.
2. **Disability** is the effect of an impairment on the ability of an individual to function in society.
3. **Environmental epidemiology** is the study of environmental toxins and their effects on populations.
4. **Environmental Protection Agency (EPA)** is an agency established as a separate branch of the government in 1970 to provide research, standard setting, and enforcement to "protect human health in the environment."
5. **Epidemiology** is the study of disease in populations.
6. **Ergonomics** is the study of the interaction of human beings and an engineered environment.

Table 12-1. Distribution of the Work Force in 1979 and 1984 as Reported by the Labor Department

	Percentage of Labor Force	
	1979	**1984**
Manufacturing	21.1%	18.5%
Service	19.4%	22.4%
Agriculture	3.3%	3.1%
Trade	22.0%	22.7%

7. **Impairment** is the objective description of the loss of function of the human body.
8. **Medical surveillance** is periodic medical testing designed to identify adverse health effects of environmental substances prior to the point at which they cause permanent disability.
9. **National Institute for Occupational Safety and Health (NIOSH)** is an agency established in 1970 as part of the United States Department of Health and Human Services to provide for research, professional training, and advice to the Occupational Safety and Health Administration concerning the science of occupational safety and health.
10. **Occupational disease** is any disease caused in whole or in part by exposure in the work environment, usually excluding accidental trauma.
11. **Occupational medicine** is the diagnosis and treatment of human pathology caused in whole or in part by an individual's work environment.
12. **Occupational Safety and Health Administration (OSHA)** is an agency established in 1970 as part of the United States Labor Department to "assure safe and healthful working conditions" for American workers. It is charged with establishing, enforcing, and educating the public concerning workplace health and safety standards.
13. **Permissible exposure limit (PEL)** is a term that was created by OSHA to identify the maximum legally allowable exposure of a toxic substance in the workplace.
14. **Threshold limit value (TLV)** is an airborne concentration of substances established by the ACGIH to represent conditions under which nearly all workers may work without adverse effects.
15. **Time weighted average (TWA)** is an average concentration of airborne substances usually calculated on an 8- or 10-hour workday.
16. **Toxicology** is the study of external substances and their effects on humans.
17. **Toxin** is a substance in the environment with the potential for causing human disease or injury.
18. **Workman's Compensation** is a series of state laws that establish a no-fault insurance system for workers disabled on the job.

II. OCCUPATIONAL HISTORY. Occupational diseases frequently present as common medical conditions, such as asthma, lung cancer, atopic dermatitis, peripheral neuropathy, and psychiatric disorders. A key factor in a physician's ability to recognize an occupational disease is the occupational history.

A. Screening the patient. A schema that can be used routinely by all practicing physicians, regardless of specialty, to assist in the detection of occupational and environmental diseases follows. Screening questions related to work exposure should be asked of all patients and should include:

1. **A chronological list of all jobs.** This is important because work exposures in the past may be etiologic factors in diseases presenting years later.
2. **A description of any temporal relationships between a work exposure and a presenting illness.** This relationship may provide clues as to the etiology of disease. It is important to ascertain, for example, if the patient's condition improves on weekends or vacations.
3. **Known hazards in the workplace.** As part of a review of systems, the patient should always be asked questions about exposure to fumes, dusts, chemicals, loud noise, or radiation in the workplace.

B. Screening the employer. Additional information may be required to establish the degree of exposure when an occupational disease is suspected. In addition to seeking occupational information from the patient, it may be useful to obtain information from the employer, OSHA records, the labor union, or by a site visit to the workplace, remembering that these activities must be performed *only* with the consent of the patient to avoid a breach of patient confidentiality. Questions that focus on a specific hazard or job thought to be related to the patient's condition include:

1. **General conditions of the workplace**, such as the size of the work area, location and adequacy of ventilation, location of changing rooms and showers, and any history of citations for violations of workplace standards.

2. **The specifics of the patient's exposure**, such as the distance from the toxin and the route of absorption.
3. **Personal protective devices**, such as the types of respirators used, the frequency of respirator use, the adequacy of fit, and the availability of replacement filters.
4. **The presence of disease in co-workers**.
5. **The chemical composition of the toxin and the levels of exposure**.

III. OCCUPATIONS that exemplify (not exhaust) the hazards, associated diseases, and target organs relevant to occupational health are discussed below.

A. Foundry workers. There are approximately 340,000 foundry workers in the United States who work in the metal casting industry. Important hazardous exposures in this industry include:

1. **Silicon dioxide**, which is a crystalline silica that is used in the molding process. It is capable of causing silicosis.
2. **Asbestos**, which is used in forming gates and riser sleeves of molds and in the linings of furnaces and ladles. It is associated with:
   - **a.** Lung cancer (and other cancers).
   - **b.** Mesothelioma.
   - **c.** Asbestosis.
   - **d.** Pleural disease.
3. **Polycyclic aromatic hydrocarbons**, which are formed from the burning of fossil fuels and the heating of oil binders. They are associated with:
   - **a.** Lung cancer.
   - **b.** Skin cancer.
4. **Formaldehyde and isocyanate compounds**, which are used in binding resins. They are associated with:
   - **a.** Irritation of the mucous membranes and eyes.
   - **b.** Asthma.
5. **Noise**, which is associated with:
   - **a.** Hearing loss.
   - **b.** Hypertension.
6. **Metal dusts and fumes**, such as beryllium, nickel, chromium, lead, and zinc. They are associated with:
   - **a.** Metal fume fever.
   - **b.** Cancer.
   - **c.** Nervous system, hematologic, and renal diseases.
7. **Carbon monoxide**, an asphyxiant gas, which is a product of the decomposition of binder systems and burning of carbonaceous substances. Carbon monoxide strongly binds with hemoglobin and may seriously compromise the oxygen-carrying capacity of blood.
8. **Heat**, especially excessive heat near ovens and furnaces, which may produce:
   - **a.** Heat exhaustion.
   - **b.** Heat stroke.
   - **c.** Burns.
9. **Nonionizing** (ultraviolet and infrared) **radiation**, which is associated with:
   - **a.** Cataracts.
   - **b.** Photoallergic reactions and burns of the skin.

B. Painters. There are over 200,000 painters and allied tradesmen in the United States. Occupational exposures include:

1. **Solvents.** These agents may cause neural behavioral abnormalities and skin conditions, such as chronic dermatitis secondary to defatting of the skin.
2. **Pigments.** Chromate pigments have been associated with elevated lung cancer risks. Lead oxide was a serious hazard in the past, but its use has been limited in recent years; however, removing old paint can be a lead hazard.
3. **Polyurethane paints and acrylic paints.** These materials have caused asthma in exposed workers.

C. Welders. Gas and electric arc welding are common occupations throughout the United States. Important hazardous exposures associated with these occupations include:

1. **Ultraviolet light.** Excessive exposure may cause skin burns, and short-term exposure of the eyes may cause a painful conjunctivitis known as "flash burn."
2. **Heat.** Excessive heat stress may cause:
   a. Heat exhaustion.
   b. Heat stroke.
   c. Skin burns.
3. **Metal fumes.** Welders may be exposed to the fumes of iron, chrome, nickel, vanadium, copper, zinc, lead, tungsten, and cobalt, depending on the composition of the metals being welded, the welding rods, and the flux. These substances are toxic to the respiratory system and may cause:
   a. Pneumoconiosis.
   b. Bronchitis or bronchiolitis.
   c. Metal fume fever.
4. **Gases.** Chlorine and phosgene gases, which are hazardous respiratory irritants that cause pneumonitis and pulmonary edema, may be present when welding is done in an atmosphere of degreasing solvents. Carbon monoxide, an asphyxiant gas, and ozone, an irritant gas that causes mucous membrane and respiratory irritation, are commonly present in the welding environment.
5. **Noise, ionizing radiation, and electrical hazards.**

D. Artists. Modern painters and sculptors use a wide variety of materials, many of which are new and untried. A partial list of hazardous substances used by artists includes:

1. **Solvents**, which are used as diluents and thinners. These materials are associated with:
   a. Irritation of the skin and mucous membranes.
   b. Neural behavioral abnormalities.
2. **Synthetic resins**, such as acrylics, polyvinyl chloride, and polyvinyl acetate, which are hazardous during formulation and heating. These resins are associated with:
   a. Mucous membrane irritation.
   b. Allergic skin and respiratory reactions.
3. **Dusts.** While working with siliceous stone, such as quartz and granite, or wood, sculptors may be exposed to silica dust and wood dust, which are associated with:
   a. Pneumoconiosis.
   b. Asthma.
   c. Nasopharyngeal cancer.

E. Office workers. Occupational disorders that afflict office workers have only recently been recognized. These disorders can result from:

1. **Video display terminals.** Workers who must spend a large portion of their time working with video display terminals commonly complain of:
   a. Eye strain.
   b. Musculoskeletal discomfort.
2. **Repetitive trauma.** Repetitive tasks like mail sorting may produce such conditions as:
   a. Carpal tunnel syndrome.
   b. Tendonitis.
3. **Indoor air pollution.** The "tight building syndrome," which results from office work in modern, energy-efficient buildings with reduced outside air exchange, can produce:
   a. Headache.
   b. Nausea.
   c. Eye irritation.
4. **Stress.** Isolation, confinement, overload, or an inability to control the work load or work conditions can produce stress, leading to:
   a. Anxiety.
   b. Depression.
   c. Drug and alcohol abuse.
   d. Cardiovascular disease.
   e. Peptic ulcer disease.

F. Health care workers. There are more than 3 million hospital employees in the United States. Due to the technological complexity of health care and the risks inherent in caring for sick members of society, there are a great many health hazards to which health care workers are exposed, including:

1. **Safety hazards**, such as:
   a. Lifting obese patients.
   b. Electrical shocks.
   c. Needle sticks.
   d. Accidents caused by long work hours.
2. **Ethylene oxide.** This commonly used gas sterilant can cause:
   a. Skin and mucous membrane burns.
   b. Neuropathy.
   c. Leukemia.
3. **Waste anesthetic gases.** More than 50,000 operating room personnel are exposed to anesthetic gases in trace concentrations, which are associated with:
   a. Spontaneous abortion.
   b. Teratogenesis.
   c. Mutagenesis.
   d. Carcinogenesis.
   e. Liver disease.
4. **Infectious diseases**, such as:
   a. Hepatitis B and C.
   b. Tuberculosis.
   c. Herpes simplex virus.
   d. Acquired immune deficiency syndrome.
5. **Cytotoxic agents.** Chemotherapeutic agents are administered to an estimated 200,000 to 400,000 people annually. Although undocumented as yet, chronic effects in workers who administer these agents may include:
   a. Reproductive abnormalities.
   b. Cancer.
   c. Irritation to mucous membranes, eyes, and skin (nitrogen mustard).

G. Machinists. Machine tools, such as drill presses, milling machines, and lathes are in general use in many workshops. Common hazards include:

1. **Noise**, which is associated with hearing loss.
2. **Safety hazards.** Injuries occur when hair or clothing becomes entangled in machines or when safety mechanisms have not been installed or used correctly. Common injuries include:
   a. Finger loss.
   b. Lacerations.
   c. Musculoskeletal strain.
3. **Cutting and cooling oils.** Conditions associated with use of these oils include:
   a. Skin cancer.
   b. Oil acne.
   c. Eczematous dermatitis.
   d. Febrile illness (Pontiac fever).

IV. POTENTIALLY HAZARDOUS EXPOSURES

A. Metals

1. **Arsenic**
   a. **Uses.** Arsenic is used in metallurgy and pesticides and is produced as a by-product of smelting ores.
   b. **Exposure**
      (1) Inhalation
      (2) Skin absorption (especially organic forms and arsenic trichloride)
      (3) Ingestion
   c. **Toxicity.** Exposure to arsenic fumes or dust may produce:
      (1) Nasal septal ulceration and perforation.

(2) Skin disorders, such as hyperpigmentation, hyperkeratosis, and gangrene of the fingers and toes.
(3) Lung cancer in gold miners and others after chronic exposure.
(4) Peripheral neuropathy, particularly after repeated high-dose exposure.

d. Special tests to aid in the diagnosis of toxicity include:
(1) Urinary arsenic levels.
(2) Hair and nails for arsenic.

2. Beryllium

a. Uses. Beryllium is used as a hardening agent in alloys.

b. Exposure is by inhalation.

c. Toxicity

(1) Acute. Exposure to the soluble salts of beryllium can cause pneumonitis and inflammation of:
(a) Conjunctivae.
(b) Nasal pharynx.
(c) Trachea.
(d) Bronchi.

(2) Chronic. Granulomas of the skin and lung may be accompanied by chronic debilitating disease with:
(a) Dyspnea.
(b) Dry cough.
(c) Anorexia.
(d) Fatigue.
(e) Malaise.
(f) Weight loss.

d. Special tests to aid in the diagnosis of toxicity include:
(1) Assay of tissue samples for the levels of beryllium.
(2) Analysis of blood samples to detect lymphocyte blast transformation, indicating sensitization to beryllium salt.

3. Cadmium

a. Uses. Cadmium is used in electroplating, as an aluminum solder, and in nickel cadmium batteries.

b. Exposure is by inhalation.

c. Toxicity

(1) Acute. Cadmium dust and fumes are severe pulmonary irritants, which may result in:
(a) Pneumonitis.
(b) Pulmonary edema.

(2) Chronic. Repeated exposure to low levels of cadmium may result in:
(a) Chronic lung disease.
(b) Renal tubular damage.
(c) Osteomalacia-like disease.
(d) Prostatic cancer.
(e) Respiratory tract cancer.

d. Special tests
(1) Elevated urinary cadmium levels indicate exposure only.
(2) Low molecular weight proteinuria may be an early sign of renal toxicity.

4. Lead

a. Uses. Lead is used in batteries, paint, ceramics, and ammunition.

b. Exposure
(1) Inhalation
(2) Ingestion

c. Toxicity, which is usually manifested in the adult after chronic exposure, results in:
(1) Nervous system abnormalities, such as:
(a) Motor weakness, including paralysis of the extensor muscles of the wrists.
(b) Nerve conduction abnormalities.
(c) Neural behavioral abnormalities, including weakness, lassitude, and insomnia.
(2) Hematologic abnormalities, such as anemia secondary to impaired heme synthesis.
(3) Nephropathy, including hyperuricemia (saturnine gout).
(4) Reproductive tract abnormalities, such as:
(a) Fetal toxicity.
(b) Abnormal sperm.

d. Special tests to aid in the diagnosis of toxicity include:
(1) Analysis of whole blood for lead content.

(2) Assay of free erythrocyte porphyrin or zinc protoporphyrin levels in blood to assess the body's burden of lead.
(3) Injection of calcium disodium EDTA and measurement of urinary lead content for further assessment of the body's burden of lead.

5. Mercury

a. Uses. Mercury is used in industrial instruments, pesticides, electrical apparatus, and dental amalgams.

b. Exposure
(1) Inhalation
(2) Ingestion
(3) Skin absorption

c. Toxicity
(1) Neurologic disturbances (as exhibited by the Mad Hatter in *Alice in Wonderland*)
(a) Incoordination
(b) Tremor
(c) Psychic disturbances, including insomnia, irritability, and indecision
(d) Visual field abnormalities
(2) Renal abnormalities, such as proteinuria
(3) Skin and mucous membrane abnormalities
(a) Stomatitis
(b) Gingivitis
(c) Skin irritation
(4) Pulmonary difficulties
(a) Pneumonitis
(b) Bronchitis

d. Special tests to aid in the diagnosis of toxicity include assaying the amount of mercury in a 24-hour urine sample.

6. Nickel

a. Uses. Nickel is used in electroplating, in the production of catalysts, in nickel cadmium batteries, and in alloys.

b. Exposure is by inhalation.

c. Toxicity
(1) "Nickel itch" is a dermatitis that results from sensitization to nickel. Asthma has also been described from inhalation of nickel sulfate.
(2) Chronic exposure has been associated with cancer of the paranasal sinuses and lungs in workers in nickel refineries.

7. Zinc

a. Uses. Zinc chloride is used as a soldering flux. Zinc oxide is produced when elemental zinc is heated at high temperatures, such as in the manufacturing of bronze and in galvanizing.

b. Exposure is by inhalation.

c. Toxicity. Zinc is an essential element in human metabolism; however, inhalation of zinc oxide fumes may cause an influenza-like illness termed "metal fume fever."

B. Solvents are a very large and heterogeneous group of chemical substances, which are used to dissolve other materials. In general, common usage refers to organic and inorganic solvents, which cause both acute and chronic health effects, including toxicity to the central and peripheral nervous systems and dermatologic, renal, hepatic, cardiovascular, and hematologic systems. Common organic solvents are listed below.

1. Aliphatic hydrocarbons [e.g., n-hexane, which should not be confused with common hexane (C_3H_6)].

a. Uses. Aliphatic hydrocarbons are solvents that are used in quick drying rubber cements and inks as well as in oil extraction processes.

b. Exposure is by inhalation.

c. Toxicity
(1) Upper respiratory irritation
(2) Central nervous system depression
(3) Peripheral neuropathy

2. Aromatic hydrocarbons (e.g., benzene)

a. Uses. Aromatic hydrocarbons are used as chemical intermediates in the production of other organic chemicals. They are used in solvents, unleaded gasoline, and paint removers.

b. Exposure
(1) Inhalation
(2) Skin absorption

c. Toxicity. There is clinical and epidemiologic data linking benzene with:
(1) Leukemia, especially the acute myeloblastic type.
(2) Central nervous system depression.
(3) Hematopoietic system depression.

3. Cyclic hydrocarbons (e.g., cyclohexane)

a. Uses. Cyclic hydrocarbons are used as chemical intermediates and in solvents for rubber, waxes, resins, oils, and fats.

b. Exposure is by inhalation.

c. Toxicity
(1) Irritation of the skin and mucous membranes
(2) Central nervous system depression
(3) Possible liver and kidney damage

4. Alcohols (e.g., methanol)

a. Uses. Alcohols are used in paints, varnishes, cements, and in the production of formaldehyde, inks, and dyes.

b. Exposure
(1) Inhalation
(2) Skin absorption

c. Toxicity
(1) Optic neuropathy
(2) Metabolic acidosis

d. Special tests
(1) Measurement of formic acid levels in urine
(2) Measurement of acid-base balance, such as arterial blood gas determinations

5. Nitrohydrocarbons (e.g., nitroethane)

a. Uses. Nitrohydrocarbons are used for organic chemical synthesis and as solvents.

b. Exposure is by inhalation.

c. Toxicity
(1) Irritation of the mucous membranes and respiratory system
(2) Possible central nervous system depression
(3) Liver toxicity with high-dose exposures

6. Glycols (e.g., ethylene glycol)

a. Uses. Glycols are used in antifreeze and hydraulic fluids.

b. Exposure is by ingestion. Respiratory exposures are not considered to be toxic.

c. Toxicity
(1) Central nervous system depression
(2) Renal failure related to the formation of glycolic and oxalic acids after ingestion

7. Esters (e.g., ethyl acetate)

a. Uses. Esters are used as lacquer solvents.

b. Exposure is by inhalation.

c. Toxicity
(1) Mucous membrane irritation
(2) Eczematous eruptions
(3) Possible central nervous system depression
(4) Anemia
(5) Pulmonary irritation with high exposures

8. Ethers (e.g., ethylene glycol monoethyl ether)

a. Uses. Ethers are used as solvents for lacquers and alkyl resins in the dyeing of textiles and leather and as cleaners and varnish removers.

b. Exposure
(1) Inhalation
(2) Skin absorption

c. Toxicity
(1) Mucous membrane irritation
(2) Possible bone marrow disorders
(3) Lung and renal injuries with high doses

9. Ketones (e.g., methyl ethyl ketone)

a. Uses. Ketones are used as solvents for resins, gums, synthetic rubber, lacquers, varnishes, and lubricating oils.

b. Exposure is by inhalation.
c. Toxicity
(1) Mucous membrane irritation
(2) Possible central nervous system depression with high exposure

10. Aldehydes (e.g., formaldehyde)
a. Uses. Aldehydes are used in urea formaldehyde, phenol formaldehyde, and other plastics, as a disinfectant and a fumigant, and in paper, rubber, and dye manufacturing.
b. Exposure is by inhalation.
c. Toxicity. Formaldehyde is mutagenic and carcinogenic in animal species and is being investigated as a human carcinogen.
(1) Strong irritation to mucous membranes and the respiratory system
(2) Sensitization dermatitis of the eczematous type
(3) Possible asthma

11. Halogenated hydrocarbons (e.g., carbon tetrachloride)
a. Uses. Halogenated hydrocarbons are used as solvents for lacquers, varnishes, waxes, resins, oils, and fats. Carbon tetrachloride has been used for degreasing, cleaning, and in the past, as a fire extinguisher.
b. Exposure
(1) Inhalation
(2) Skin absorption
c. Toxicity
(1) Central nervous system depression
(2) Severe damage to the liver and kidneys with necrosis of the liver and renal tubular necrosis.

C. Dusts

1. Inorganic dusts
a. Asbestos
(1) **Uses.** Asbestos is used as insulation, in fireproofing and roofing materials, and in automotive parts.
(2) **Exposure** is by inhalation; however, ingestion may be a factor in malignancy.
(3) **Toxicity**
(a) Interstitial lung disease (asbestosis)
(b) Benign pleural effusion
(c) Pleural thickening and calcification
(d) Mesothelioma
(e) Gastrointestinal cancer
(f) Laryngeal cancer
(g) Lung cancer
b. Coal
(1) **Uses.** Coal is used as a heating fuel and in the manufacture of coke.
(2) **Exposure** is by inhalation.
(3) **Toxicity.** Coal workers' pneumoconiosis is characterized by coal macules, which appear as small, rounded opacities on chest radiograph. Progressive massive fibrosis may develop. Coal workers may also have an increased risk of gastric cancer.
c. Hard metals (e.g., tungsten carbide and cobalt)
(1) **Uses.** Hard metals are used for high-speed cutting tools and drills and armor plating.
(2) **Exposure** is by inhalation.
(3) **Toxicity.** A diffuse interstitial pulmonary fibrosis may occur, which produces fine linear opacities on chest film. Also, asthma and fibrosing alveolitis have been described.
d. Iron
(1) **Uses.** Iron is used in welding and casting and in steel structures.
(2) **Exposure** is by inhalation.
(3) **Toxicity.** Siderosis results from inhalation of iron oxide fume or dusts. This pneumoconiosis differs from coal, silica, and asbestos in that there is little or no functional impairment of the respiratory system, although the chest film may reveal impressive rounded opacities.
e. Silica
(1) **Uses.** Silica is used as a blasting abrasive in molding sands in metal casting, pottery, porcelain, glass, granite cutting, grinding, and tunneling.
(2) **Exposure** is by inhalation.
(3) **Toxicity.** Crystalline silica or silicon dioxide has been associated with three forms of lung disease:
(a) Acute silicoproteinosis

(b) Accelerated silicosis, especially in sand blasters and often associated with atypical *Mycobacteria*

(c) Chronic silicosis, which is a pneumoconiosis characterized by silicotic nodules in the lungs and rounded opacities on chest film

f. Talc

(1) **Uses.** Talc is used in paint, pharmaceuticals, cosmetics, ceramics, rubber, roofing, and paper.

(2) **Exposure** is by inhalation.

(3) **Toxicity**

(a) Diffuse interstitial pulmonary fibrosis with nodular or irregular opacities on chest film

(b) Pleural thickening and calcified pleural plaques

2. Organic dusts

a. Cotton dust

(1) **Uses.** Cotton is used for yarns and fabric.

(2) **Exposure** is by inhalation.

(3) **Toxicity.** Byssinosis is a bronchospastic respiratory condition that begins as occasional chest tightness on the first day of the work week but may progress to permanent respiratory disability with severe irreversible impairment of lung function.

b. Thermophilic mold spores

(1) **Uses.** The genuses of *Thermoactinomyces*, *Penicillium*, *Cryptostroma*, and *Micropolyspora* may contaminate moldy hay, moldy sugar cane stalks (bagasse), maple bark, and a variety of other organic materials.

(2) **Exposure** is by inhalation.

(3) **Toxicity.** Hypersensitivity pneumonitis as a result of allergic sensitization to the mold spore antigens has been described. A variety of names has been attached to this condition, depending on the nature of the exposure and the type of mold responsible, such as farmer's lung, bird fancier's lung, bagassosis, mushroom worker's lung, and maple bark stripper's disease.

D. Pesticides are chemical substances designed to kill, repel, or otherwise control populations of organisms considered pests to man. These may be grouped as insecticides, fungicides, herbicides, and vertebrate poisons.

1. Insecticides

a. Organophosphorus compounds

(1) **Exposure**

(a) Inhalation

(b) Skin absorption

(c) Ingestion (accidental or deliberate)

(2) **Toxicity.** This group of compounds inhibits acetylcholinesterase and produces continuous stimulation of cholinergic fibers, resulting in muscarinic or nicotinic manifestations of toxicity.

(3) **Special tests**

(a) Measurement of serum cholinesterase levels

(b) Measurement of cholinesterase levels in red blood cells

b. Carbamate compounds

(1) **Exposure**

(a) Inhalation

(b) Skin absorption

(c) Ingestion

(2) **Toxicity.** The carbamate insecticides, such as carbaryl, are short-acting acetylcholinesterase inhibitors. Their toxicity is similar to the organophosphorus pesticides.

(3) **Special tests**

(a) Measurement of cholinesterase levels in red blood cells

(b) Measurement of serum cholinesterase levels

c. Organochlorine compounds

(1) **Exposure**

(a) Inhalation

(b) Skin absorption

(c) Ingestion

(2) **Toxicity.** Organochlorine compounds, such as chlorophenothane (DDT), dieldrin, lindane, and chlordane, currently have very limited use. They accumulate in fat stores and may remain in the environment for long periods of time. They probably interfere with axionic transmission of nerve impulses and have produced liver and kidney dis-

ease in animals. Several of them have been carcinogenic, teratogenic, and mutagenic in animal models.

d. Pyrethrins
- **(1) Exposure** is by inhalation.
- **(2) Toxicity**
  - **(a)** Dermatitis
  - **(b)** Occasional pulmonary sensitization

2. Fungicides

a. Organic mercury compounds
- **(1) Exposure**
  - **(a)** Inhalation
  - **(b)** Skin absorption
  - **(c)** Ingestion
- **(2) Toxicity.** The alkylmercury compounds, such as methylmercury and ethylmercury chloride, may cause central nervous system dysfunction and irritation of the skin, eyes, and mucous membranes. Severe intoxication results in paresthesias of the lips, hands, and feet; ataxia; dysarthria; impairment of vision and hearing; emotional disturbances; and spasticity. Dermatitis may also occur.

b. Creosote and other phenols
- **(1) Exposure**
  - **(a)** Rapid skin absorption
  - **(b)** Inhalation
  - **(c)** Ingestion
- **(2) Toxicity**
  - **(a)** Irritation of the skin, eyes, and upper respiratory system
  - **(b)** Hyperpyrexia and heat stroke
  - **(c)** Chloracne
- **(3) Special tests** include urine testing for pentachlorophenol.

c. Dimethyldithiocarbamate compounds
- **(1) Exposure** is by inhalation.
- **(2) Toxicity**
  - **(a)** Irritation of the eyes and respiratory tract
  - **(b)** Dermatitis in sensitized individuals
  - **(c)** Antabuse-like effect after ethanol ingestion

d. Organotin compounds
- **(1) Exposure**
  - **(a)** Inhalation
  - **(b)** Skin absorption
- **(2) Toxicity**
  - **(a)** Irritation of eyes, mucous membranes, and skin
  - **(b)** Hepatic necrosis
  - **(c)** Cerebral edema

3. Herbicides

a. Chlorophenoxy compounds
- **(1) Exposure** is by inhalation.
- **(2) Toxicity**
  - **(a)** Chloracne
  - **(b)** Peripheral neuropathy
  - **(c)** Liver dysfunction
  - **(d)** Adverse reproductive effects
  - **(e)** Soft tissue sarcoma and other cancers

b. Paraquat
- **(1) Exposure**
  - **(a)** Inhalation
  - **(b)** Skin absorption
  - **(c)** Ingestion
- **(2) Toxicity.** Ingestion has been associated with:
  - **(a)** Rapid progressive pulmonary fibrosis.
  - **(b)** Myocardial, hepatic, and renal dysfunction.
  - **(c)** Irritation of eyes, skin, and mucous membranes.

4. Rodenticides

a. Warfarin
- **(1) Exposure**
  - **(a)** Inhalation

(b) Skin absorption
(2) **Toxicity**
(a) Hypoprothrombinemia
(b) Vascular injury resulting in hemorrhage

b. Yellow phosphorus
(1) **Exposure**
(a) Inhalation
(b) Ingestion
(c) Skin absorption
(2) **Toxicity**
(a) Direct contact may result in deep thermal burns. Prolonged direct absorption may cause necrosis of the maxilla and mandible (phossy jaw).
(b) Ingestion results in severe injury to the gut and peripheral zonal necrosis of the liver.
(c) Inhalation results in strong irritation to mucous membranes.

5. Nematocides

a. Dibromochloropropane
(1) **Exposure**
(a) Inhalation
(b) Skin absorption
(2) **Toxicity**
(a) Oligospermia
(b) Aspermia

b. Ethylene dibromide
(1) **Exposure**
(a) Inhalation
(b) Skin absorption
(2) **Toxicity**
(a) Severe irritation of the mucous membranes and respiratory system
(b) Central nervous system depression
(c) Central lobular necrosis of the liver
(d) Focal proximal tubular damage in the kidney

E. Irritant gases. Several gases can produce acute and chronic damage to the air passages and pulmonary parenchyma.

1. Water soluble gases. Gases that are highly water soluble, such as sulfur dioxide, ammonia, and chlorine, cause intense irritation to mucous membranes and unless trapped, workers should immediately remove themselves from exposure. Chlorine, an example of a soluble irritant gas, has the following characteristics.

a. Uses. Chlorine is used for water purification and in chemical manufacturing of pesticides, bleach, disinfectants, and household cleaners.

b. Exposure is by inhalation.

c. Toxicity. Severe irritation of mucous membranes, eyes, and skin at high concentrations may result in burns to these areas. Tracheobronchitis, pulmonary edema, and pneumonitis may occur after inhalation of high concentrations. Chronic effects include prolonged airflow obstruction and mild hypoxemia.

2. Insoluble gases. Gases that are less water soluble, such as phosgene, nitrogen dioxide and ozone, may be inhaled deeply into the lungs without warning or a cough reflex. Nitrogen oxide (NO_2), an example of an insoluble irritant gas, has the following characteristics.

a. Uses. Nitrogen oxide is a by-product of silo filling, welding, and combustion of nitrogen-containing materials, such as explosives, chemical manufacturing, space flight, and nitric and sulfuric acid production.

b. Exposure is by inhalation.

c. Toxicity. Pulmonary edema may occur within 1 to 2 hours after heavy exposure. However, a late, recurrent pulmonary edema may occur as late as 2 to 3 weeks after exposure. Of those who survive the acute injury, chronic pulmonary disease with bronchiolitis obliterans may develop.

3. Other irritant gases include:

a. Acetaldehyde, which is used in the manufacture of plastics, synthetic rubber, acetic acid, and disinfectants.

b. Acrolein, which is used in the manufacture of pharmaceuticals, resins, and food supplements.

c. **Ammonia**, which is used in refrigeration, the manufacture of fertilizers, nitric acid, plastics, and explosives.
d. **Hydrogen chloride**, which is used in pickling of steel, the manufacture of chlorinated organic chemicals, and in dyes.
e. **Hydrogen fluoride**, which is used in etching of glass, manufacturing of aluminum, fluorocarbons, and in alkylation processes.
f. **Ozone**, which is a by-product of photochemical smog, welding, and high-voltage electrical equipment.
g. **Phosgene**, which is a by-product of combustion of chlorinated compounds.
h. **Phosphine**, which is used in fumigation, acetylene gas production, and flares.
i. **Sulfur dioxide**, which is used in the manufacture of sulfuric acid, bleaches, fumigation, refrigeration, and is a by-product of petroleum refining and combustion of fossil fuels.

F. Asphyxiant gases. Any gas in high enough concentration can displace oxygen and cause asphyxiation due to oxygen deprivation. The gases listed below, however, are especially toxic and have caused many deaths because of the direct effect they have on oxygen transport processes within the body.

1. Carbon monoxide

a. **Uses.** Carbon monoxide is a by-product of the incomplete combustion of carbonaceous substances.
b. **Exposure** is by inhalation.
c. **Toxicity.** Carbon monoxide has an affinity for hemoglobin about 240 times greater than oxygen. This binding with hemoglobin interferes with the release of oxygen from hemoglobin and affects such critical tissues as the myocardium and central nervous system.
d. **Special tests** include measurement of blood carboxyhemoglobin levels.

2. Hydrogen cyanide

a. **Uses.** Hydrogen cyanide is used in fumigation, annealing of steel, and the purification of gold and silver.
b. **Exposure**
  (1) Inhalation
  (2) Skin absorption
  (3) Ingestion
c. **Toxicity.** Cyanide ion inhibits many enzyme systems, particularly the cytochrome oxidase system, thereby inhibiting cellular respiration.
d. **Special tests** include measurement of blood and tissue cyanide levels.

3. Hydrogen sulfide

a. **Uses.** Hydrogen sulfide is used in leather tanning and is a by-product of sewage and petroleum.
b. **Exposure** is by inhalation.
c. **Toxicity**
  (1) Irritation of the mucous membranes and eyes
  (2) Respiratory paralysis
  (3) Inhibition of respiratory enzymes

G. Physical stressors

1. Noise

a. **Exposure**
  (1) Decibel (db) is a unit of measure of sound intensity. A scale between 0 and 140 is logarithmic—for example, 10 times 1 db and 20 db is 100 times 1 db.
  (2) Hertz (cycles per second) is a unit of measure of pitch or frequency.
b. **Toxicity** to the auditory system usually is manifested after chronic exposure to at least 90 db.
  (1) Acoustic trauma. Bone or tissue damage can result from exposure to a high pressure wave (e.g., an explosion).
  (2) Noise-induced hearing loss. A sensorineuronal deficit involving the hair cells of the cochlea can be produced by loud, sustained noise.
    (a) Temporary threshold shift is a loss of hearing that recovers within the first 24 hours after exposure but may also show improvement over a 7-day period.
    (b) Permanent threshold shift is a loss of hearing that occurs first in the 4000 hertz frequency range, extending gradually with continued exposure through the higher frequencies and finally in the lower frequencies as well. These changes are irreversible.
  (3) Noise levels of 90 dbA (decibels recorded reflecting the attenuation produced by the human ear) of the average workplace will cause a 25% 1000–3000 hertz hearing loss in

approximately 25% of individuals exposed over a 40-year period. A similar loss will be caused by 85 dbA in 10%–15% and 80 dbA in 0%–5%.

c. Special tests include audiometric hearing testing at intervals between 500 and 8000 cycles per second (hertz).

d. Treatment. None

2. Heat

a. Exposure. The American Conference of Governmental Hygienists recommends that for an 8-hour day, 40-hour week, light work should not be performed at higher than 86°F in a humid environment and heavy work, at no more than 77°F.

b. Toxicity

(1) Acute

(a) Heat fatigue

(b) Heat cramps characterized by muscle spasm

(c) Heat exhaustion characterized by:

(i) Volume depletion

(ii) Fatigue

(iii) Occasional emesis

(iv) Light headedness

(d) Heat stroke resulting in:

(i) Hyperthermia of over 106°F

(ii) Dry flushed skin

(iii) Confusion progressing to coma

(2) Chronic toxicity is poorly defined by the literature.

c. Treatment. Heat stroke is treated with rapid cooling, intravenous fluids, and treating any electrolyte abnormalities. All other reactions can be treated with rest, removal from the hot environment, and oral fluids.

3. Cold

a. Exposure. Workers should not be exposed to environments that do not permit the body to maintain its core temperature.

b. Toxicity

(1) Hypothermia is characterized by:

(a) Decreased core temperature.

(b) Confusion progressing to coma.

(c) Cardiac arrhythmias on rewarming.

(2) Frostbite is characterized by frozen tissue with irreversible cellular damage.

(3) Chilblains is characterized by swelling of exposed skin after prolonged cold exposure.

4. Acute trauma disorders, the most common occupational health problem, include:

a. Fractures.

b. Dislocations

c. Strains.

d. Abrasions.

e. Lacerations.

5. Cumulative trauma disorders, a consequence of repetitive awkward motions, include:

a. Bursitis.

b. Tenosynovitis.

c. Carpal tunnel syndrome.

d. Degenerative joint disease.

6. Barotrauma

a. Exposure. Workers who are employed in occupations below sea level, such as divers, tunnel diggers, and others, may experience barotrauma.

b. Toxicity

(1) Air emboli

(2) Nitrogen emboli (bends)

(3) Bone necrosis

c. Treatment is by repressurizing and surfacing slowly to allow for reacclimatization.

H. Radiation

1. Ionizing radiation includes x-rays, gamma rays, alpha particles, and beta particles.

a. Exposure. The average annual dose equivalent for occupationally exposed workers in the United States is 0.3 rem; the maximum allowable dose is 5 rem. A chest x-ray produces gamma radiation equivalent to 0.017 rem and an abdominal film, 0.485 rem.

b. Toxicity
- **(1) Acute high dosage** produces:
  - **(a)** Leukopenia.
  - **(b)** Purpura.
  - **(c)** Hemorrhage.
  - **(d)** Fever.
  - **(e)** Diarrhea.
  - **(f)** Electrolyte disorders.
  - **(g)** Convulsions.
  - **(h)** Ataxia.
  - **(i)** Lethargy.
- **(2) Chronic low level exposure** produces cancer of many organs.

2. Nonionizing radiation includes radio frequency, infrared, microwaves, and visible frequencies.
- **a. Exposure** is ubiquitous.
- **b. Toxicity.** High-dose directed exposure to microwaves will produce cataracts. Long-term effects to a variety of organ systems have not been well documented.

I. Biologic hazards

1. Bacterial diseases
- **a. Brucellosis**, a bacterial disease that causes fever, sweats, malaise, and weight loss, is most apt to affect veterinarians, animal attendants, farmers, packinghouse workers, rendering-plant workers, tanners, and laboratory workers.
- **b. Tularemia**, a bacillary disease associated with skin ulcerations and a systemic syndrome, affects outdoor workers, hunters, trappers, foresters, veterinarians, and laboratory workers.
- **c. Leptospirosis**, which is characterized by fever, headache, meningeal inflammation, and an immune second phase, affects farmers, construction workers, sewer workers, veterinarians, and packinghouse workers.
- **d. Anthrax**, a bacillary infection that manifests as skin ulcerations but may cause hemorrhagic mediastinitis, is almost exclusively seen in handlers of imported hides, wool, and goat hair.
- **e. Erysipeloid**, which is caused by a gram-positive bacillus that produces a local cellulitis or meningitis, affects butchers, kitchen workers, fish handlers, and tanners. It is contracted by contact with infected swine, cattle, sheep, fish, dogs, and rabbits.
- **f. Tetanus**, which produces muscle spasms, affects agricultural workers in particular.
- **g. Plague**, which may cause adenitis or pneumonia, affects shepherding families, farmers, ranchers, hunters and geologists in sparsely populated areas of the Western United States.
- **h. Tuberculosis**, which frequently manifests as a pulmonary infection, affects physicians, nurses, and laboratory workers.
- **i. Cutaneous granulomas** from *Mycobacterium marinum (balnei)* is seen primarily in fish handlers.
- **j. Psittacosis**, an influenza-like illness, affects individuals who raise and process poultry, pet shop workers, bird fanciers, and zoo attendants.

2. Rickettsial and chlamydial diseases
- **a. Rocky Mountain spotted fever and Colorado tick fever**, which are transmitted by tick bites and cause malaise, irritability, fever, muscle aches, and anorexia that may be severe and fatal, affect outdoorsmen, foresters, rangers, ranchers, farmers, trappers, and construction workers.
- **b. Q fever**, a self-limiting influenza-like illness that is associated with pneumonia, affects dairy farmers, ranchers, stockyard workers, and slaughterhouse workers.

3. Viral diseases
- **a. Hepatitis**, especially type B, which is often contracted by contaminated needle sticks, is seen most often in health care workers, including dentists, dialysis technicians, blood bank workers, and physicians.
- **b. Rabies**, which is produced by animal bites, affects outdoor workers, especially in rural areas.
- **c. Cat scratch disease**, a regional lymphadenitis followed by skin lesions, affects dog and cat handlers.
- **d. Orf**, which is characterized by skin ulcers and regional lymphadenopathy, affects sheep and goat handlers.
- **e. Milker's nodules**, subcutaneous nodules caused by a pox virus, affect dairy farmers who contract them by milking cows with mastitis.
- **f. New Castle disease** is an influenza-like illness found in poultry handlers.

4. **Fungal diseases**
   a. **Coccidioidomycosis**, an infection usually limited to the lungs but which may affect all organs, affects migrant farmers and other agricultural workers, construction workers, military personnel in endemic areas, and laboratory workers.
   b. **Histoplasmosis**, a systemic infection that produces lung granulomas, affects chicken farmers, pigeon breeders, laboratory personnel, and workers who clear old silos or clean up bird and bat excreta.
   c. **Candidiasis**, a common infection between the fingers and around the nails, is seen in workers whose hands are frequently wet and prone to maceration, such as dishwashers, housewives, bakers, waiters, bartenders, goose pluckers, and poultry packers.
   d. **Aspergillosis**, a pneumonia occasionally presenting as a fungus ball, affects farmers, grain mill workers, and bird handlers who handle grain and other decaying and fermenting vegetation.
   e. **Sporotrichosis**, a systemic disease precipitated by a thorn scratch and local ulceration, affects horticulturists, florists, gardeners, and others who work with sphagnum moss.

V. ORGAN SYSTEM APPROACH TO OCCUPATIONAL DISEASES

A. Pulmonary diseases

1. **Pneumoconioses**
   a. **Asbestosis**, a pleural and parenchymal fibrotic disease, affects insulation workers, pipe fitters, and construction workers.
   b. **Coal workers' pneumoconiosis**, a nodular interstitial disease, is seen in coal miners.
   c. **Baritosis** (barium) affects chemical workers.
   d. **Hard metal diseases** (tungsten, cobalt) affect welders and toolmakers and are primarily characterized by nodules on chest film.
   e. **Mixed dust fibrosis** (i.e., several fibrogenic dusts together) affects welders and foundry workers.
   f. **Siderosis**, an interstitial disease with little effect on pulmonary function, results from iron oxide exposure and is seen primarily in welders.
   g. **Silicosis**, a progressive interstitial disease, results from silicon dioxide exposure and is seen in sandblasters, tunnelers, and foundry workers.
   h. **Talcosis** (talc) affects rubber workers, talc miners, and millers.

2. **Asthma**, or reversible bronchospasm, has been observed following exposure to:
   a. Isocyanates in polyurethane foam and paint workers.
   b. Enzymatic detergents in detergent manufacturing workers.
   c. Flour dusts in bakers.
   d. Platinum salts in jewelers and dentists.
   e. Aluminum solder flux in electronics workers.
   f. Nickel in metallurgists and electroplaters.
   g. Chromium in electroplaters and welders.
   h. Wood dusts in furniture workers.
   i. Cotton dusts in cotton mill workers and card room workers who straighten the cotton fibers.

3. **Bronchitis**, which is characterized by a daily cough with sputum production, is prevalent in:
   a. Coal miners.
   b. Welders.
   c. Foundry workers.

4. **Hypersensitivity pneumonitis** (extrinsic allergic alveolitis), which produces an acute, febrile, 48-hour pneumonia, occurs as a result of exposure to:
   a. Moldy hay.
   b. Moldy bagasse.
   c. Mushroom compost.
   d. Cork dust.
   e. Maple bark.
   f. Redwood dust.
   g. Wood pulp.
   h. Moldy barley.
   i. Isocyanates.
   j. Pigeon droppings.
   k. Wheat flour.

5. **Lung cancer** has been epidemiologically associated with exposure to:

a. Arsenic in ore smelters and pesticide manufactures.
b. Acrylonitrile in acrylic fiber manufactures.
c. Asbestos in insulators, pipe fitters, and construction workers.
d. Cadmium in metal refiners, electroplaters, and battery manufacturers.
e. Beryllium in aerospace and electronics workers.
f. Chloromethyl ethers in ion exchange resin workers.
g. Chromates in chrome smelters and refining workers.
h. Coke oven emissions in coke oven workers.
i. Fluorspar in fluorspar miners.
j. Hematite in iron and hematite miners.
k. Mustard gas in the manufacture of mustard gas.
l. Nickel in battery makers, welders, and chemists.
m. Uranium in uranium mining.
n. Vinyl chloride in polyvinyl chloride makers.

6. **Infectious diseases** may be related to occupational exposures in special situations as indicated below.
   a. An increased rate of **tuberculosis** has occurred in patients with silicosis and in health care workers.
   b. **Q fever** can occur in farmers, veterinarians, and slaughterhouse workers.
   c. **Anthrax** can occur in tanners and animal hair workers.
   d. **Coccidioidomycosis** can occur in construction workers in endemic areas.
   e. **Histoplasmosis** has occurred in farmers.
   f. **Leptospirosis** has occurred in longshoremen.

B. Cardiovascular diseases

1. **Coronary artery disease** has been associated with exposure to:
   a. Carbon disulfide in viscose rayon workers.
   b. Nitroglycerin in munitions and pharmaceutical workers.
   c. Carbon monoxide.
2. **Cardiac arrhythmias** can occur as a result of exposure to:
   a. Fluorocarbons in refrigeration workers.
   b. Halogenated hydrocarbons.
3. **Peripheral vascular disease** manifests as vibration white finger syndrome in air hammer users.

C. Hepatic diseases

1. Health care workers are at increased risk for **hepatitis B and non-A, non-B hepatitis.**
2. **Hepatic necrosis** can occur as a result of occupational exposure to:
   a. Carbon tetrachloride and other chlorinated hydrocarbon solvents in chemical workers.
   b. Yellow phosphorus in pesticide workers.
   c. Trinitrotoluene in munitions workers.
3. **Intrahepatic cholestasis** has been observed following exposure to methylene dianiline in plastic resin workers.

D. Musculoskeletal disease. Low back pain is one of the leading causes of time lost from work, second only to the common cold. The causes of low back pain include:

1. **Acute trauma disorders**, such as:
   a. Fractures.
   b. Dislocations.
   c. Strains.
2. **Cumulative trauma disorders**, such as:
   a. **Bursitis**, including:
      (1) Olecranon bursitis (miners' elbow).
      (2) Infrapatellar bursitis (housemaid's knee).
      (3) Subcalcaneal bursitis (policeman's heel).
   b. **Tenosynovitis**, including:
      (1) De Quervain's disease (trigger thumb), which is seen in typists and switchboard operators.
      (2) Lateral epicondylitis (tennis elbow).
   c. **Carpal tunnel syndrome** (median neuropathy), which is seen in manual workers and mail sorters.

d. **Degenerative joint disease**, including:
(1) Osteoarthritis of the elbow and shoulders, which is seen in pneumatic drill operators.
(2) Osteoarthritis of the feet, which is seen in construction workers and dancers.

E. **Reproductive disorders.** Reproductive health hazards are agents that cause reproductive impairment in adults and developmental impairment or death in the embryo, fetus, or child.

1. **The scope of the problem** of reproductive health hazards is illustrated by the following statistics.
   a. Birth defects, the causes of which are unknown in 60%–70% of cases, affect 7% of liveborn infants in the United States.
   b. Over 60% of married women over age 20 work at some time during the 12 months prior to the birth of their children; of these, over 17% work in industries in which they face potential exposure to a teratogen.
   c. Approximately 8.4% of couples in the United States in which the wife is of childbearing age are infertile.

2. **Mechanisms of action** of reproductive stressors
   a. Agents that adversely affect human reproduction may be chemical, physical, or biologic.
   b. Toxic agents may affect the male reproductive system by acting directly on spermatogenesis or by acting on accessory organs of reproduction.
   c. Toxic agents may affect the female reproductive system by causing ovulatory dysfunction, acting directly on the early conceptus, or by disrupting the intrauterine environment.
   d. Adverse effects on the fetus include:
      (1) Mutagenic alteration of inherited DNA.
      (2) Teratogenic or generative alteration of organogenesis.
      (3) Embryotoxic or fetotoxic degenerative damage to the developing fetus.
      (4) Carcinogenic damage resulting in cancer in the child.
   e. The effect on the fetus is determined by the:
      (1) Timing of exposure. The fetus is susceptible to the effects of various teratogens only during "critical windows" of organogenesis.
      (2) Dosage of the toxin.
      (3) Ability of the mother and fetus to metabolize the toxin.
      (4) Ability of the toxin to cross the placenta.

3. **Examples of occupational reproductive hazards**
   a. Lead exposure in women has been associated with menstrual disorders, infertility, spontaneous abortion, stillbirths, and neonatal deaths. Lead exposure in men has been associated with abnormalities in sperm.
   b. Maternal ingestion of fish contaminated with methylmercury resulted in congenital Minamata disease in their children.
   c. Maternal ingestion of rice oil contaminated with polychlorinated biphenyl resulted in congenital Yusho disease in their children.
   d. Dibromochloropropane production workers complaining of infertility were found to have dose-related reductions in sperm counts.
   e. Health care workers exposed to waste anesthetic gases in operating rooms have been found to have increased rates of spontaneous abortion.

F. **Cancer.** See Tables 12-2 and 12-3.

VIII. OCCUPATIONAL MEDICAL SERVICES

A. **Corporate services** either in plants or on a contractual basis with community hospitals or outpatient facilities include:

1. Pre-employment physical examinations to assess the ability of employees to perform required tasks.

2. Periodic medical examinations and biologic testing to monitor the adverse effects of toxins to which workers are exposed—for example, pulmonary function testing for workers exposed to silica dust.

3. Recommendations concerning preventive programs to control toxins in the plant environment.

4. Acute medical therapy for injuries and illnesses.

5. Advice to personnel departments as to work restrictions for partially incapacitated employees.

Table 12-2. Cancer Sites for Which Relationships with Occupational Exposures Are Well Established

Cancer Sites	Carcinogens

Bladder	Benzidine
	β-Naphthylamine
	4-Aminobiphenyl
	Dyes
	  Auramine
	  Magenta

Blood (leukemia)	Benzene Radiation (x-rays)
Bone	Radium Mesothorium
Larynx	Ethanol (ethyl alcohol)* Isopropyl alcohol* Mustard gas Asbestos
Liver (angiosarcoma)	Arsenic† Vinyl chloride

Lung and bronchus	Arsenic
	Asbestos
	Bis (chloromethyl) ether
	Chromium compounds
	  Coal carbonization processes
	  Coal tar pitch volatiles
	Iron ore mining
	Mustard gas
	Nickel refining
	Radiation

Nasal cavity and sinuses	Isopropyl alcohol* Mustard gas Nickel refining Radium Mesothorium Woodworking
Peritoneum (mesothelioma)	Asbestos
Pharynx	Mustard gas
Pleura (mesothelioma)	Asbestos

Skin (epithelioma)	Arsenic†
	Coal tar products
	  Coal tar
	  Creosote
	  Pitch
	  Soot
	Mineral oils
	  Shale
	  Coal
	  Petroleum
	Radiation (x-rays)

Adapted with permission from Decoufle P: Occupation. In *Cancer Epidemiology and Prevention*. Edited by Schottenfeld D, Fraumeni JF. Philadelphia, Saunders, 1982.

*Manufacture by strong acid process.

†Inorganic compounds.

6. Advice to personnel departments on an employee's ability to return to work following an illness.
7. Disability evaluations.
8. Identification and communication with medical consultants concerning workers suffering illness or injury on the job.
9. Communicating an understanding of the workplace environment to community physicians involved in the treatment of employees.
10. Policy development for collective bargaining and legislation.

Table 12-3. Occupational Groups Associated with High Risks for Cancer

Groups	Types of Cancer
Benzoyl chloride manufacturers	Lung
Chemists	Brain Lymphatic tissues Hematopoietic tissues Pancreas
Coal miners	Stomach
Coke by-product plant workers	Colon Pancreas
Foundry workers	Lung
Leather workers	Bladder Larynx Mouth Pharynx
Metal miners	Lung
Petrochemical workers	Brain Multiple myeloma Stomach Leukemia Esophagus Lung
Painters	Leukemia
Printing workers	Lung Mouth Pharynx
Rubber industry workers	Bladder Leukemia Brain Lung Prostate Stomach
Textile workers	Nasal cavity Sinuses
Woodworkers	Lymphatic tissue (Hodgkin's disease)

Adapted with permission from Decoufle P: Occupation. In *Cancer Epidemiology and Prevention*. Edited by Schottenfeld D, Fraumeni JF. Philadelphia, Saunders, 1982.

B. Hospital, group practice, or primary care services provide many of the services outlined in section VIII A above on a contract basis.

C. Government services include:

1. Laboratory, clinical, and epidemiologic research to expand the knowledge of occupational medicine and toxins.
2. Advice to local, state, and federal government policymakers concerning safety standards to protect the health of workers.
3. Epidemiologic and laboratory evaluation of new chemicals.
4. Consultation to health professionals concerning occupational health problems.
5. Publication of scientific reports on occupational toxins.
6. Reviewing university research for the purposes of funding and training in all disciplines of occupational health.

D. Independent university or hospital services include:

1. Clinical evaluations of patients thought to be suffering from occupational diseases for physicians, lawyers, companies, or governmental agencies.
2. Epidemiologic and laboratory evaluations of newly suspected toxins supported by grants from the government or private industry.
3. Preventive advice to industries or unions on occupational health.
4. Expert medical testimony in toxic injury litigation.

E. Labor union services include:

1. Advice concerning design and content of health and safety educational programs for the membership.
2. Hazard evaluation and literature review concerning local union plant health and safety problems.
3. Advice to the union concerning health and safety policy development both for collective bargaining and legislation.
4. Aiding the membership in epidemiologic or toxicologic study of problems.

BIBLIOGRAPHY

Levy BS, Wegman DH: *Occupational Health*. Boston, Little, Brown, 1983

NIOSH Pocket Guide To Chemical Hazards, US Department of Health and Human Services, Public Health Service, Centers for Disease Control, National Institute for Occupational Safety and Health, September, 1985

Parmeggiani L: *Encyclopaedia of Occupational Health and Safety*, 3rd ed. Geneva, International Labour Office, 1981

Rom, WN: *Environmental and Occupational Medicine*. Boston, Little, Brown, 1983

STUDY QUESTIONS

Directions: Each question below contains five suggested answers. Choose the **one best** response to each question.

1. Health care workers are at risk for developing which of the following diseases because of occupational exposure?

(A) Silicosis
(B) Byssinosis
(C) Pneumoconiosis
(D) Bagassosis
(E) Hepatitis

2. All of the following cancers have been associated with occupational exposure EXCEPT

(A) bladder cancer
(B) lung cancer
(C) hematopoietic cancer
(D) breast cancer
(E) liver cancer

3. Which of the following properties best describes carbon monoxide?

(A) It is a cellular toxin that causes tracheobronchitis
(B) It interferes with hemoglobin's ability to carry oxygen
(C) It is a hepatotoxin
(D) It smells like rotten eggs
(E) None of the above

Directions: Each question below contains four suggested answers of which **one or more** is correct. Choose the answer

A if **1, 2, and 3** are correct
B if **1 and 3** are correct
C if **2 and 4** are correct
D if **4** is correct
E if **1, 2, 3, and 4** are correct

4. Pesticides, chemicals designed to control organisms considered pests to man, include which of the following?

(1) Insecticides
(2) Herbicides
(3) Vertebrate poisons
(4) Fungicides

5. Foundry workers may suffer which of the following diseases as a result of occupational exposure?

(1) Silicosis
(2) Asbestosis
(3) Lung cancer
(4) Hearing loss

Directions: The group of questions below consists of lettered choices followed by several numbered items. For each numbered item, select the one lettered choice with which it is most closely associated. Each lettered choice may be used once, more than once, or not at all. Choose the answer

A if the item is associated with **(A) only**
B if the item is associated with **(B) only**
C if the item is associated with **both (A) and (B)**
D if the item is associated with **neither (A) nor (B)**

Questions 6–9

For each metal listed below, select the condition that is most likely to result from chronic exposure to it.

(A) Cancer
(B) Nervous system dysfunction
(C) Both
(D) Neither

6. Lead
7. Beryllium
8. Mercury
9. Arsenic

ANSWERS AND EXPLANATIONS

1. The answer is E. (*III F 1 c, 4 a–d*) There are more than 3 million hospital employees in the United States, some of whom are at risk for developing diseases, such as hepatitis B and non-A, non-B hepatitis, tuberculosis, herpes simplex virus, and acquired immune deficiency syndrome. Hepatitis B or non-A, non-B hepatitis can develop following needle sticks or other contact with the bodily fluids of infected patients. Byssinosis is a disease of textile workers. Silicosis and pneumoconiosis are interstitial dust diseases of the lung. Bagassosis is a hypersensitivity pneumonitis of sugar cane workers, which results from the inhalation of the dust of bagasse, the waste of sugar cane.

2. The answer is D. (*Table 12-2*) Bladder cancer is associated with exposure to leather dyes, β-naphthylamine, benzidine, and 4-aminobiphenyl. Lung cancer is associated with exposure to asbestos, arsenic, chromium compounds, iron ore, mustard gas, nickel, and radiation. Leukemia is associated with exposure to benzene and radiation. Liver cancer is associated with exposure to arsenic and vinyl chloride. Breast cancer has yet to be connected to any occupational exposure.

3. The answer is B. (*IV F 1*) Any gas in high enough concentration can displace oxygen and cause asphyxiation due to oxygen deprivation. However, carbon monoxide is especially toxic and has caused many deaths as a result of interfering with the ability of the lungs to oxygenate hemoglobin and the ability of the blood to release oxygen due to its high affinity for the hemoglobin molecule. It is a colorless and odorless gas.

4. The answer is E (all). (*IV D 1–4*) Pesticides are chemicals that are designed to kill, repel, or otherwise control organisms considered pests to man. They may be grouped as insecticides, fungicides, herbicides, and vertebrate poisons. They can be further classified according to mode of entry, the pest that they kill, or chemical composition.

5. The answer is E (all). (*III A 1–6*) Foundry workers who work in the metal casting industry are exposed to several hazardous substances. Silicon dioxide, which is used in the molding process, is capable of causing silicosis. Asbestos, which is used in forming gates and riser sleeves of molds as well as in the linings of furnaces and ladles, is associated with lung cancer, mesothelioma, asbestosis, and pleural disease. Noise in the foundries is associated with hearing loss and hypertension. Additional hazardous exposures include polycyclic aromatic hydrocarbons, metal dusts and fumes, formaldehyde and isocyanate compounds, carbon monoxide, heat, and nonionizing radiation.

6–9. The answers are: 6-B, 7-D, 8-B, 9-C. (*IV A 1 c, 2 c, 4 c, 5 c*) Lead poisoning causes diffuse central nervous system dysfunction, which may manifest as an encephalopathy. Cancer is not associated with lead exposure.

Acute exposure to the soluble salts of beryllium can cause pneumonitis and inflammation of the conjunctivae, nasal pharynx, trachea, and bronchi. Chronic exposure results in granulomas of the skin and lung, which manifest as a chronic debilitating respiratory disease.

Mercury is a neurotoxin that causes neurologic disturbances, renal abnormalities, irritation of the skin and mucous membranes, and pulmonary difficulties, such as pneumonitis and bronchitis.

Arsenic is also a neurotoxin and a lung carcinogen. In addition, exposure to arsenic fumes or dust may produce skin disorders, such as hyperpigmentation, hyperkeratosis, gangrene of the fingers and toes, and nasal septal ulceration and perforation.

13
Environmental Health Issues

Samuel L. Rotenberg

I. INTRODUCTION

A. Toxicity. All chemicals are toxic under some conditions of exposure. Toxicity depends on the exposure level and the dose at which various toxic effects occur. Because contact or exposure to our environment and to chemicals within that environment occur all the time, it is important to understand as much as possible about both the toxic effects that chemicals can cause and the doses at which these toxic effects are observed. The following examples show how chemicals that are normally assumed to be nontoxic or safe produce toxic effects in humans under certain exposure conditions.

1. Oxygen, which is present in the atmosphere at a concentration of about 20%, is essential for respiration in higher organisms. However, oxygen causes vasoconstriction of the retinal vascular system of premature infants and can lead to permanent damage if oxygen exposure levels remain above atmospheric levels.
2. Nitrogen—the major component of air (about 78%)—is chemically inert. However, at concentrations higher than those found in the atmosphere, nitrogen acts as a simple asphyxiant by excluding oxygen from the lungs. Nitrogen is also toxic when it is released into the bloodstream of divers who surface too rapidly.
3. Water—a major component of the environment—is essential to life. Mammals are composed of more than 50% water by weight, and it is generally considered that man can survive only a few days without water. However, water in the lungs blocks oxygen uptake and results in drowning, the cause of hundreds of deaths each year.

B. Exposure. Toxicity to a chemical cannot occur without exposure. An exposure pathway is a description of how a chemical in an environmental medium leads to human exposure. Understanding an exposure pathway can help to limit or reduce human exposure if appropriate controls or management of chemicals entering the environment are employed.

C. Risk assessment is the process by which risks to humans are estimated from known toxicologic data. Although some chemicals in the environment pose very significant risks to the environment or to other species, the strongest action to restrict chemical exposure occurs because of the effects on human health.

D. Managing and preventing risks to humans from chemicals present in the environment are two very difficult challenges facing our technological society today.

II. TOXIC EFFECTS OF CHEMICALS.

It is important to determine if the toxic effects of a chemical exposure (or other insult) demonstrate a threshold because of the different ways in which risk is estimated for threshold and nonthreshold effects.

A. Nonthreshold and threshold effects. A chemical or insult is said to produce a nonthreshold effect if any exposure results in the effect. No safe dose or exposure can be established—that is, any exposure is associated with some risk.

1. **Carcinogenesis** is the most important nonthreshold effect for man. The causes of cancer and

Note.—This chapter was written by Samuel L. Rotenberg, Ph.D., in his private capacity. No official support or endorsement by the Environmental Protection Agency or any other agency of the federal government is intended or should be inferred.

the changes in cancer incidence are important public health concerns. Cancer is a severe disease, one that is associated with pain, suffering, and death. One-sixth of the annual deaths in the United States are attributed to cancer.

2. **Mutagenesis** is an effect for which no threshold can be assumed. At present, it is not possible to estimate the significance of mutagenic effects of chemicals in humans.

3. **Teratogenesis and reproductive disorders** as a result of chemical exposures are considered threshold effects. This is a reasonable assumption if the chemical acts by a nongenetic interaction that alters fetal development or reproductive function. A nongenetic interaction is one that does not involve the genetic material DNA.

B. Toxic effects of chemicals can be classified as threshold and nonthreshold effects (see II A) or according to the duration and route of exposure, reversibility of effects, and toxic end points.

1. **Duration of exposure**
   a. **Acute effects** are considered the initial effects of an exposure to very high doses as well as the effects that result from a single exposure rather than the most severe effects that can occur.
   b. **Chronic effects** refer to either lifetime exposures or the longest period of exposure time needed to produce an effect. Chronic does not reflect the persistence or reversibility of the effect but simply the length of exposure.
   c. **Subchronic effects** refer to all exposures intermediate in length of exposure between acute and chronic.

2. **Reversibility of effects.** Reversibility refers to the inherent ability of the biologic system to return to normal function upon recovery; it does not refer to the ultimate toxic effect of an unlimited exposure. Many, if not most, of the toxic effects that occur in humans are fully reversible.
   a. **Reversible effects** occur when no permanent change is made in the biologic system. However, the mechanism of reversibility depends on the chemical and the toxic effect. For example, cyanide acts by complexing with cytochrome a_3 in the respiratory chain to prevent utilization of oxygen as an acceptor of electrons. If sufficient cyanide binds to the cytochrome, completely blocking oxygen use, then death results. However, if only a portion of the cytochrome a_3 is affected, the cyanide complexed to cytochrome gradually decreases over time, and the organism will survive. After complete recovery from cyanide poisoning, the organism will respond as if no past exposure had occurred.
   b. **Irreversible effects** occur when the biologic system does not return to its former state after removal of the toxic insult; some permanent change has occurred as a result of the chemical interaction.
   c. **Cumulative effects** occur when the chemical is sequestered (usually in a target organ) and does not affect the organ system until a critical body burden is present.

3. **Toxic end points.** The threshold or safe dose of toxic end points can be estimated by a number of methods, depending on the available data base. Because a chemical has many toxic effects, a safe dose or acceptable daily intake level must be based on the most sensitive toxic end point and the most sensitive human population at risk. There are an unlimited number of toxic end points that have been the subject of toxicity testing, ranging from toxic effects, such as death, to subtle effects, such as neurotoxicity. Some examples of tests, observations, research, and toxic end points of chemicals in animals and man follow.
   a. Physical observation
   b. Irritation
   c. Analytic tests
   d. Pathologic and histologic tests
   e. Teratogenic tests
   f. Reproductive toxicity
   g. Mutagenesis
   h. Carcinogenesis
   i. Immune system function
   j. Organ function tests
   k. Neurologic tests
   l. Behavioral toxicology
   m. Metabolic pathways
   n. Mechanism of toxicity

C. Carcinogens

1. **Human epidemiologic studies.** Most of the human epidemiologic studies involving cancer-

causing chemicals are **workplace exposure** studies. Occupational exposures have two of the important factors necessary for a successful study in humans: relatively high exposure as compared to the general public and an exposed population that can be followed for long time periods.

a. **Positive studies.** The correlation of increased cancer incidence with exposure is directly applicable to other human populations. However, positive epidemiologic studies are most often limited to chemicals that either are very potent carcinogens or cause rare or unusual cancers.

b. **Negative studies.** Studies that show no correlation may mean that the chemical is not a carcinogen. However, there are a number of confounding factors.

(1) **Long latency periods** for many human carcinogens result in many negative epidemiologic studies.

(a) The latency period is defined as the time between the beginning of exposure and the appearance of cancer.

(b) Typical latency periods for human carcinogens are measured in years and decades as shown in Table 13-1. If a chemical has a 20-year latency period, an epidemiologic study must follow workers for more than 20 years after the exposure before measurable increases in cancer incidence are seen.

(2) **Small numbers of individuals** in an exposed group limits the ability to detect carcinogens other than those that are potent or cause rare tumors. Because cancer incidences in nonexposed populations are appreciable, it is difficult to show a statistically significant increase in cancer in an exposed group of small numbers.

(3) **Lack of lifetime study follow-up** for an exposed group limits the ability to detect chemical carcinogens. When animals exposed to carcinogens are sacrificed and examined for tumors at times less than their full lifetime, the cancer incidence is markedly decreased. Thus, negative human studies where most of the individuals are still alive may not validly conclude that the observed exposure did not cause an increased cancer incidence.

(4) **Other factors** also contribute to the incidence of cancer and complicate the analysis of human studies.

(a) In most workplace situations, workers are not exposed to a single chemical or agent. In addition, workers often change occupations and thus are exposed to chemicals other than the one being studied.

(b) Genetic factors, smoking, diet, medication, and other life-style factors confound the analysis of human cancer rates.

2. **Animal bioassay tests** for animal carcinogens are typically 2 years in length, which is the life span of the rats or mice used in the test. Exposure is by ingestion or inhalation, and all tissues are examined at the conclusion of the study.

a. **High doses** used in animal bioassay tests are constantly criticized. It has been argued that the high dose itself is the reason that an animal bioassay is positive and that the chemical would not be carcinogenic at a low dose.

(1) This argument ignores the fact that **most chemicals are not carcinogens**, no matter how large the dose. Large doses of chemicals may be toxic, but they do not necessarily cause cancer.

(2) Guidelines adopted by the Environmental Protection Agency (EPA) for carcinogenic testing require that the highest dose used does not shorten the life span of the test species. Scientific justification for the use of high doses is both logical and practical.

(a) It has been demonstrated that the latency period is reduced at high doses. Since the life span of rats and mice is about 2 years, it is important that the cancer-causing effect show up within the 2-year life span.

Table 13-1. Approximate Latency Periods for Human Carcinogens

Chemical	Cancer Site	Latency Period (Years)
Arsenic	Skin and lung	20
Asbestos	Pleura and peritoneum	15–20
Benzene	Blood	10–20
Benzidine	Bladder	16
Chromium (VI)	Lung	10–20
Bis-chloromethylether	Lung	8
Nickel	Lung and nose	20
Vinyl chloride	Liver angiosarcoma	15

(b) Experiments using animal species with a longer life span, such as dogs, cats, or monkeys, would take decades to complete and would be costly because the animals are larger and live longer than mice and rats. Additionally, longer bioassay experiments would lengthen the time to determine if a chemical were a carcinogen.

(c) There is no significant scientific advantage in knowing that a chemical causes cancer in animals higher than a rodent.

b. A high-dose response in some cases is not indicative of the cancer-causing potential of a chemical—that is, a high dose of a chemical could alter the response at the target site and lead to cancer that would not occur at a low dose as a result of:

(1) **Metabolism of the chemical** to the active carcinogenic species. If a chemical is metabolized by a different pathway at high doses and one of the metabolites along the high-dose pathway is the actual carcinogen, then low doses would not be expected to cause cancer because the cancer-initiating metabolite is not produced.

(2) **Nonspecific or physical carcinogenesis.** If a physical irritant such as bladder stones were produced by high doses but not by low doses, then the presence of the bladder stones may be directly responsible for bladder cancer.

c. Route of exposure for many animal bioassays is by ingestion. However, because exposure to chemicals in the environment (and workplace) is usually by inhalation, the validity of ingestion experiments has been questioned. The predominent difference between ingestion and inhalation exposure is the degree of absorption. Some chemicals are known animal carcinogens by both inhalation and ingestion experiments.

(1) **Inhalation.** A chemical absorbed into the bloodstream from the lungs passes directly to the heart and then into the systemic circulation.

(2) **Ingestion.** Chemicals absorbed from the stomach and intestines pass through the liver before entering the heart.

(a) Since the **liver is the predominent organ of metabolism** for most chemicals, ingested chemicals are metabolized faster then inhaled chemicals.

(b) For some chemicals, the metabolized form is more toxic than the original chemical, while for other chemicals the converse is true.

(c) Unless *all* of an ingested chemical is metabolized by the liver after absorption, some will be carried back to the heart and into the systemic circulation.

(d) Ingestion experiments are easier to control than inhalation experiments, so many of the early (1970s) experiments were performed by gavage tube.

d. Advantages of animal studies include the following:

(1) The exposure can be limited to a single chemical being tested.

(2) Several doses of a chemical can be used.

(3) Negative results from well-conducted studies in several species increase the likelihood that the chemical does not present a carcinogenic risk.

e. Disadvantages of animal studies include the following:

(1) Positive animal tests do not prove that the chemical is a human carcinogen. It is possible for a chemical to be carcinogenic in animals and not humans because the chemical is not metabolized to the carcinogenic metabolite in humans as it is in animals. Although this possibility exists in theory, it is not at all likely for most animal carcinogens.

(2) Estimating human cancer risks from animal cancer data requires converting animal exposure information and extrapolating and modeling dose-response information.

3. Genotoxic tests. Short-term tests have been developed to measure the ability of a chemical to interact with or alter genetic material (DNA). Positive genotoxic test results are not considered sufficient to classify a chemical as a known carcinogen; however, positive results are suggestive and thus are often used to select chemicals for animal bioassays.

a. Point mutations are measured as an end point designed to test the ability of a chemical to cause a mutational event.

(1) **The Ames test**, the most well known and widely used of all short-term tests, measures the ability of a chemical to mutate a specific gene in *Salmonella typhimurium*. Because *S. typhimurium* is a bacterium, a chemical is tested in the presence and absence of a mammalian enzyme fraction to determine if a metabolic event (activation) is required for mutagenesis:

(a) **Advantages of the Ames test**

(i) About 90% of the chemicals that test positive in the Ames test are also carcinogenic in animal bioassay tests.

(ii) It is a short-term, low-cost test that is easy to perform.

(b) **Disadvantages of the Ames test** include the following:

(i) Negative test results are common for metals and some chlorinated organics.

(ii) It is difficult to test volatile compounds.
(iii) Mutagenesis is not directly equated with carcinogenesis.

(2) **Other point mutation tests** use bacteria, yeast, or animal cell systems.

b. **Chromosome effects** are measured as changes in the structure or number of chromosomes, or the production of chromosome fragments. Many cell types are used and exposure to the chemical can occur in vivo or in vitro.

c. **DNA damage** is measured as either direct breaks in DNA or the inability of a cell system to repair such breaks. Both bacterial and mammalian cell systems are used for DNA damage tests.

d. **Mammalian cell transformations** are changes in cells exposed to a chemical that cause the cell to induce tumors in recipient animals. Transformation is often accompanied by characteristic morphologic changes in the transformed mammalian cell.

4. **Structural similarities.** In the absence of animal or human data, structural similarities can be important in determining the likelihood that a chemical is a carcinogen.

a. An untested nitrosamine or benzidine derivative would be expected to be carcinogenic since so many different nitrosamines and benzidines have tested positive in animal bioassay tests.

b. The three dichlorobenzene isomers would be expected to be carcinogens because the most highly chlorinated benzene, hexachlorobenzene, is an animal carcinogen, and benzene itself is a human carcinogen. Thus, it is logical, but not proven, that the dichlorobenzenes are carcinogens.

5. **Weight of evidence classification**, an integration of all of the relevant scientific data for a chemical, describes the probability that the chemical is a human carcinogen. The classification system used by the EPA to classify chemical carcinogens is summarized in Table 13-2.

a. The **qualitative** conclusion that a chemical is a possible, probable, or definite human carcinogen is simply a yes or no answer to the likelihood of the chemical causing cancer in man. Only after a determination is made that a chemical is carcinogenic can the question of how carcinogenic be asked.

b. The **quantitative** estimation of potency for a carcinogen is separate from the qualitative weight of evidence conclusion concerning its carcinogenicity.

c. Negative animal or human studies are often cited as reasons to modify a qualitative weight of evidence conclusion or quantitative potency determination. As a rule, negative studies are not factored into the weight of evidence conclusion unless all studies are negative.

(1) For human studies, see section II C 1 b for some of the reasons that studies can be negative, yet the chemical could still be a carcinogen.

(2) For animal studies, there are many experimental design problems that can result in a negative study.

(3) It is more difficult to make errors in an experimental protocol that shows a chemical to be carcinogenic when it is not than vice versa.

(4) In determining potency, a well-done negative epidemiologic study can establish an upper limit of risk for a chemical that is a known animal carcinogen. However, to date no human study has been used to modify the potency of a chemical determined to be an animal carcinogen.

Table 13-2. Environmental Protection Agency Weight of Evidence Classification System for Carcinogens

Group	Description	Comment
A	Human carcinogen	Sufficient evidence in epidemiologic studies to support causal association
B1	Probable human carcinogen	Limited evidence of carcinogenicity in humans
B2	Probable human carcinogen	Sufficient evidence of carcinogenicity in animals
C	Possible human carcinogen	Limited evidence of carcinogenicity in animals
D	Not classified	Inadequate evidence of carcinogenicity in animals
E	No evidence of carcinogenesis for humans	No evidence of carcinogenicity in animals or humans

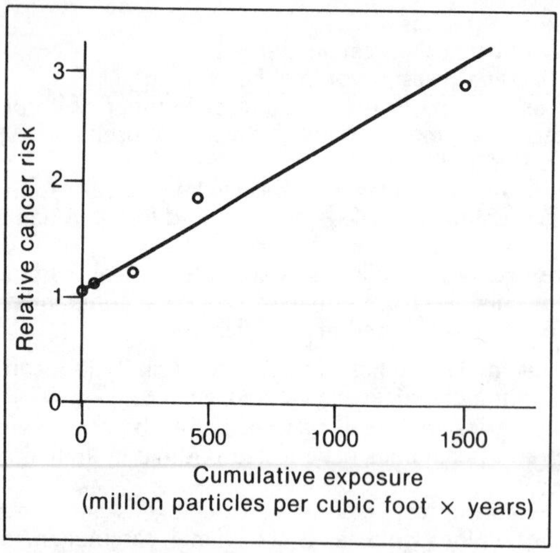

Figure 13-1. The dose-response curve for respiratory cancer mortality in a group of asbestos workers.

III. DOSE-RESPONSE EVALUATION

A. Carcinogens

1. Carcinogenesis

a. Asbestos-induced cancer mortality is shown in Figure 13-1 for a group of asbestos workers. The relative risk of cancer death is plotted against the cumulative exposure to asbestos.

(1) If a threshold existed, the plot would be expected to show a relative risk of 1 for some exposures greater than 0, and it apparently does not.

(2) Since these data show relative risk, the actual shape of the curves may not be meaningful.

(3) These data are consistent with no threshold for asbestos-induced cancer deaths or no safe dose of asbestos exposure.

b. 2-Acetylaminofluorene (2-AAF) exposure in mice at various levels in the diet and the resultant bladder and kidney cancers are shown in Table 13-3. The cancer incidence rates are plotted in Figure 13-2.

(1) This experiment was performed to determine if a threshold could be seen for an animal carcinogen by lowering the dose and using larger numbers of animals in each exposure group.

(2) The data for bladder cancer may or may not be consistent with a threshold model of carcinogenesis.

(3) The liver tumor data clearly are not consistent with a threshold model.

c. Radiation-induced cancers show dose-response curves that are consistent with no threshold.

(1) Radiation exposure is not identical to chemical exposure. However, radiation acts at the level of the genetic material, as do chemical carcinogens, and radiation-induced cancers show latency periods in man as do chemical carcinogens.

Table 13-3. Incidence of Bladder and Liver Tumors in Mice Fed 2-Acetylaminofluorene

Dose (ppm)	Tumor Response*			
	Bladder	%	Liver	%
0	2/759	0.26	20/762	2.62
30	9/2105	0.43	164/2109	7.78
35	5/1357	0.37	128/1361	9.40
45	4/881	0.45	98/888	11.0
60	6/756	0.79	118/758	15.6
75	13/586	2.22	118/587	20.1
100	51/297	17.2	76/297	25.6
150	236/313	75.4	126/314	40.1

*Response is reported as the number of animals with the tumor compared with the total number of animals in the dose group and the calculated percent response.

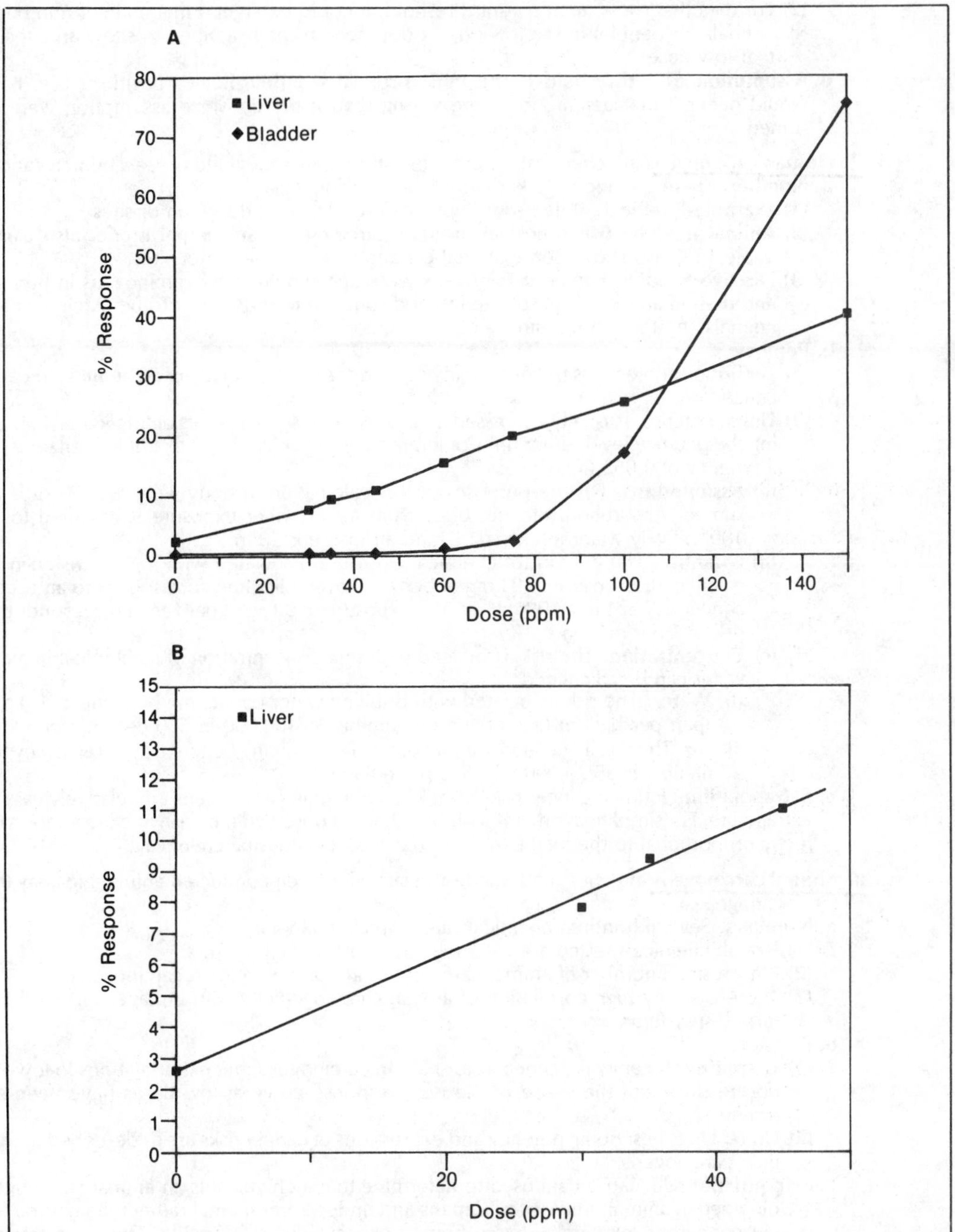

Figure 13-2. Liver and bladder tumor response in mice fed 2-acetylaminofluorene. (*A*) Dose-response curve. (*B*) Low-dose range of dose-response curve for liver tumors.

(2) Lack of an apparent threshold for radiation-induced cancers in man is circumstantial evidence for lack of a threshold for chemical carcinogens.

(3) Radon is a chemically inert gas that enters the human body via inhalation. It is also a radioactive element, breaking down to a high-energy alpha particle, which is responsible for the cancer-causing properties of radon.

d. The existence or absence of a threshold cannot be proved scientifically.

(1) For data that show no apparent threshold, it could be argued that data at lower doses need to be analyzed to show no effect at lower doses.

(2) For data that show an apparent threshold, it could be argued that a larger number of animals (or people) in the low-dose group need to be examined to show an effect at that low dose.

e. **Assumption of a threshold is the most protective public health position**. Less harm would occur if that assumption were wrong than if the converse assumption were assumed.

2. **Human carcinogens** are chemicals or other insults that are thought to cause a human cancer.

a. **Number.** There are about 30 known human carcinogens.

(1) **Examples.** Table 13-4 lists some human carcinogens and the tumor sites.

(2) **Animal models. For almost all human carcinogens, an animal model also exists.** Table 13-4 also shows some animal carcinogens and the tumor sites.

(3) **Discovery.** Some human carcinogens were first shown to be carcinogens in humans and then in animals (e.g., benzene), and some were shown first to be carcinogens in animals and then in humans (e.g., vinyl chloride).

b. **Potency**

(1) **Definition.** Potency is the quantitative description of the ability of a chemical to cause cancer.

(2) **Units.** Potency is usually expressed as a cancer rate slope in units of $(mg/kg/day)^{-1}$. Using the potency level, other units of interest can be derived. For example, benzene has a potency of 0.052 $(mg/kg/day)^{-1}$.

(a) **Assumptions.** For the purposes of this calculation, a body weight of 70-kg is assumed. Absorption into the body from air or water exposure is assumed to be 100%. Daily water intake is 2 L, and air intake is 20 m^3.

(b) **Quantity.** The amount of chemical exposure associated with a given risk can be calculated. Exposure to 93 mg of benzene over a lifetime corresponds to an excess cancer risk of 1 in a 1000. Likewise, exposure to 93 μg of benzene corresponds to a risk of 1 per million.

(c) **Concentration.** The risk associated with unit concentration of a chemical in air or water can be calculated.

(i) **Water.** The risk associated with drinking water containing benzene at 1.0 ppb (part per billion) [μg/1] over a lifetime is 55/100,000 or 550 per million.

(ii) **Air.** The risk associated with inhaling air containing benzene at 1.0 $\mu g/m^3$ over a lifetime is 55/10,000, or 5500 per million.

c. **Extrapolation.** Human cancer risks from known human carcinogens are relatively easy to extrapolate. For simplification, it is assumed that the observed increase in cancer rate is directly proportional to the total exposure to the cancer-causing chemical.

3. **Animal carcinogens** are chemicals that test positive in a well-conducted animal bioassay test for carcinogenesis.

a. **Numbers.** Several hundred chemicals are animal carcinogens.

(1) Not all chemicals tested are carcinogenic; most, in fact, are not.

(2) Only a small number of animal carcinogens are proven human carcinogens.

(3) There is a very high correlation of animal carcinogenicity with mutagenicity in short-term test systems.

b. **Potency.**

(1) **Definition.** Potency is defined as for human carcinogens, but extrapolations to low-exposure dose and the shape of the dose-response curve at low doses have been assumed.

(2) **Units.** Units describing potency and expressions of cancer risks are as described for human carcinogens.

c. **Extrapolations.** Because data used to determine that a chemical is an animal carcinogen are obtained in animals and not in humans and under experimental rather than natural exposure conditions, extrapolations to human exposure must be made. There are several

Table 13-4. Tumor Sites of Chemical Carcinogens in Humans and Animals

	Target Organ and Route of Exposure	
Chemical	**Humans**	**Animals**
Aflotoxins	Liver (oral and inhalation)	Liver, stomach, colon, and kidney (oral)
Benzidine	Bladder (oral and inhalation)	Liver (oral)
Diethylstilbestrol	Uterus and vagina (oral)	Mammary gland (oral)
Mustard gas	Lung and larynx (inhalation)	Lung (inhalation)
Vinyl chloride	Liver, brain, and lung (inhalation)	Lung, liver, mammary gland, and kidney (inhalation)

possible ways, as described below. In the absence of data to the contrary, the EPA assumes a surface area equivalency for conversion of doses in animal species to doses in man.

(1) **Body weight equivalency.** Assume that a given dose in mg/kg yields identical toxicologic effects in all species.

(2) **Air exposure equivalency.** Assume that an air level in $\mu g/m^3$ yields identical toxicologic effects in all species.

(3) **Food equivalency.** Assume that a food concentration in ppb yields identical effects.

(4) **Water equivalency.** Assume that a water concentration in ppb yields identical effects.

(5) **Surface area equivalency.** Assume that a given dose in mg/surface area yields identical toxicologic effects in all species.The pharmacologic basis for this assumption is that metabolic rate of different species is more closely associated with surface area than with body weight.

d. **Low-dose models.** Exposure of animals in a bioassay test are at doses higher than a likely environmental exposure. The extrapolation of the expected dose responses at low doses has been another area of scientific discussion.

(1) **Numbers.** The absence of low-dose exposure and response data has resulted in many models or hypotheses of cancer mechanism and methods for extrapolating to low-dose ranges.

(2) **Models.** Risks predicted at low doses from some of the more common models are shown in Table 13-5, and graphs of the dose-response curves are shown in Figure 13-3.

(3) **Assumption.** As a protective public health assumption, the EPA currently uses a multistage model that essentially assumes a linear dose response from the lowest observable data point.

B. Noncarcinogens

1. **Determining thresholds.** Thresholds or safe doses can be estimated for any required period of time, but the usual estimate of a safe dose is one that is safe for a lifetime exposure. In some circumstances, a 1-day or 10-day safe dose might be determined for a state or local health department to help them respond to an exposed population from a contamination incident.

a. **Lifetime safe dose.** The lifetime safe dose is a daily dose that is expected to produce no adverse health effects in all humans exposed to that dose over a lifetime of exposure.

b. **Most sensitive toxic effect.** A lifetime safe dose that protects a human population against the toxic effects that occur at the lowest exposure will also protect that same population against the toxic effects that occur at a higher exposure. Therefore, it is important that the most sensitive toxic effect or end point be used for the threshold determination of a safe dose.

c. **Carcinogens.** A lifetime safe dose from the noncarcinogenic effects of carcinogens can also be determined, and this estimate does not invalidate the concept of no safe dose for carcinogens. Rather, threshold and nonthreshold effects are separated with respect to determining a safe dose for a chemical.

d. **No observed versus no adverse effect.** The most sensitive toxic effect may not be easily determined, in part because our understanding of toxic effects is constantly changing. However, there is often reference to an adverse effect in the literature. This implies a judgment about what observed changes are in fact significant. Without questioning the integri-

Table 13-5. Dose-Response Relationships Extrapolated to Low-Dose Levels for Some Models

	Proportion Responding within Each Model				
Dose	**Multihit***	**Weibull**	**Multistage**	**Single Hit**	**Log Logistic**
16	. . .	. . .	. . .	0.999	0.998
8	. . .	1.00	1.00	0.977	0.992
4	0.99	0.995	0.998	0.848	0.963
2	0.850	0.850	0.850	0.610	0.850
1	0.500	0.488	0.468	0.376	0.551
0.5	0.210	0.210	0.210	0.210	0.210
0.25	0.07	0.0798	0.0933	0.110	0.0544
0.125	. . .	0.0289	0.0431	0.0572	0.0123
0.0625	. . .	0.0103	0.0206	0.029	0.00269
0.01	0.00050	0.000657	0.00315	0.00470	0.0000473
0.001	0.0000035	0.0000206	0.000313	0.000470	0.000000294
0.0001	0.000000001	0.000000645	0.0000312	0.0000470	0.000000002

Note.—Parameters for models were chosen to produce identical responses at a dose of 0.5 and, if possible, at 2.0.
*Proportion responding was not calculated for all doses for this model.

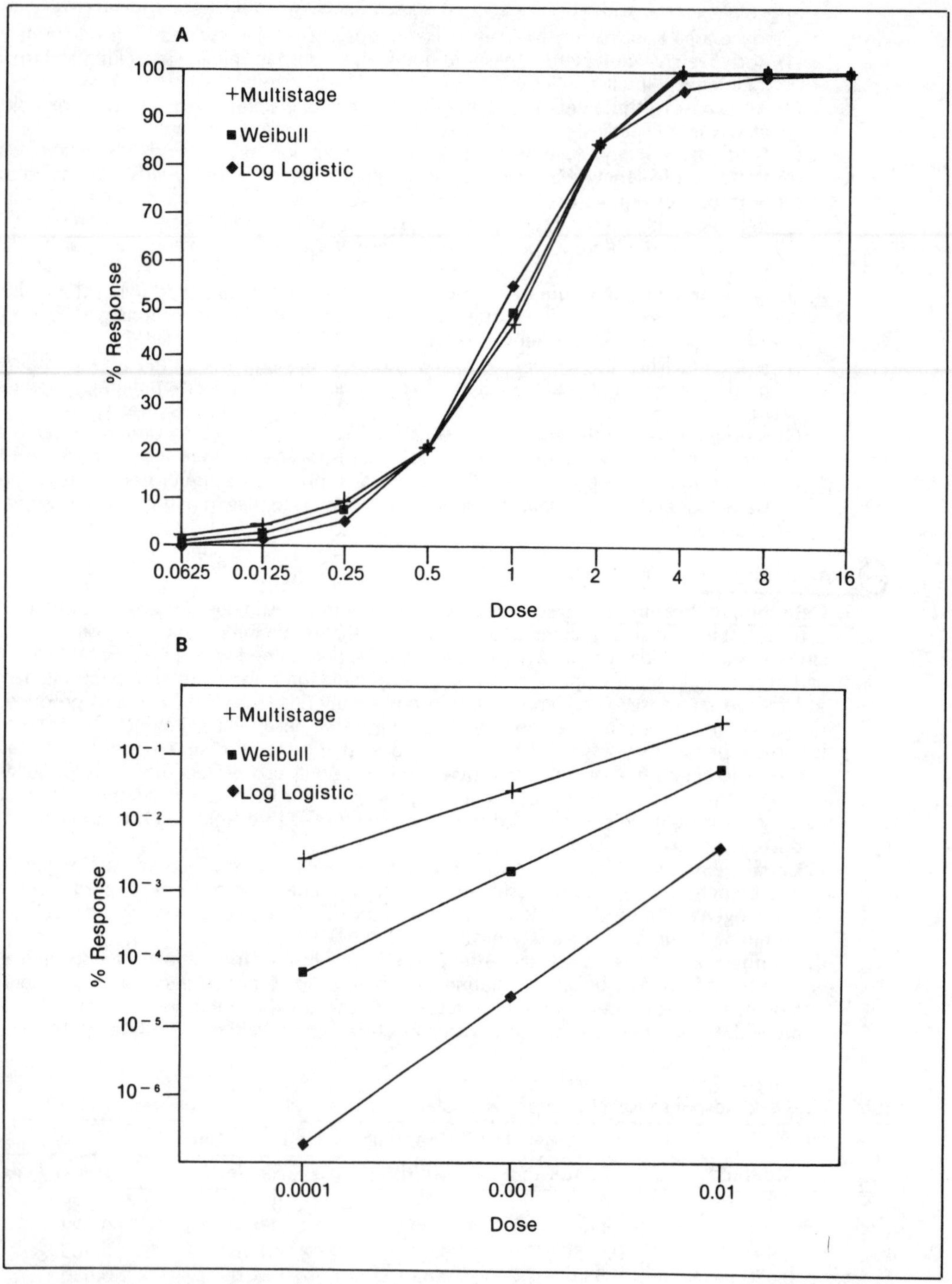

Figure 13-3. Dose-response curves for selected models. (*A*) Dose response at high doses. (*B*) Predicted dose response at low doses.

ty of the observers and judgments made in the past, any observed change caused by a chemical may decrease the ability of the person to respond to changes usual to their environment. Thus, observed changes that are the result of a chemical exposure need to be considered as the toxic effect itself.

2. **Uncertainty factors** are used to reduce an exposure level or safe dose to humans to reflect some condition other than the original exposure conditions.

a. **Sensitive population.** If an experiment has used a healthy population, an uncertainty factor of 10 is used to convert that exposure to a sensitive population exposure. This uncertainty factor is used typically in evaluation of occupational exposure information or human experimental information (in both situations where the exposed population is healthier than the general population).
b. **Animal population.** An uncertainty factor of 10 is used to convert the results of animal studies to results in humans. A portion of this factor may be the surface area to body weight dose issue discussed previously, but another consideration is that humans may be more sensitive than the animal species used for the tests.
c. **Short term.** An uncertainty factor of 10 is used to convert short-term toxicologic test results to long-term results.
d. **Adverse effect.** An uncertainty factor of 2 to 10 is used to decrease the exposure when an adverse exposure is converted to a no adverse effect exposure.
e. **Numbers.** Some cynics would observe that the number 10 more closely agrees with the number of fingers or toes humans possess than any better scientific reason.

3. **Human exposure data.** In evaluating human exposure, many factors must be considered.
   a. **Route of exposure.** The route of exposure is important in evaluating human exposure because many chemicals are not absorbed equally efficiently by all routes. When data using human studies are evaluated, the actual amount of chemical is most important for systemic toxicity. For irritation effects, the concentration in the environment is needed.
   b. **Workplace recommendations.** Human workplace exposure recommendations [National Institute for Occupational Safety and Health (NIOSH) or Occupational Safety and Health (OSHA)] may be used to estimate safe doses.
      (1) Workplace exposures are for only 40 hours a week, so exposure limits need to be reduced by the factor 40/168 to correct for constant exposure.
      (2) Uncertainty factors of 10 for exposure to a healthy population and 10 for a "no adverse effect exposure" to a "no observed effect exposure" are used.
      (3) Thus, a probably safe dose for the general population would necessitate division of the recommended level by 420. Conservative toxicologists would probably reduce this further by a factor of 2, while industrialists would probably increase it by a factor of 5.
      (4) NIOSH recommendations are health based, while those of OSHA may be based on other factors, such as cost or politics.
      (5) Air exposure limits in the workplace [i.e., threshold limit values (TLVs)] have historically been reduced with time.
   c. **Experimental human exposure.** For some chemicals, short-term human exposure data are available. Where the toxicologic end points are relevant (such as behavioral or neurologic changes) rather than not (lung function or liver function), such data are useful starting places to estimate safe doses.
      (1) Advantages
         (a) The effects that are observed are obviously relevant to humans.
         (b) Observations of toxic effects in humans at high doses are useful in indicating research directions for animal toxicity experiments.
      (2) Disadvantages
         (a) Lack of long-term controlled exposure for experiments conducted with human volunteers limits the usefulness of some human exposure data.
         (b) Inability to control confounding factors and other chemical exposures complicates analysis of cause and effect.

4. **Animal exposure data.** As with human data, many factors must be considered for animal exposure information.
   a. **Route of exposure.** The actual dose to the animal depends on the route of exposure and the percent absorbed.
      (1) Ingestion studies where chemicals are added to water or food or into the animal by gavage tube are easier to control than inhalation studies.
      (2) If ingested chemicals are fed in water or food, exposure monitoring must determine that normal eating and drinking habits are not altered by the chemical.
   b. **Metabolism.** Although metabolic patterns are generally the same in all animal species, including man, it is not so for all chemicals.
   c. **Advantages**
      (1) Exposure to a single chemical is controlled.
      (2) Exposure is given in several doses.
      (3) A wide range of toxic effects are observable.
   d. **Disadvantage.** Although similar to humans in many biochemical and physiologic functions, animals are not humans, so toxic effects must be evaluated with care to determine the actual relevance to man.

5. Example. Table 13-6 shows estimates of the safe dose for toluene using the available data base. These safe-dose estimates are for the noncarcinogenic effects of toluene. Additionally, toluene has been tested for carcinogenicity in an animal bioassay study and has not been determined to be carcinogenic. The conclusion of the safe toluene dose is that the daily safe dose of toluene is not likely to be below 2020 μg/day, and that this limit is expected to be protective of children or other sensitive members of the population.

IV. ROUTES OF EXPOSURE

A. General principles

1. Environmental fate of a chemical is a description of how and to what extent a chemical is removed from one medium or transferred from one medium to another.

a. Mediums, or environmental compartments, are:

(1) Air.
(2) Water, including:
  (a) Surface water.
  (b) Groundwater.
(3) Sediment.
(4) Soil.
(5) Aquatic organisms.
(6) Plant organisms.
(7) Particulates.

b. Movement between mediums is dependent mainly on the physical and chemical properties of the chemical, the concentration of the chemical, metabolism, and chemical transformation.

(1) Physical and chemical properties describe the affinity of a chemical for one environment compared to another.

(2) Concentration of chemical in each medium is a factor controlling the rate of transfer from one medium to another. In most environmental situations, one medium normally exists without any of the chemical.

(3) Metabolism (usually by microorganisms) is important for some chemicals in some mediums.

(4) Chemical transformation may play a major role in removal of a chemical from a medium. The transformation product may also be a toxic chemical. Photo-oxidation is an example of a chemical transformation that takes place in air. Some of the parameters that could affect the rate are:
  (a) Light intensity.
  (b) Wavelength of light.
  (c) Humidity.
  (d) Temperature.
  (e) Particles.

(5) The rate of transfer between mediums can be modified by the following factors:
  (a) Mixing or aeration increases the volatile organic transfer rate from water to air.
  (b) Fish with a high fat content accumulate higher concentrations of nonpolar organics than fish with a lower fat content.
  (c) Insoluble metal precipitate slows down metal transfer from water to sediment.
  (d) Sandy soils show less differences in groundwater migration rates of water soluble and less water soluble organics.

Table 13-6. Estimates of Safe Doses of Toluene Exposure

Toxicologic Data Base or Source of Estimate	Estimated Safe Dose (μg/day)*
Human (CNS†/chronic)	2750
Rat (CNS/subchronic)	147,000
Rat (CNS/chronic)	2020
Mouse (teratogenic)	30,000
NIOSH	8980
EPA	20,200

Note.—Estimates of safe doses of toluene exposure were made by the author by using uncertainty and exposure factors to the human or animal toxicity data or to the safe exposure estimates of the National Institute for Occupational Safety and Health (NIOSH) or the Environmental Protection Agency (EPA).

*Estimated for a 70-kg adult.

†CNS = central nervous system.

(6) **Principles** that show how chemicals move between mediums follow. Examples of the values for some chemicals are shown in Table 13-7.
(a) Volatile chemicals tend to move toward air.
(b) Nonpolar chemicals tend to transfer to sediment and fish.
(c) Water soluble organics tend to move with water through soil.

c. **Physical parameters** that help to predict the environmental fate of chemicals follow.
(1) **The octanol water partition coefficient (K_{ow})** describes the partitioning of a chemical between octanol and water.
(2) **Henry's law constant (H)** describes the ratio of the concentration of a chemical in the atmosphere with that in solution.
(3) **Vapor pressure (P_v)** describes the contribution to pressure that a chemical would produce in the gas phase at a given temperature. The higher the vapor pressure, the greater tendency to volatilize.
(4) **Bioconcentration factor (BCF)** describes the affinity of the chemical for aquatic organisms. High BCF values indicate an accumulation of the chemical in fish compared to the water in which they swim.
(5) **Solubility (S_w)** describes the maximum amount of a chemical that could be dissolved in water at a given temperature.

2. **Absorption.** Physical and chemical properties and concentration determine the extent of absorption.

a. **Inhalation of chemicals**
(1) **Chemicals adsorbed onto particulates** are absorbed slowly relative to gas phase chemicals.
(a) Water solubility increases the absorption rate of chemicals on particulates.
(b) Water insoluble chemicals are absorbed by being engulfed by macrophages.
(2) **Gas phase chemicals** are absorbed into the bloodstream at rates that are a function of the polarity of the molecule.
(a) **Characteristics of polar chemicals**
(i) Water-like
(ii) High dielectric constants
(iii) Soluble in water
(iv) Insoluble in oil
(b) **Characteristics of nonpolar chemicals**
(i) Fat-like
(ii) Low dielectric constants

Table 13-7. Physical Properties of Some Chemicals

Chemical Class/Examples	Water Solubility (mg/L)	Vapor Pressure (mm Hg)	Henry's Law Constant (atm – m³/mol)	Octanol Water Partition Coefficient (ml/g)	Bioconcentration Factor (L/kg)
Volatile organics					
Benzene	1.8 E+03	9.5 E+01	5.6 E−03	8.3 E+01	5.2
Chloroform	8.2 E+03	1.5 E+02	2.9 E−03	3.1 E+01	3.8
1,1-Dichloroethylene	2.3 E+03	6.0 E+02	3.4 E−02	6.5 E+01	5.6
Toluene	5.4 E+02	2.8 E+01	6.4 E−03	3.0 E+02	1.1 E+01
Vinyl chloride	2.7 E+03	2.7 E+03	8.2 E−02	5.7 E+01	1.2
Nonvolatile organics					
Chlordane	5.6 E−01	1.0 E−05	9.6 E−06	1.4 E+05	1.4 E+04
Polychlorinated biphenyls	3.1 E−02	7.8 E−05	1.1 E−03	5.3 E+05	1.0 E+05
Metals					
Arsenic	Very dependent on specific compound				4.4 E+01
Cadmium					8.1 E+01
Chromium					1.6 E+01
Lead					4.9 E+01
Other					
Asbestos	1.0 E−11	Very low		Unknown	8.0 E−02
Cyanides	5.0 E+05	Species dependent		Very low	1.0

Note.—Numerical values in this table are notated with a two-digit number raised to some power of 10; thus, 3.4 E−02 = 3.4×10^{-2}.

(iii) Insoluble in water
(iv) Soluble in oil

b. Absorption of ingested chemicals

(1) Inhaled particles greater than 6–10 μ in diameter are trapped by the celia in the nasal passages and upper bronchial tree and enter the body by ingestion.

(2) Particles and metal compounds in general are absorbed to a lesser extent after ingestion than after inhalation.

c. Absorption through the skin or mucus membranes is possible, but environmental exposure by direct contact is usually insignificant compared to exposure by inhalation or ingestion.

(1) Nonpolar chemicals are absorbed to a much greater degree than polar chemicals because of the properties of skin.

(2) Dilute concentrations of chemicals in air or water are absorbed to a lesser degree through skin than when ingested or inhaled.

(3) Abraded skin or mucus membranes are more likely to absorb chemicals than intact skin.

(4) Absorption of chemicals is not a prerequisite for local or irritative effects. Irritants act directly by damaging the skin or exposed mucus membrane.

3. Metabolism. Alteration in the metabolic pathway or rate of metabolism can change a toxic response by affecting the amount of toxic metabolite delivered to the systemic circulation. Almost all of the metabolic transformations that occur in living systems are enzyme catalyzed reactions.

a. Metabolic pathway describes the chemical intermediates to which a chemical is converted during metabolism. In general, the metabolic pathways of a chemical are similar for most organisms. However, there are often differences in pathways in microorganisms, plants, and animals. There are sometimes differences in metabolic pathways within animal or bacterial species and even within strains of the same species.

b. Rate of metabolism describes the time course of the metabolism and is usually a quantitative statement of the disappearance of a toxic chemical or the appearance of a given metabolite. See the discussion about differences in metabolism after ingestion or inhalation exposure in section II C 2 b.

4. Target organ dose is the amount or concentration of chemical to which the systemic target is exposed; this dose can be measured if there is sufficient knowledge about the toxic mechanism and the actual target site. Such doses are measured in different units than doses describing exposures.

a. Target organ doses might use units such as mg/L (of blood supplied to organ) or mg/kg (of target organ weight) rather than an exposure dose in units such as mg/kg (of body weight).

b. Blood levels of chemicals after exposure are useful for systemic toxicants, but many samples are needed to determine the accurate time course of blood levels of a chemical after a given exposure.

c. Without detailed knowledge of how a chemical interacts at a sensitive target organ to cause a toxic effect, blood level measurements contribute little to the understanding of the toxic effect.

5. Mediums and routes of exposure

a. Routes of exposure refer to the points of entry into the body for local effects and to the points of absorption into the bloodstream for systemic effects.

b. Mediums are the materials that contain the chemical that causes the toxic effect.

(a) Air as a medium contains chemicals in the vapor or gas phase and chemicals adsorbed onto particles entrained in air.

(b) Water as a medium refers to drinking water, surface water, groundwater, or rain.

(c) Soil refers to materials mixed with or adsorbed to soil particles.

(d) Food refers to fish, plants, and animals.

c. Relationships. The medium of chemical exposure is sometimes associated with a given route of exposure. However, multiple routes of exposure should be considered.

(1) Water is associated with ingestion, but other exposures result from direct contact (bathing) and inhalation (showering).

(2) Soil is associated with direct contact, but other exposures result from inhalation (entrainment of particles) and ingestion.

B. Mediums

1. Air exposures can be classified by both space and activity.

a. Ambient air is the outdoor air surrounding us wherever we are, in the absence of any activity that might change its composition. For convenience, ambient air can be divided further into:

(1) **Gas phase components** or gases, which are chemicals in the vapor phase.

(2) **Particulates**, which are solid materials suspended in air.

b. **Indoor air** is the air present in buildings where we live or work in the absence of any industrial activity that might change the air.

(1) **Life-styles** affect exposure to toxic chemicals. For example, smoking leads to direct exposure of the smoker and indirect exposure of others in the indoor area. Exposure to the carbon monoxide in smoke reduces the ability to use oxygen for metabolism. Exposure to the polynuclear aromatic hydrocarbons (many of which are known animal carcinogens) adsorbed onto particulates is probably responsible for the increased lung cancer rates of both smokers and exposed nonsmokers.

(2) **Home maintenance activities** can contribute to chemical exposure.

(a) **Formaldehyde** offgassing, or release from improperly cured urea foam formaldehyde insulation, can result in high levels of formaldehyde that can be detected by a characteristic odor and that can cause a chronic response in humans. If the insulation is properly applied, no formaldehyde is released, and no exposure occurs.

(b) **Radon** accumulation occurs when homes are insulated or otherwise modified to reduce air exchange with the outside.

(i) Although less air exchange results in energy savings, the "air-tight" home prevents dissipation of the radon that enters through the basement slab or crawl space into the lower levels of the home.

(ii) Naturally occurring radioactive radon results from decay of radium in the soil. Radium is present in all soils, but it is more concentrated in granite and black shale.

(iii) Because radiation is a nonthreshold insult, increased lung cancer incidence is expected as a result of increased radon exposure.

(c) **Solvent exposure** from paint removal or painting activity occurs through indoor use of materials containing solvents.

(d) **Termiticide** (e.g., aldrin and chlordane) exposure can occur from the improper application of the pesticide for home termite control.

(3) **Water containing volatile organic compounds (VOCs)** can contribute to indoor air levels of those chemicals. Chloroform, an animal carcinogen, is the predominent halomethane produced by the process of chlorinating surface waters, and thus VOCs are present in much of the drinking water supplied to cities. The regulatory limit for total halomethanes in drinking water is 100 ppb. This limit is a technology-based limit rather than a health-based limit.

(a) Activities such as showering, bathing, clothes washing, cooking, and cleaning can release VOCs contained in the water.

(b) The amount of chemical released from water depends on a number of factors, such as physical and chemical properties of the VOC, concentration, temperature, and agitation of the water.

(c) Air exposure to VOCs occurs both to individuals involved in the activity releasing the chemical (e.g., the individual taking a shower) and the other occupants of the house as the chemical is dispersed in the indoor air.

(d) VOCs are removed from indoor air by the exchange with outside air.

(4) **Deterioration of asbestos insulation** in office buildings, schools, and homes can lead to exposure to asbestos fibers. Although damage by contact with water is the most common cause of asbestos exposure, removal activities can lead to very high air exposures if appropriate precautions are not taken. Asbestos is a known human carcinogen, and exposure to any concentration is associated with an increase in cancer risk.

(5) **Hobbies**, such as building model airplanes, can contribute to indoor air exposure to solvents found in glue and paint.

c. **Recreational air** exposure can lead to chemical exposure as VOCs are released from water used to fill swimming pools and from streams used by fishermen.

d. **Occupational air** exposure is important because exposure to chemicals often occurs at high concentrations and for an appreciable fraction an individual's lifetime. (Occupational health is discussed in Chapter 12 and will not be discussed here.)

2. **Water exposure** can be categorized by the source of the water or by the activity resulting in exposure to a chemical in water.

a. **Drinking water.** Most of the drinking water in the United States comes from **public water supplies**, which **are regulated** under the Safe Water Drinking Act. Some drinking water comes from **private wells**, which **are not regulated**. Public water is obtained from:

(1) Surface water (rivers).

(2) Groundwater (wells).

b. Fish and other aquatic organisms accumulate chemicals in their edible flesh; thus, ingestion of fish results in exposure of humans to these chemicals.

(1) The ratio of concentration of chemical in edible flesh to the water in which the fish lives is the BCF. BCFs refer to the concentration ratio at equilibrium or after a sufficient period of time so that no change in the ratio is observed.

(2) Typically, inorganic metals do not bioaccumulate, while organic chemicals accumulate depending on their polarity and the extent of metabolism. Table 13-7 lists the BCFs for some chemicals.

c. Direct exposure

(1) Activities that involve contact of water with skin or mucus membranes can result in absorption directly through skin. Examples of such activities are bathing and swimming.

(2) Mucus membranes and abraded skin allow more rapid transport of chemicals in water than intact skin.

(3) Chemicals adsorbed to particulates are absorbed very slowly through the skin as compared to the same chemical dissolved in water.

(4) Quantities of chemicals absorbed through the skin are usually small relative to amounts absorbed through other routes of exposure.

3. Land disposal. Waste piles, dumps, spills, releases onto land, road oiling, and land treatment are all units or activities that are classified as land disposal. Landfills should only be used to dispose of nonliquid wastes while surface impoundments are designed for liquid waste storage.

a. Direct contact. Exposures from direct contact with a solid or semisolid material containing a chemical can occur, but in general this contact is not appreciable except in special circumstances, such as high concentrations, long exposure times, or by chemicals that can damage skin.

b. Food. Uptake of chemicals by vegetables from the soil can occur.

(1) Rates of uptake or the amount of chemical accumulated in the plant depend on:

(a) The physical and chemical properties of the chemical.

(b) The species of vegetable.

(c) The soil conditions.

(2) Different parts of the vegetable accumulate chemicals from soil differently; thus, human exposure depends on what portion of the plant is normally eaten.

c. Particulates. Entrainment of particles into air from soils can be a significant route of exposure.

(1) The physical properties of the chemical in soil determine to what extent the chemical will be adsorbed to particulates that are small enough to be entrained.

(2) The factors that affect entrainment are:

(a) Particle size.

(b) Water content.

(c) Meteorology.

(d) Site topography.

(e) Vegetation.

(f) Physical activity (e.g., dirt biking).

d. Ingestion. Direct ingestion of soil and therefore the chemicals found in soil are considered significant only in young children.

(1) The actual amount of dirt or soil ingested by small children is a matter of vigorous current debate, with extremes of ingestion ranging from 0.1 to 10 g/day.

(2) Ingestion is likely to occur for only a small portion of a lifetime.

(3) Dirt could also be ingested by population groups other than small children if they work with soil and then consume food in the same area.

e. Groundwater contamination. Leaching of toxic chemicals from landfills has been the cause of chemical contamination of many public and private wells. Landfills and surface impoundments leak. Chemicals from materials and wastes placed in land disposal units eventually leak out into the soil and groundwater beneath the disposal site.

(1) Double liners that are now required for hazardous waste landfills and surface impoundments can delay the migration of hazardous constituents from the unit, but cannot prevent leaching. Typically, liners and double liners retard migration for periods ranging from decades to centuries.

(2) Past disposal practices are responsible for much of the groundwater contamination throughout the United States. Two examples of the worst kinds of poor management and lack of environmental controls are:

(a) Placing liquid wastes into unlined surface impoundments.

(b) Disposing of bulk liquid spent solvent wastes in municipal or sanitary landfills. These units are designed to bury garbage and trash. When properly designed and operated, sanitary landfills do not endanger public health or the environment.

(3) The concentration of chemicals in groundwater underneath the site is dependent on many factors, including:
(a) Waste composition.
(b) Liner integrity.
(c) Physical and chemical properties.
(d) Groundwater flow rate.
(e) Rainfall.
(f) Soil type.
(g) Other wastes present.
(h) Geology.

4. **Other exposures** to toxic chemicals can occur as by-products of everyday activities such as use of food, drugs, medications, and cosmetics.
a. **Food.** Toxic effects of exposure to foodstuffs or additives in food are commonly known.
(1) **Ethanol** is consumed as a beverage, providing calories as well as enhancing the pleasures of eating; it is also a toxic chemical affecting nearly all who consume it.
(a) Ethanol exposure can lead to liver damage as a chronic toxic effect.
(b) Traffic fatalities caused by drunk drivers can also be considered toxic effects of ethanol.
(2) **Peanut butter** contains the chemical aflotoxin, which is released by a mold that grows on the peanuts. Processed peanut butter contains some small or trace amounts of aflotoxin.
(a) Aflotoxin is an animal carcinogen, and therefore a probable human carcinogen.
(b) Consuming peanut butter is associated with some excess cancer risk compared with not eating peanut butter.
(3) **Food additives** have known toxic effects, although many are indeed safe to almost all individuals at the levels used in food.
(a) **Monosodium glutamate (MSG)** is used as a flavor enhancer in Oriental cooking and causes a characteristic headache in some individuals who consume Chinese food prepared with MSG.
(b) **Sulfite** used to preserve fruit can result in a severe allergic reaction in a small group of people.
b. **Drugs, medicines, and cosmetics are** other examples of materials that can cause some toxic effects in humans because they are chemicals or because they contain chemicals.

V. EXPOSURE EVALUATION

A. **General principles.** Physical presence and exposure are not synonymous. A chemical may be present in a medium at very high concentrations yet pose no health hazard because exposure cannot occur from the medium due to the physical or chemical state of the chemical.

1. **The chemical state of an element** refers to its oxidation state or valence. Because physical properties of an element or compound depend on the oxidation state, release of the chemical into a medium may be affected by its oxidation state.
a. Inorganic elements often have many oxidation states in the environement, while organic chemicals generally have a single oxidation state.
b. Changes in the oxidation state of a chemical may affect availability of that chemical to a given medium.
(1) Chromium in the hexavalent state, Cr(VI), is a human carcinogen, while trivalent chromium, Cr(III), is not. Many industries use the trivalent form of chromium in manufacturing processes, and wastes from these processes contain chromium. If the chromium is in the Cr(III) form and oxidation to Cr(VI) is prevented, exposure presents no cancer risks.
(2) Lead in the ionic state (Pb^{2+}) is extremely toxic to small children, impairing nervous system development. Elemental lead (Pb) is the lead used in automobile batteries and in lead bullets.
(a) Lead from battery crushing operations (reclamation) can migrate to groundwater because the concentrated sulfuric acid used in batteries oxidizes lead from Pb to Pb^{2+}, which can then leach to groundwater; therefore, drinking water may contain lead.
(b) In the absence of a source of concentrated acid, lead from bullets used at a practice range is very unlikely to migrate into groundwater and pose a health problem. Lead bullets are not oxidized to ionic lead to any appreciable degree.
(c) Acid from acid rainfall events is more than 100-fold less acidic than the acid used in car batteries.

2. **The physical form of a chemical** refers to its physical association with other materials or to some property of the chemical.
   a. **Binding and trapping** of a chemical can prevent its release. Asbestos insulation used to protect structural steel against collapse during a fire or to insulate pipes contains 30%–60% asbestos. If the insulation is intact, no asbestos fibers are released into the air, no exposure can occur, and no increased cancer risk results. Contact with water from leaking roofs and pipes results in the release of asbestos into the air, resulting in exposure and an increased cancer risk. If there is no damage to the insulation, no exposure occurs even though asbestos is present in large quantities.
   b. **Lack of solubility** can retard the release of a chemical. Many of the common salts of lead are relatively insoluble in water. For example, the concentration of $Pb(SO_4)_2$ [lead sulfate] in water of pH = 9 is 1 μg/L. However, as the pH drops and the medium becomes more acidic, the solubility increases; at pH = 5.5, the solubility is 10 g/L. Thus, solid lead sulfate spilled into water dissolves very slowly at a pH above 9 but dissolves rapidly at a pH less than 6.
   c. **Containment** is another method that makes a chemical unavailable to a medium.
      (1) Transformers most often contain a mixture of polychlorinated biphenyls (PCBs) and chlorobenzenes. Exposure to these substances cannot occur unless the transformer ruptures in use or the insulating fluid leaks or spills during normal operation and maintenance.
      (2) Solvents stored in 55 gallon drums are not an exposure source if the drums are always closed during management.

B. Chemical analysis

1. **Analytic methodology.** Analytic techniques determine concentrations of contaminants in all mediums and materials. Analyses of air, water, soil, and sediment are routine while analysis of fish tissue is less common.
   a. **Priority pollutants.** There are 129 chemicals or classes of chemicals that are designated as priority pollutants. These chemicals are commonly used in commercial processes or are unusually toxic. Chemicals most relevant to the environment are listed in Table 13-8. This list was developed to settle the 1976 lawsuit against the EPA by the Natural Resources Defense Council (NRDC).
   b. **Analysis of organic and inorganic compounds** is by methods that are highly specific to the organic or inorganic compound measured.
      (1) **Gas chromatography** is the basic method for analyzing organic compounds.
      (2) **Atomic absorption** is the basic method for analyzing inorganic heavy metals.
   c. **The detection limit** is the minimum amount of a chemical that can be positively identified by an analytic method.
      (1) In aqueous samples, the detection limit is about 1 ppb for most chemicals.
      (2) In air and soil, detection limits are higher.
      (3) In special situations, detection limits are lower than routinely obtained (e.g., stack sampling for determining hazardous waste incinerator permit conditions or soil testing for PCBs, dibenzodioxins and dibenzofuranes). Low detection limits raise analytic costs.
   d. **The units of measurement** for determining the concentration of chemicals in various mediums are as follows:
      (1) **Air levels** are generally stated as:
         (a) Parts per million or billion (ppm or ppb) on a volume per volume basis.
         (b) Milligrams or micrograms per cubic meter (mg/m^3 or $\mu g/m^3$) on a weight per volume basis.

Table 13-8. Priority Pollutants

Category/Description	No.	Examples
Metals	13	Arsenic, lead, and silver
Pesticides	7	Chlordane, chlorophenothane (DDT), and toxaphene
Inorganics (other)	2	Asbestos and cyanides
Polyaromatic hydrocarbons	5	Naphthalene
Benzenes	7	Benzene, dichlorobenzene, and dinitrotoluene
Phenols	7	Phenol and pentachlorophenol
Chlorinated volatiles	14	Haloethers, trichloroethylene, and vinyl chloride
Chlorinated nonvolatiles	3	Dioxins and polychlorinated biphenyls
Miscellaneous organics	7	Acrylonitrile, benzidine, and nitrosamines

(2) **Water concentrations** are generally given as ppm or ppb on a weight per weight basis. Because 1 ml of water weighs about 1 g at temperatures found in the environment, ppm is equivalent to mg/L and ppb to μg/L.
(3) **Soil concentrations** are usually given as ppm or ppb, and these are equivalent to mg/kg soil or μg/kg soil, respectively. Note that the soil is not dried to remove water before analysis.
(4) **Particulate concentrations** in air are measured as mg/m^3 or $\mu g/m^3$, which represent the amount of particulate material contained in 1 m^3 of air.

2. **Environmental monitoring** involves sampling and analysis.
   a. **Monitoring environmental mediums** such as water, air, fish, or soil for chemicals has direct implications for humans exposed to those mediums.
   b. **Monitoring materials** such as spent solvent, used oil, asbestos insulation, waste streams, or chemical ingredients for chemicals usually has an indirect relationship to exposure and represents a potential for a chemical to be released into a medium.

3. **Monitoring individuals.** Monitoring individuals for parameters of exposure is divided into three areas. For each area, appropriate sampling and analytic methods are important.
   a. **Sampling the air** around an individual for chemicals or using a radiation sensitive badge are ways in which to measure individual exposure.
   b. **Measurement of tissue or body fluid levels** of a chemical or metabolite can verify exposure.
   (1) Blood and urine are the most common body fluids analyzed. Fat biopsy for chemicals is occasionally used; however, it is much more difficult to obtain a fat sample than it is to obtain blood or urine.
   (2) A metabolite may need to be measured rather than the original chemical because chemicals are often metabolized by the body.
   (3) The relationship of body fluid levels to exposure is known for relatively few chemicals. Usually the relationship is known only if the chemical is used industrially where medical surveillance, including body fluid analysis, occurs and if the chemical is of low acute toxicity.

   c. **Body functions can also be measured.** For example, blood cholinesterase measurements used to determine pesticide exposure. However, usually blood cholinesterase levels are used only to indicate a need for therapy or to stop a known exposure. Rarely can functional tests measure the amount of exposure.

C. **Models** are a set of assumptions used to estimate exposures. As such, models estimate exposures for individuals to the extent that the assumptions made are accurate. Models are useful because of the ability to determine the change in exposure when one of the assumptions is changed. Thus, individual variation in exposure can be obtained.

1. **Assumptions** that are used to estimate exposures must be as accurate and reasonable as possible since they directly affect the exposure estimate. Assumptions are sometimes deliberately made to protect public health. **Common assumptions** used for the models are listed below:
   a. **Body weight** is 70 kg for adults and 10 kg for children.
   b. **Life span** is 70 years for humans.
   c. **Water consumption** is 2 L/day for adults and 1 L/day for children.
   d. **Air inhalation** is 20 m^3/day for adults.
   e. **Particles** larger than 10 μ in diameter are ingested, particles less than 0.1 μ in diameter are exhaled, and particles of intermediate size are retained in the lungs.
   f. **Fish consumption** is 6.5 g/day of edible flesh.
   g. **Soil ingestion** is 0.1 g/day.

2. **Models in mediums**
   a. **Models for air exposure** to a chemical are determined by using air levels of the chemicals obtained by modeling or monitoring combined with exposure assumptions.
   (1) **Inhaled volume** of 20 m^3/day is a total volume per day and is summed over all daily activities. The inhaled volume of air per individual varies with:
   (a) Age.
   (b) Health status.
   (c) Body weight.
   (d) Work output or physical activity.
   (2) **Absorption** of a chemical in air into the bloodstream is measured in inhalation exposure. Absorption is determined from existing experiments, estimated from structurally similar chemicals, or assumed to be complete. Absorption of chemicals adsorbed to particles deposited in the lungs is assumed to be 100%.

b. **Models for drinking water exposure** use a daily volume of water consumed and an absorption factor determined by experiment or assumption.

c. **Models for fish ingestion** depend on the amount and species of fish ingested.

(1) The average amount of fish consumed daily in the United States in 1980 was 6.5 g/day of edible flesh.

(2) The fat content of the edible flesh is directly related to the amount of chemical that has accumulated. BCFs are standardized to a weighted fat content of 3.0%. Table 13-9 shows the fat content of some selected fish species.

d. **Models for direct exposure** are not commonly used because this route usually contributes much less to the total exposure than inhalation and ingestion.

e. **Models for dirt ingestion** use an estimate of dirt consumed and an absorption factor determined by experiment or assumption.

(1) The assumed amount of dirt ingested is 0.1 g/day. However, young children are known to ingest a significant amount of dirt. More representative estimates for children are 1 g/day; however, some observers have estimated up to 10 g/day.

(2) Children are assumed to be exposed for only a portion of their 70-year life span; it is commonly estimated that exposure takes place for 10 years.

(3) Exposure may not occur every day, and sometimes exposure for a certain number of days a year is assumed.

D. **Modeling** is a procedure by which concentrations of a chemical released into air, water, or land are estimated from knowledge of emission or release rates and assumptions about the movement and fate of the chemical in the environment.

1. **Air dispersion modeling** can be used to estimate concentrations of a chemical at various locations around a point of emission. A variety of modeling approaches are reasonable, and choice depends on the characteristics of the emission source, terrain, and meteorology. Air modeling can be used for particulates as well as gas phase chemicals.

a. **Factors affecting the concentration of a chemical** include:

(1) Emission rate.
(2) Temperature.
(3) Chemical and physical properties of emitted chemical.
(4) Meteorology.
(5) Stack height.
(6) Terrain.
(7) Environmental fate.

b. **Examples of environmental releases.** Air modeling has successfully approximated actual measured concentrations of:

(1) VOCs released from sewage treatment plants.
(2) Solvent releases from vented storage tanks.
(3) Particulate releases from smelters.
(4) Chemical releases from industrial processes.

c. **Outputs of air modeling** are typically concentration isopleths for the chemical averaged over some time period. Modeling can also identify the location or point of maximum air concentration of the chemical.

2. **Surface water modeling** is used to estimate concentration of a chemical in surface water after releases into the water.

a. The three most common releases are by:

(1) Direct discharge into the water.
(2) Groundwater discharge into the surface water.
(3) Sediment or soil release of adsorbed chemicals.

b. **Factors affecting the concentration of chemical** at a given location in surface water include:

(1) Emission rate.
(2) Chemical and physical properties.
(3) Environmental fate.
(4) Velocity of water flow.
(5) Temperature.
(6) Dilution.
(7) Treatment.

c. **Examples of environmental releases.** Surface water modeling approximates the actual water concentrations measured in:

(1) Solvent released into a stream as a spill.
(2) Acid waste discharge allowed by an environmental permit.
(3) PCBs released from sediments in a river.

Table 13-9. Fat Content of Edible Flesh of Some Fish Species

Ocean		Freshwater		Shellfish	
Species	**Percent Fat**	**Species**	**Percent Fat**	**Species**	**Percent Fat**
Bluefish	3.3	White perch	4.0	Soft clam	1.9
Cod	0.3	Yellow perch	0.9	Crab	1.9
Eel	18.3	Brook trout	2.1	Crayfish	0.5
Tuna	4.1	Lake trout	10.0	Lobster	1.9
Atlantic		Rainbow trout	11.4	Mussel	2.2
Herring	11.3	Lake whitefish	8.2	Octopus	0.8
Mackerel	12.2			Eastern oyster	7.8
Ocean perch	1.2			Western oyster	2.2
Salmon	13.4			Scallop	0.2
Pacific				Shrimp	0.8
Herring	2.6			Squid	0.9
Mackerel	7.3				
Ocean perch	1.5				

d. Surface water modeling results are water concentration of a chemical and its variation with time at a given point, usually a public drinking water supply intake.

3. Groundwater modeling is used to estimate concentrations in groundwater from chemical releases onto or into land or soil. The groundwater could be used for private or public drinking water wells, or it could become surface water as it is discharged into streams.

a. Factors affecting the concentration of a chemical in groundwater include:

(1) Emission rate.
(2) Physical and chemical properties.
(3) Groundwater flow rate.
(4) Soil type.
(5) Environmental fate.
(6) Geology.

b. Examples of releases to soil. Groundwater modeling successfully approximates concentrations of chemicals in groundwater monitoring wells in:

(1) Solvent tanks leaking directly into soil.
(2) PCBs released into a river by groundwater flow from material spilled onto and buried in soil.

c. Groundwater modeling results are expressed as:

(1) Concentration of a chemical at various locations.
(2) A variation of concentrations with time.

VI. REGULATION OF CHEMICALS IN THE ENVIRONMENT.

Chemicals in the environment are regulated on a programmatic basis that includes environmental mediums and end uses.

A. Air. The Clean Air Act (CAA) is the most important federal law protecting the air that we breathe. It establishes ambient air standards for six pollutants and emission standards for those six and other chemicals. The CAA does not have jurisdiction over workplace exposure.

1. Concentration standards

a. Criteria pollutants. Six noncarcinogenic pollutants have been labeled "criteria" pollutants. Because none of the six are carcinogens, threshold or safe levels can be established. These criteria pollutants are:

(1) Carbon monoxide.
(2) Lead.
(3) Nitrogen dioxide.
(4) Ozone.
(5) Particulates.
(6) Sulfur dioxide.

b. Sources. Both mobile and stationary sources are regulated under the CAA. Exemptions from regulations exist for some sources based on the industrial process and the amount of the pollutant emitted.

(1) Emissions from automobiles contribute significant amounts of all criteria pollutants, except sulfer dioxide.
(2) Stationary sources, including utility boilers, manufacturing processes, and chemical storage, emit many chemicals.

c. **Right-to-know laws.** Some states or local jurisdictions have right-to-know laws or similar legislation that establish local ambient air standards.

2. **Emission controls**
   a. **Hazardous air pollutants** are chemicals that may "reasonably be anticipated to result in an increase in mortality or an increase in a serious reversible illness."
      (1) **Identity.** Table 13-10 shows the hazardous air pollutants that are identified by the EPA. Most are animal or human carcinogens.
      (2) **Controls.** The CAA requires the EPA to identify sources and set emission standards with an "ample margin of safety to protect the public health."
         (a) The EPA has identified the industrial processes that emit large quantities or result in high ambient concentrations of each hazardous air pollutant.
         (b) Since any exposure to a carcinogen is associated with some risk of cancer (see section III A 1), risk assessments have been conducted for each source of a hazardous air pollutant.
         (c) Risk management decisions are made for each emission from each source. The decision is based on the risk to the individual and the total population, and on the possible potential reduction of risk with available technology.
   b. **Criteria pollutants** emitted from many sources are regulated.
   c. **Unregulated chemicals.** The EPA has virtually no authority to regulate releases of chemicals other than criteria and hazardous air pollutants.
      (1) **Toxic chemical releases** are currently unregulated except for a small number of sources of hazardous air pollutant releases. Both "normal" process releases or losses and emergency or accidental releases require tight environmental controls.
      (2) **Indoor air quality** is currently unregulated. Radon accumulation, VOCs from drinking water, formaldehyde, and carbon monoxide are examples of chemicals that are not controlled in indoor air.
      (3) **Air releases** from environmental cleanup activities, such as sewage treatment plants, hazardous waste incinerators using solvents as fuels, or air stripping of VOC contaminants from groundwater, are usually not controlled.

B. Water. The Clean Water Act (CWA) and the Safe Drinking Water Act (SDWA) are the two federal laws responsible for protecting water as an environmental medium.

1. **Drinking water standards.** Public drinking water is regulated by establishment of standards. Private wells used by single families are not regulated. Public drinking water can be pumped from either groundwater or surface water. Only the finished water is regulated, not the water source prior to treatment.
   a. **Regulated contaminants** include:
      (1) Microorganisms.
      (2) Radioactivity.
      (3) A group of eight heavy metals.
      (4) A group of six pesticides.
      (5) Some inorganic anions.
      (6) Total haloforms.
   b. **Unregulated toxic organic chemicals.** Regulatory concentrations for many VOCs and other organic chemicals have been proposed and will probably result in some maximum contamination level (MCL).
      (1) **For noncarcinogens**, the proposed MCLs are protective of the most sensitive human population.
      (2) **For carcinogens**, the levels proposed would result in no greater lifetime risk than 10^{-5} or 1 in 100,000.

2. **Effluent standards** are limits for discharge into waters of the United States; they regulate many industries that discharge priority pollutants and other chemicals.
   a. **Sources.** Most discharge sources are regulated, for example:
      (1) Industrial manufacturing process discharges.
      (2) Cooling water tower discharges.

Table 13-10. Hazardous Air Pollutants

Asbestos
Benzene
Beryllium
Mercury
Radionuclides
Vinyl chloride

(3) Storm water runoff.
(4) Chemical industry discharges.
(5) Groundwater treatment discharges.
(6) Municipal sewage treatment plant effluents.

b. Effluent limitations

(1) The first set of effluent standards were developed in the early 1970s and were based on controlling the conventional pollutants shown in Table 13-11. Discharge permits do not usually govern individual chemical contaminants but instead limit only conventional pollutants.
(2) Effluent permits currently being issued by the EPA and the states limit amounts of priority pollutants discharged and require that dischargers use the best available treatment technology. Thus, regulation of effluent discharges is technology based, not health based.

c. Unregulated chemicals

(1) There are no concentration limitations for chemical constituents for current or future use of:
(a) Groundwater.
(b) Recreational water.
(c) Streams.
(d) Lakes and ponds.
(2) Underground injection wells, which are a potential source of groundwater contamination, are also unregulated.
(3) Health-based standards rather than technology-based standards are needed for drinking water.

C. Land. The Resource Conservation and Recovery Act (RCRA) and the Comprehensive Environmental Response, Compensation, and Liability Act (CERCLA or Superfund) are the two federal laws governing regulation of present and future land disposal practices and cleanup.

1. Land disposal units include:

a. Landfills for:
(1) Municipalities or sanitation.
(2) Hazardous wastes.
(3) Industrial residues.
(4) Infectious or pathologic materials.

b. Surface impoundments or lagoons for:
(1) Wastewater treatment.
(2) Hazardous waste treatment or storage.
(3) Equalization basins.
(4) Storm water runoff.

c. Waste piles used for accumulating any noncontainerized solid nonflowing materials.

d. Land treatment for waste application onto or incorporation into the soil surface.

2. Waste management practices

a. Liners used for any land disposal units eventually fail.
(1) Recent regulations require two liners and a leachate collection system between the double liners. However, many of the existing surface impoundments and landfills do not have any liners.
(2) Originally liners were compacted from clay available near the site; however, synthetic plastic liners are the liners of choice for almost all waste materials.

b. Liquids are not suitable for landfill disposal.

c. Inorganic wastes are generally more suitable for landfill disposal than organic wastes.
(1) Organic compounds can cause synthetic liners to fail because they are sometimes incompatible with the liner.
(2) Inorganic materials that have been removed (mined) from the earth cause mimimal problems of containment when placed back into the earth.

d. Treatment by encapsulation or similar processes can retard the mobilization of soluble

Table 13-11. Conventional Water Pollutants

Suspended solids
Oil and grease
Extremes of pH
Fecal coliform
Biologic oxygen demand

constituents for many years, thus delaying and diluting the appearance of a chemical in groundwater beneath the land disposal unit.

3. Standards

a. Prohibitions. Hazardous wastes that may not be disposed of in landfills include:
- **(1)** Liquid hazardous wastes.
- **(2)** Solvents.
- **(3)** Some dioxin-containing wastes.
- **(4)** Other selected organic wastes.

b. Emissions. Releases from land disposal units are controlled.
- **(1)** Groundwater monitoring is required for all land disposal units.
- **(2)** Indicator parameters are used to determine if a unit is leaking.
- **(3)** Remedial activity is required for releases.

c. Closure. Requirements for clean closure are part of all land disposal permits issued.
- **(1)** Removal of all wastes and contaminated residues is required for storage or treatment surface impoundments.
- **(2)** Capping and groundwater monitoring is required for 30 years for all landfills.

4. Cleanup activities range from emergency removal of waste materials at sites where an imminent and substantial danger exists to a remedial activity planned and executed over a several year period. Although both RCRA and CERCLA have provisions for cleaning up sites:

a. CERCLA is usually implemented when a responsible party does not exist, as in bankruptcy, or chooses not to cooperate.

b. RCRA is used with responsible parties that initiate cleanup.

5. Unresolved land disposal issues

a. Lack of adequate enforcement of existing standards and regulations is the most significant land disposal problem.

b. Developing new treatment techniques to treat waste materials to reduce the reliance of societies on land disposal is a significant technological challange.

c. Lack of public confidence in the government's commitment to protect public health is one of the obstacles in siting hazardous waste management facilities.

d. Lack of adequate capacity for hazardous and nonhazardous wastes.

D. Food. The Food and Drug Administration (FDA) regulates levels of chemicals in food through the authority of the Food, Drugs, and Cosmetics Act. Several thousand substances are regulated.

1. Food additives serve many purposes, such as to:

a. Flavor.
b. Color.
c. Preserve.
d. Sweeten.
e. Emulsify.
f. Anticake.
g. Stabilize.
h. Bleach.
i. Enhance flavor.

2. Classifications

a. Substances can be classified according to how the additive gets into food.

(1) Intentional food additives are added during some part of the commercial or home preparation of the food. Examples of intentional food additives are:
- **(a)** Sodium benzoate, which is used as a food preservative.
- **(b)** Monosodium glutamate (MSG), which is used as a flavor enhancer.
- **(c)** Agar-agar, which is used as a stabilizer.
- **(d)** Vanillin, which is used as a flavor.
- **(e)** Caramel, which is used to add color.

(2) Unintentional food additives are substances that are not deliberately added, but are in the food as a result of the growth process or from harvesting or storage. Examples of unintentional food additives are:
- **(a)** Antibiotics, which are used to control diseases.
- **(b)** Residues of pesticides, which are used to control insects.
- **(c)** Chemicals, which are used for storage or packaging purposes.
- **(d)** Radioactivity from fallout after nuclear weapons testing.

b. Substances can also be classified according to the degree of regulation.

(1) Hundreds of additives are Generally Recognized As Safe (GRAS) because of historic use in food and the lack of reports of adverse health effects. This group is the least regulated of all substances added to food.

(2) Substances in the GRAS group have been evaluated for toxicity using modern toxicologic methods, resulting in the removal of some chemicals from the GRAS group.
(3) All remaining food additives are stringently regulated.

3. **Carcinogens** are banned as intentional food additives because of the Delaney Amendment to the Food Additive Amendment of 1958. This farsighted amendment prohibits the FDA from considering as "safe" any chemical that has caused cancer in humans or animals.
   a. Cyclamate was banned as an artificial sweetener because it caused bladder cancer in animals.
   b. Saccharin was banned for the same reason, but the United States Congress stayed the ban.
      (1) One argument made for allowing saccharin use is that the risk of adverse health effects of obesity and of diabetes outweighs the risk of cancer.
      (2) In 1977, when the saccharin ban was proposed by the FDA, no other artificial sweetener was considered safe. Thus, saccharin was the only low-calorie sweetener used by the general public as an aid to controlling weight.

4. **Action levels** are chemical concentrations at which the FDA will take action to remove a food containing that chemical from the market. The FDA has set action levels for more than 20 chemicals in various foodstuffs. Over half of these chemicals are pesticides. Action levels:
   a. Are not permissible levels of contamination where that contamination is avoidable. They represent the maximum concentration of unavoidable contamination, resulting from growth, harvest, storage, and preparation.
   b. Apply to selected foods. For a given chemical, separate action levels are set in each food or foodstuff; for example:
      (1) Endrin has an action level of 0.05 ppm in asparagus and 0.3 ppm in fish and shellfish.
      (2) Chlordane has an action level of 0.8 ppm in rendered animal fat and 0.3 ppm in fish.

E. Consumer products. The Consumer Product Safety Commission (CPSC) administers several laws developed to protect consumers from unsafe products that are otherwise unregulated.

1. Tris(2,3-dibromopropyl)phosphate (TRIS) was used to make children's sleepwear fire-resistant. The requirement for fire-resistant sleepwear is part of the Flammable Fabrics Act. After TRIS was determined to be a potent animal carcinogen, the CPSC banned its use and required that treated garments be removed from the market.

2. Formaldehyde is a gas that is produced when urea foam formaldehyde insulation is improperly formulated. Formaldehyde is an animal carcinogen that produces nasal cancer in rats.
   a. The insulation requires preparation at the site of installation, and when properly formulated, does not result in offgassing of formaldehyde. In a small percentage of installations, the insulation is not mixed properly. When this happens, the insulation does not produce the desired polymer, and formaldehyde is released into the interior of the home.
   b. The CPSC banned the use of urea foam formaldehyde insulation because of the potential for improper formulation. However, the ban was rescinded by court order after an industrial lawsuit.
      (1) The use of urea foam formaldehyde insulation has declined dramatically because of the publicity accompaning the CPSC ban.
      (2) Existing urea foam formaldehyde insulation that was properly formulated and has "set up" or polymerized will not produce formaldehyde and did not do so when first installed.

F. Toxic chemicals. The Toxic Substances Control Act (TSCA) is the federal law that regulates production and use of new chemicals and previously unregulated chemicals.

1. TSCA applies to all chemicals except foods, drugs, cosmetics, and pesticides.

2. Before a new chemical can be produced for industrial or commercial use, the EPA must review the available toxicologic data base. The EPA has the power to regulate any chemical judged to pose an unreasonable risk of injury to human health or to the environment. Regulatory options that have been used under TSCA include:
   a. Banning.
   b. Labeling requirements.
   c. Disposal requirements.
   d. Exposure precautions.
   e. Informational requirements.

3. Specific chemicals regulated under TSCA are:
   a. **Asbestos.** TSCA requires notification of the public if friable (crumbly) asbestos is found in public schools and establishes removal and disposal requirements.

b. PCBs. TSCA regulates the use, treatment, and disposal of PCBs.
c. Dioxins. TSCA regulates the disposal of dioxin-containing waste.

G. Radiation and radioactive materials. The Atomic Energy Act is the single most important federal law regulating radioactive substances. This Act is administered by the Nuclear Regulatory Commission for nonmilitary purposes while the Department of Defense is responsible for military controls. Also, some radioactivity in environmental mediums is controlled by various laws administered by the EPA.

1. Sources
- **a. Ionizing radiation** occurs naturally or is man-made and includes:
  - **(1)** Cosmetic irradiation incident to the earth's surface.
  - **(2)** Naturally occurring radionuclides in the earth's crust.
  - **(3)** Radiation from medical diagnostic or treatment machines.
  - **(4)** Radionuclides prepared for medical, technical, or scientific uses.
  - **(5)** Nuclear power reactors.
  - **(6)** Nuclear weapons.
- **b. Nonionizing radiation** that occurs naturally is ultraviolet light, a component of sunlight.

2. Effects. Both ionizing and nonionizing radiation can cause cancer. Since cancer is a non-threshold effect, cancer incidence is directly proportional to exposure.

3. Controls
- **a. Concentration standards** exist for radioactivity in some media, such as:
  - **(1)** Drinking water.
  - **(2)** Milk.
- **b. Emission standards** or controls exist for releases into:
  - **(1)** Air.
  - **(2)** Groundwater.
  - **(3)** Surface water.
- **c. Radiation exposure is** controlled for:
  - **(1)** Workplaces.
  - **(2)** Medical x-rays.
- **d. Radioactive material exposure** is controlled for:
  - **(1)** Nuclear power generation.
  - **(2)** Nuclear weapons production and storage.
  - **(3)** Scientific and medical research.

H. Workplace. The Occupational Safety and Health Act (OSHA) is the single most important federal law regulating workplace exposure. Because occupational exposure to chemicals is discussed in a separate chapter of this volume (see Chapter 12), only a few areas of concern are noted here.

1. The OSHA includes significant exemptions for some occupational groups of workers and for workplaces employing small numbers of workers.

2. Other laws also control some workplace exposures, and these regulate:
- **a.** Air. The EPA may act if a pollution source is presenting an imminent and substantial danger to anyone.
- **b.** Hazardous waste management. The EPA may act to protect workers health.
- **c.** State or local jurisdictions.
- **d.** Chemicals in commerce. The EPA may act to protect workers.

3. Occupational standards are intended to assure that an employee shall suffer no material impairment of health or functional capacity even if exposed throughout his or her working life. However, occupational standard setting is as much a political process as scientific and medical processes. Historically, workplace standards have been made more stringent as our scientific and medical data bases increase.

I. Drugs and cosmetics. The Food, Drug, and Cosmetics Act administered by the FDA is the major federal law regulating drugs and cosmetics. Although exposure to drugs and cosmetics is voluntary, the routes of exposure differ. Cosmetic exposure is by direct contact, and absorption of chemicals by this route is much slower than drug absorption via ingestion or inhalation.

1. Drugs are chemicals that are used because of specific effects that they cause in humans.
- **a. Doses or exposure to drugs** must be high enough to produce the desired effect, and such high doses often cause other effects that are considered toxic side effects. Side effects are not unusual because chemicals can interact at many sites in humans.

b. Use of a drug is an example of a risk management decision. The benefits of the drug therapy must be considered in conjunction with:

(1) The risks of not using the drug.

(2) The risks of side effects.

(3) The risks and benefits of alternate available therapies.

c. The classification of drug use as licit or illicit is not relevant in considering toxic effects.

d. Drug abuse is the excessive use of a drug because of nonmedicinal effects of the drugs. Chemicals that are not drugs can also be abused, and such abuse differs only in that the chemical is not regulated as a drug (e.g., glue sniffing where the chemical is the solvent toluene). Although drug abuse occurs with licit and illicit drugs, most of the public focus on drug abuse is on the illegal use of narcotics, barbiturates, amphetamines, cocaine, and psychedelic drugs. However, the most abused drugs in our society are legal drugs—ethanol and tobacco.

2. Cosmetics. Because exposure to chemicals in cosmetics is by direct application to skin or mucus membranes, only small amounts of chemicals are expected to pass through the skin into the systemic circulation. Thus, toxic effects from cosmetic application are usually confined to effects on the skin or mucus membranes.

VII. MANAGEMENT OF ENVIRONMENTAL RISKS

A. Risks

1. Definition

a. Risk is the likelihood of a given toxicologic end point resulting from a specified exposure situation. Environmental risks are often associated with exposure to chemicals but are also the result of exposure to other insults, such as microorganisms or radiation.

b. Safety is the opposite of risk and is the probability that a given toxicologic end point will *not* occur as a consequence of a specified exposure.

2. Voluntary and involuntary risks

a. Voluntary risks are those accepted by individuals or society with some knowledge that the activity involved has risks; however, the extent or severity of the risks may not be accurately or fully understood. Causes, consequences, and probabilities for some voluntary risks are listed in Table 13-12.

b. Involuntary risks are those risks about which individuals or society have no knowledge or control and are usually imposed on the individual or groups. Examples of involuntary risks are listed in Table 13-12.

Table 13-12. Voluntary and Involuntary Risks

Cause/Activity	Consequence	Individual Lifetime Risk*	Lifetime Risk* per Million Population
Involuntary			
Home accidents	Death	1/1190	840
Traffic accidents (using seat belts)‡	Death	1/114	8750
Struck by lightning	Death	1/28,500	35
Pneumonia	Death	1/45	22,300
Outdoor exposure to radon	Lung cancer	1/2000	500
Voluntary			
Coal mining accidents†	Death	1/17	58,500
Coal mining black lung disease†	Death	1/3	369,000
Traffic accidents (without seat belts)‡	Death	1/114	8750
Truck driving accidents†	Death	1/220	4500
Smoking one cigarette per week	Lung cancer	1/3500	285
Smoking one cigarette per day	Lung cancer	1/500	2,000
Smoking one pack of cigarettes per day	Lung cancer	1/25	40,000

*Lifetime risks are shown in two equivalent ways: the lifetime risk of death for an individual and the lifetime risk per million population.

†Lifetime risk assumes a 70-year lifetime exposure; however, the occupational exposure of coal miners and truck drivers is 45 years.

‡Risk is the excess risk of death in a traffic accident when not using seat belts. The seat-belt use and the non–seat-belt excess risk were determined from the total traffic accident risk using the assumption that half of the deaths would be prevented by the use of seat belts. The total risk of death from traffic accidents is the sum of the seat belt use risk and the non–seat-belt use excess risk; this total is 1/57 or 17,500 per million.

3. **Risk assessment** is the scientific determination of the identity and probability of adverse human health effects from exposure to a chemical or insult.
   a. **Components.** Information from scientific and technical disciplines are integrated into a complete risk assessment.
      (1) **Hazard identification** is the identification of the health effects or toxicologic end points that result from exposure to a chemical or insult.
      (2) **Dose-response evaluation** is the quantitative relationship between exposure and toxic effect.
      (3) **Exposure evaluation** is the quantitative estimate of population and individual exposure to the chemical or insult.
      (4) **Risk characterization** is the integration of all of the toxic effects, dose-response, and exposure evaluation information.
   b. **The results** of risk assessments for carcinogens and noncarcinogens are expressed differently.
      (1) **Noncarcinogens.** A risk assessment for noncarcinogens results in an estimate of the exposure to the noncarcinogen compared to a threshold or safe exposure. If the ratio of exposure to threshold is less than 1, then a toxic effect is not expected or likely to occur. Conversely, if the ratio is greater than 1, a toxic effect may occur in the exposed individual.
      (2) **Carcinogens.** A risk assessment for chemical carcinogens results in an estimate of the maximum excess cancer risk from exposure to the carcinogen. Because of the uncertainties and protective public health assumptions, the cancer risk derived is the upper limit of the true risk. This means that the actual risk is not likely to be greater than the estimated risk and may in fact be much less.

4. **Scientific policy.** Risk assessment for most chemicals or insults is not an exact quantitative science because the scientific data base is rarely sufficient. In the absence of sufficient data to determine a relationship, scientific policy decisions are made. These decisions combine the available data with protective public health assumptions. Scientific policy decisions have been made in the following areas.
   a. Animal studies are valid indications of human carcinogenic potential.
   b. Animal bioassay tests using high doses are valid predictors of human response.
   c. Benign tumor formation in animal bioassays is considered a cancer-producing response.
   d. Both inhalation and ingestion routes of exposure are valid methods for animal bioassays.
   e. The most sensitive animal bioassay response is valid to estimate human cancer potency.
   f. No threshold is a valid assumption for carcinogenesis.
   g. Dose conversions between species use surface area equivalence.
   h. High- to low-dose extrapolation models predicting linearity at low doses are valid.

5. **Uncertainties.** Because some of the inputs to quantitative risk assessments include assumptions that are protective of public health, there are some uncertainties associated with the resulting risk assessment. These uncertainties can be classified into two groups:
   a. Those that are the result of scientific policy decisions.
   b. Those that are the result of assumptions about human exposure. In general, the area of human exposure has the greatest uncertainty for risk assessments.

6. **Risks of living.** Life is not risk free. Individual and societal decisions involving risk affect the cause and time of death but not the end result.
   a. **Daily life.** The lifetime risk of death from "normal" activities is shown for a few examples in Tables 13-12. and 13-13.
   b. **Chemical exposure.** Exposure and associated cancer risks for a few selected chemicals are shown in Table 13-13. Note that the chemical concentrations used are those actually measured in an ambient environmental medium.
   c. **Radiation exposure.** Exposure and associated cancer risks from radiation are also shown in Table 13-13.

B. **Risk management** is the process of choosing between regulatory or risk reduction options. Risk assessments are important to risk management decisions. Without some human health risk, there would be little need for a risk management decision.

1. **General issues.** Almost all risk management decisions can be categorized into the following categories:
   a. **Legal or regulatory.** Regulations and laws often require or prohibit certain actions.
   b. **Health.** Public or individual health consequences of a risk management action is the "pure" risk assessment contribution to risk management.
   c. **Ethical.** Individuals (e.g., physicians or toxicologists) and social institutions (e.g., hospitals or government agencies) often have ethical considerations that affect risk management decisions.

Table 13-13. Cancer Risks from Chemical or Radiation Exposure

Chemical or Radiation	Exposure Conditions (Concentration)	Individual Lifetime Risk*	Lifetime Risk per Million Population
Benzene	Rural ambient air (4.5 μg/m³)	1/29,900	33
Benzene	Urban ambient air (8.9 μg/m³)	1/15,100	66
Benzene	Self-service gasoline station (780 μg/m³)†	1/349,000	3
Chloroform	Rural ambient air (0.20 μg/m³)	1/250,000	4
Chloroform	Urban ambient air (0.49 μg/m³)	1/102,000	10
Chloroform	Chlorinated surface drinking water supply (10 μg/L)‡	1/49,900	20
Chloroform	Chlorinated surface drinking water supply (75 μg/L)‡	1/6670	150
Chloroform	Daily shower using surface water supply (75 μg/L)§	1/7660	130
Asbestos	Office building with friable asbestos (58 ng/m³)‖	1/22,900	41
Radon	Indoor exposure (1 pCi/L)**	1/514	1940
Radiation	Yearly chest x-ray	1/20,000	50
Arsenic	Remote ambient air (0.0004 μg/m³)	1/175,000	6
Arsenic	Urban ambient air (0.003 μg/m³)	1/23,400	43
Arsenic	Ambient air near smelters (0.03 μg/m³)	1/2340	428
Arsenic	Occupational exposure at smelter (1 μg/m³)‖	1/370	2700
Arsenic	Occupational exposure at smelter (10 μg/m³)‖	1/37	27,000
Polychlorinated biphenyls	Eating bluefish (2.0 ppm)††	1/1430	696
Chlordane	Private home air levels after misapplication (2.1 μg/m³)**	1/1770	564
Saccharin	Drinking two cans of diet soda per day	1/3330	300

*Lifetime risks are shown in two equivalent ways: the lifetime risk of death for an individual and the lifetime risk per million population. Exposure is assumed to 70 years.
†Assumes a 5 minute per week exposure.
‡Environmental Protection Agency limits for total haloforms in drinking water are 100 μg/L.
§Exposure was modeled by the author, assuming one 15-minute shower per day.
‖Occupational exposure is based on a 40-hour work week, 46 weeks per year for 45 years.
**Assumes a 14 hour per day exposure.
††Assumes an ingestion of one 6-ounce portion of bluefish per month.

d. Practical. Good management is usually the most important consideration for activities that are unregulated but pose some risk.

e. Other. In addition to human health considerations, other concerns are integrated into risk management decisions, including:

(1) Economics.
(2) Politics.
(3) Public expectations.
(4) Social considerations.
(5) Technical feasibility.

C. Health professional risk management. The response of health professionals and government officials to environmental exposures most often concern exposure to chemicals that are carcinogens or that pose other serious health consequences.

1. Present exposure

a. Treat the symptoms, if present.

b. Verify exposure.

(1) If analytic results show the presence of the chemical in a medium and if exposure is likely, it is reasonable to assume that exposure has occurred.

(2) If analytic results are not available nor likely to be available, and a simple and inexpensive blood or urine test can yield an unequivocal result, then body fluid samples should be analyzed. If the results of a test will not alter treatment or reduce exposure, do not perform any tests; simply assume that exposure has occurred.

c. Reduce presumed exposure by whatever means necessary.

2. Past exposure

a. Treat the symptoms, if present.

b. Assume that exposure has occurred for purposes of determining potential health effects.
c. Recommend a test of environmental medium of body fluids only if a test result would alter some action to be taken.

3. **Toxic end points** of special concern are carcinogenesis, teratogenesis, and reproductive effects. Uncertainties exist in estimating risks or effects from carcinogens and teratogens. It is important that these risks and uncertainties be communicated to patients.
   a. **Carcinogenesis.** Exposure to a cancer-causing chemical will at most increase the lifetime cancer risk of the individual. For many chemical exposures, estimates (risk assessments) show that the excess cancer risk is quite small, on the order of 10^{-6} or 1 in a million lifetime risk. For other chemical exposures the risks estimated may be appreciable, such as 10^{-4} or 1 in 10,000 lifetime risk. Whatever the actual number, it is reassuring to know what the risk is rather than worrying about what it might be. Since risk assessments estimate the maximum likely risk and represent an upper bound or limit, the actual risk may be much smaller.
   b. **Teratogenesis and reproductive effects.** Exposure to chemicals that cause teratogenic or reproductive effects are not likely to result in those effects unless the exposure is massive. Society places a special value on protecting the developing fetus and the process of reproduction. However, these toxic effects are likely threshold responses. Therefore, safe doses or thresholds exist. Generalization cannot substitute for data, but exposure to chemicals that are teratogens or affect reproduction must be within an order of magnitude of the exposure needed to show acute effects directly. Thus, it is unlikely that many exposures result in doses high enough for reproductive or teratogenic effects to occur.

STUDY QUESTIONS

Directions: Each question below contains five suggested answers. Choose the **one best** response to each question.

1. Volatile organic chemicals tend to concentrate in

(A) surface water
(B) air
(C) sediment
(D) edible fish tissue
(E) soil

2. A positive dose-related response in the Ames test shows that the chemical or metabolite can cause

(A) cancer
(B) mutational events
(C) teratogenic effects
(D) behavioral effects
(E) vasodilation

Directions: Each question below contains four suggested answers of which **one or more** is correct. Choose the answer

A if **1, 2, and 3** are correct
B if **1 and 3** are correct
C if **2 and 4** are correct
D if **4** is correct
E if **1, 2, 3, and 4** are correct

3. True statements about modeling and monitoring include which of the following?

(1) Results are measured in the same concentration units
(2) Emission rate and environmental fate must be measured
(3) Chemical species is the same for both
(4) Estimates of the maximum potential concentration in the medium must be made

4. Polychlorinated biphenyls appear in appreciable concentrations in

(1) groundwater
(2) sediment
(3) air
(4) edible fish tissue

5. Trichloroethylene (TCE) is a known animal carcinogen. Which of the following are potential shortcomings of a negative epidemiologic study describing TCE production workers?

(1) Small group size
(2) Lack of quantitative TCE exposure information
(3) Less than lifetime follow-up
(4) Exposure to other chemicals

ANSWERS AND EXPLANATIONS

1. The answer is B. (*IV A 1 b, c; Table 13-7*) Volatile organic chemicals (VOCs) such as benzene, trichloroethylene (TCE), and vinyl chloride have high vapor pressures compared to other organic chemicals or metals and have low octanol water partition coefficients (K_{ow}) and bioconcentration factors (BCFs) compared to other organic chemicals. Thus, VOCs will concentrate in air but not in water or soil because they have high vapor pressures. Also, VOCs cannot be transferred from water to sediment or fish tissue because of the low K_{ow} and BCF values. VOCs are found in both groundwater and soil at sites where there has been a spill. The upper layers of soil often have a lower VOC concentration than lower layers due to volatilization to air and migration down into lower soil layers.

2. The answer is B. [*II C 3 a (1)*] The Ames test is a short-term genotoxic test that determines the ability of a chemical to cause (point) mutations. Thus, a chemical that is positive in the Ames test is a mutagen. Although cancer requires interaction with genetic material and the correlation between carcinogens and the Ames test is more than 90%, a positive Ames test is not considered sufficient to classify a chemical as a carcinogen. Neither are teratogenic, behavioral, and vascular system effects measured by the Ames test, although a chemical that is a mutagen could possibly also cause any of the other systemic effects.

3. The answer is B (1, 3). (*V B 2, C–D*) The essential difference between modeling and monitoring is that modeling makes use of reasonable assumptions about environmental fate and movement of chemicals while monitoring simply measures the chemical concentration in a medium. Both yield estimates of the concentration of the given chemical species in an environmental medium. However, monitoring results are not (necessarily) estimates of the maximum concentration because the results are obtained at the time of measurement and not at the time of likely maximum concentration. Wind speed and directions can alter measured air levels, and increased flow and agitation can alter surface water measurements. Monitoring results are not dependent on factors such as emission rates or environmental fate because monitoring results express only what is present and measurable, no matter how the chemical got there. However, results from modeling are very dependent on the emission rate and environmental fate assumptions.

4. The answer is C (2, 4). (*IV A 1 b–c; V C 2 c*) Polychlorinated biphenyls (PCBs) have high octanol water partition coefficients (K_{ow}) and high bioconcentration factors (BCFs) relative to other classes of organic chemicals and metals. The K_{ow} describes the partition of a chemical between oil-like and water-like mediums, while the BCF describes the uptake of chemicals into fish tissue from the surrounding water. PCBs tend to move from water into sediment because of the organic content of sediment and the high value of K_{ow} (5×10^5). PCBs tend to move from water to edible fish tissue because of the high BCF value (10^5). Neither groundwater nor air should contain appreciable concentrations of PCBs because of low water solubility (about 30 ppb) and low vapor pressure.

5. The answer is B (1, 3). [*II C 1 b (1)–(4)*] Negative human epidemiologic studies are quite common for many known animal carcinogens. Assuming that the study is well designed, a study is usually negative because of small group size. The chemical carcinogen is often not sufficiently potent to produce an excess of cancer incidence that can be observed in small groups of exposed workers. Another common reason is that the exposed group is often examined at times much less that full lifetime, and thus some cancers may not have had sufficient time to appear in the human population. Exposure to other chemicals may be a reason for high cancer incidence in controls or for cancer responses that are not dose related to trichloroethylene (TCE) but are not a reason for negative studies. A lack of quantitative exposure information can make quantitative estimation of potency of a carcinogen difficult but that is not related to negative studies in humans.

14
Legal Aspects of Medical Practice and Community Medicine

Arnold J. Rosoff

I. INTRODUCTION. Health care practice is more regulated today than ever before. Therefore, it is important that health care providers have a basic knowledge of the law and its applications to assure their own legal safety and that of their institutions, to control their practice environment, and to take an active role in shaping future legal developments through the political process.

Health care regulation takes many forms:

A. Medical malpractice litigation brought by private parties is a form of regulation that focuses on the quality of care. The incidence of such litigation, which reached crisis levels in the early 1970s, is again rising precipitously.

B. State regulation of practitioners, facilities, practice organizations [e.g., Health Maintenance Organizations (HMOs)], and health financing programs is widespread, even in states where trends to limit government intervention in the private sector are strong.

C. Federal regulation through publicly funded programs (e.g., Medicare and Medicaid) is a potent regulator. Although the conditions required for participation in these federally funded programs are rigorous, few health care institutions or providers can survive without the service revenues generated by such participation.

II. THE UNITED STATES LEGAL SYSTEM

A. Precedent. The common law system is based on case precedent. Except in special circumstances, legal principles established in one case are followed in similar cases in the same jurisdiction.

1. The principle of adhering to precedent is referred to as *stare decisis*, Latin for "let the decision stand."

2. Cases do not have to follow precedent if they can be distinguished as significantly different from the precedent-setting case.

3. Case precedents are not **binding** upon courts in other jurisdictions (i.e., in other states) or upon higher courts in the same jurisdiction. However, even if a precedent is not binding, it may be persuasive—that is, it may influence the development of the law.

B. Civil versus criminal suits. The same act may constitute grounds for both a civil suit and a criminal prosecution. However, these two legal actions are independent, and the outcome of one has little or no impact on the outcome of the other.

1. **Civil suits** are those involving individuals, groups, or other parties acting in a nonpublic capacity.
   a. **Plaintiffs** (i.e., individuals who begin the suit) in civil suits generally seek to obtain **compensation** for injuries suffered through the wrongful acts of **defendants** (i.e., individuals who are being sued). A suit may have multiple plaintiffs and defendants. A decision pertaining to one plaintiff or defendant does not necessarily pertain to other plaintiffs or defendants in the same suit.
   b. A defendant who loses a civil suit is said to be **liable** for damages. The term **guilty** is not technically applicable to a civil suit.

2. **Criminal suits** are those brought by the federal, state, or local government to enforce laws that exist for the protection of society at large.
   a. Criminal actions are brought to **punish** the wrongdoer with a fine, imprisonment, or both.

b. The principal purpose of punishing convicted criminals is **deterrence**.
c. A defendant who loses a criminal suit is said to be **guilty**.

C. **Burden of proof.** The standard of proof required in criminal prosecutions is higher than the standard required in civil litigation.

1. **The plaintiff in a civil suit must prove his or her case by a preponderance of evidence**—that is, the court must be persuaded that the material elements of the case **more likely than not** are in favor of the plaintiff.
2. **The prosecution in a criminal case must prove its case beyond a reasonable doubt**. This is consistent with the presumption by our legal system of innocence until one is proven guilty.
3. **The party bringing the suit**, the plaintiff or the prosecutor, generally **bears the burden of proving all material elements in the case**. Special circumstances may shift the burden of proof of certain elements to the defendant; however, this is an infrequent occurrence.

D. **Jury versus nonjury trials**

1. A right to trial by jury exists for most civil and criminal claims under federal and state constitutions, but a jury trial is not automatic. Unless one of the parties makes a request, the case is **docketed** (i.e., scheduled) for a nonjury trial. In fact, most cases are tried before a judge alone.
2. Issues in **equity**, a special subset of the law, must be heard by a judge alone—for example, cases of mental incompetence or guardianship.

E. **Functions of judge and jury**

1. **Jury.** The function of the jury is to decide disputed **issues of fact**, where such exist. A **summary judgment** will be entered by the judge, without resort to a jury, when there are no factual issues to be decided.
2. **Judge.** The function of the judge is to control the trial's **procedural aspects**, to supply the applicable law, and to decide disputed **issues of law**. If a jury is used, it may announce the **verdict**, but it is bound to apply the law as instructed by the trial judge.

F. **Statute of limitations**

1. **Definition.** A statute of limitations is a procedural rule that establishes a maximum period of time during which a legal suit may be initiated. After the statutory period is over, a suit cannot be initiated regardless of how strong the case may be.
2. **Purpose.** A statute of limitations serves two purposes.
   a. It requires parties to bring their suits to court while evidence is still fresh so that factual issues can be accurately determined.
   b. It provides a cutoff date after which parties can be confident that no suit can be brought.
3. **Length of the statutory period**. The period allowed for initiating suit may vary from jurisdiction to jurisdiction for suits concerning similar legal matters. It may also vary within a given jurisdiction for suits concerning different legal matters. For example, the statute of limitations for contract actions is commonly 4–6 years and for personal injury actions, 1–3 years. The statute of limitations can be **tolled** (i.e., stopped from running) in special circumstances—for example, if the defendant is absent from the state or is mentally incompetent and, therefore, unable to be sued. The beginning of the statutory period for medical malpractice actions is defined variously as the date:
   a. The alleged malpractice took place.
   b. The physician-patient relationship was terminated.
   c. The patient discovered the alleged malpractice.
   d. The patient discovered, by exercise of due care, or should have discovered the alleged malpractice. (This is the most commonly used definition.)

G. **Measure of damages**

1. Determining the appropriate measure of damages is as important, and sometimes just as difficult, as determining whether the defendant is liable. A number of different measures may be used either separately or in combination.
   a. **Compensatory damages** compensate the plaintiff financially for the tangible harm caused by the defendant. Tangible economic losses, such as expenses for remedial care, loss of wages, and future loss of earnings due to physical impairment, are the principal elements of compensatory damages.

b. **Pain and suffering, mental ànguish, and loss of consortium** attempt to provide dollar compensation for losses that are real and discernible but that cannot be readily measured in financial terms.

c. **Punitive damages**—that is, damages in excess of normal compensation—may be awarded against a defendant who acted in a grossly negligent manner or with deliberate wrongful intent. Their purpose is to punish wrongdoers and to deter them, and others, from acting similarly in the future. The defendant must pay punitive damages to the plaintiff along with any other damages awarded. The amount is generally computed with regard for the degree of culpability of the defendant's actions and the defendant's ability to pay.

d. **Nominal damages** are awarded when the plaintiff has been able to establish the defendant's negligence and, thus, his liability but has not been able to prove that he, the plaintiff, suffered any monetary loss. A small sum, such as one dollar, is awarded as a symbolic acknowledgment that the plaintiff won the suit.

2. Under the American legal system, each party bears its own legal expenses, regardless of who won the litigation. By contrast, in Britain the winning party can recover reasonable attorneys' fees from the losing party. However, court costs *are* assessed against one or the other or both parties at the discretion of the court.

III. TORT LAW

A. **Definition.** Torts are civil wrongs—that is, injuries to an individual's person, property, or reputation. Torts can be **deliberate** or **negligent**. Under **absolute** or **strict liability**, certain undesirable acts may be considered torts even when the **tortfeasor** (i.e., the individual who committed the tort) acted neither deliberately nor negligently. **Remedies** in tort suits generally are meant to **compensate** the aggrieved party in order to restore as nearly as possible the position the victim would have enjoyed had the tort not been committed. When a tortfeasor's conduct is particularly culpable, punitive damages may be awarded.

B. **Negligent torts.** Most of the litigation relating to failures of medical care involves alleged negligence by health care providers.

1. **Negligence liability.** An individual can sue for damages when he or she has been the victim of tortious conduct. However, unless the following four conditions (the four D's) are satisfied, there can be no recovery for the negligent tort.

a. **Duty.** A duty is an obligation recognized by the law and for the breach of which the law imposes sanctions.

(1) To recover damages, the plaintiff must establish that he or she was owed a duty and the nature and extent of that duty.

(2) The duty, or standard of care, generally must be established by **expert testimony** as to common practice within the relevant professional community.

b. **Dereliction.** The plaintiff must prove that the defendant performed significantly below the legally required standard of care.

c. **Damage.** The plaintiff must prove that he or she was harmed and establish the nature and extent of that harm.

(1) In medical malpractice litigation, damages may be based on physical injury, psychologic harm, and reputational loss.

(2) Economic losses suffered by the plaintiff generally are not recoverable unless they are coupled with some other harm suffered. For example, the costs incurred by the patient for tests or hospitalization that were determined to be unnecessary cannot be recovered from the physician who prescribed the care unless the patient suffered harm other than economic waste.

d. **Direct causation.** There can be no liability unless the defendant's negligence was the **proximate cause** of the plaintiff's injuries.

(1) A proximate cause is a factor without which the harm would not have occurred. It must be the predominant factor.

(2) In medical malpractice cases, proximate cause is often hard to establish since bad outcomes can occur even in the absence of negligence.

(3) Under the so-called **loss of a chance theory**, some courts have begun to award damages if the plaintiff can establish that the defendant's acts significantly reduced the patient's chances of survival or recovery. This liberal definition of causation makes it easier to recover damages in cases of medical malpractice.

2. **Standard of care**

a. **Reasonable care.** The care usually required is that degree of care that a reasonably prudent individual would exercise in similar circumstances. The standard of care is generally fixed by reference to the customary practice of a given profession. Because the judge and jury cannot possibly know the customary practice of all professions, this must be established in court by **expert testimony**.

(1) Participation as an **expert witness**, which must be voluntary, is secured through negotiation of a witness fee. In contrast, testimony as to one's **factual observations** can be compelled through use of a **subpoena**.

(2) It is widely claimed, especially by plaintiffs' attorneys, that a **conspiracy of silence** among physicians makes it difficult to obtain expert testimony on behalf of plaintiffs in medical malpractice cases.

b. The locality rule followed in some jurisdictions is being replaced by a new approach— **national standards** for health care practice.

(1) **Strict locality rule** requires that expert testimony on the standard of care be drawn from the geographic community in which the alleged malpractice occurred. In the late 1800s, courts recognized that customary medical and surgical practices in isolated areas were not on par with those in progressive urban areas, and a differential standard of care was allowed.

(2) **Same or similar community standard** measures the defendant's performance by reference to closely comparable medical communities. This liberalization of locality rule makes it easier for plaintiffs to obtain expert testimony in support of their cases.

(3) **National standards** have been adopted by some jurisdictions, especially in cases where specialty care is rendered by board-certified practitioners. Some states also apply national standards set by the Joint Commission on Accreditation of Hospitals to measure hospital care (*Shilkret v. Annapolis Emergency Hospital*, Maryland, 1975).

c. Generalist versus specialist standards

(1) When a physician claims the ability to provide the type of care that normally is rendered by a specialist, the standard of care applied is that of the appropriately trained specialist.

(2) Under emergency circumstances in which specialty care is not available, a general practitioner may provide care that normally is rendered by a specialist. In such cases, a generalist standard should be applied to measure the adequacy of the care rendered.

(3) Failure to refer a patient to a specialist when specialty care is indicated subjects the attending physician to liability, a case sometimes characterized as **negligent nonreferral**.

d. Court-imposed standards of care. The standard of care legally required may be fixed by a court at a level higher than that of prevailing professional practice.

(1) In *Helling v. Carey* (Washington, 1974), the state's highest court held that customary professional practice is not absolutely determinative of reasonably prudent care. In this case, two ophthalmologists were held liable for not using a tonometer test for glaucoma even though it was not customary to use this test on patients of the plaintiff's age unless there was an indication of a visual field disorder.

(2) Although Washington's legislature enacted a reform measure intended to overrule the *Helling* precedent, the state supreme court has resisted application of the new law (*Gates v. Jensen*, Washington, 1979).

(3) The *Helling* precedent has not been widely followed, but it is generally thought to be sound. Under proper (i.e., clear-cut) circumstances, other courts can be expected to use a similar approach.

3. Proof of dereliction

a. Whether or not the defendant performed up to the required standard of care is a factual matter, generally requiring proof.

(1) Although expert witnesses cannot be compelled to testify, they can be required to testify as to factual matters they directly observed in the care of the patient (plaintiff).

(2) Care may have been so deficient that a judge or lay jury may infer negligence even in the absence of expert testimony under the doctrine of ***res ipsa loquitur***, Latin for "the thing speaks for itself." Thus, the plaintiff is spared the burden of producing further evidence of negligence.

b. Today, some jurisdictions allow the plaintiff to introduce recognized medical texts as proof of accepted professional practice. However, some jurisdictions exclude such evidence as **hearsay** because the author of the text is not present in court, under oath, and subject to cross-examination.

C. Deliberate torts. Although most medical suits involve negligent torts, there is significant opportunity for suits charging deliberate torts. To establish the required **intent** to support such a charge, it is not necessary to show that the defendant meant to harm the plaintiff but only that the defendant deliberately performed the wrongful act. Of the possible types of deliberate torts, the following are the most significant in the medical area.

1. Battery—that is, touching an individual without his or her permission—often leads to health care suits.

a. The wrongful act to be avoided under battery is the invasion of a person's **right of bodily inviolability**.
b. A valid ground for complaint exists even if the defendant intended no harm and the patient suffered no physical damage. Monetary awards generally are small unless there is physical damage or the defendant meant to cause harm.
c. Cases of alleged **sexual assault** by physicians are considered battery actions.

2. **Fraud and deceit** are important grounds for deliberate tort suits. Cases in which a physician deliberately misrepresents facts to obtain a patient's consent for a procedure are treated as matters of fraud and deceit. These cases can be distinguished from the more common cases of **informed consent** (see section V).

3. **Breach of confidentiality** involves a disclosure of information about a patient's case without his or her permission. This theory can support a suit based on a number of specific theories, including:
   a. **Breach of an implied contract duty** to keep patient information confidential.
   b. **Invasion of privacy.**
   c. **Defamation**, in cases where the disclosure of information might have negative consequences for the patient's personal, social, or business life.
   d. **Unprofessional conduct.**

4. **Bad faith breach of contract** is an innovative approach to convert a tort action into a contract action, which has had some success to date (see section IV F).

IV. CONTRACT LAW

A. **Definition.** A contract is a **consensual agreement** between two (or more) parties whereby each undertakes defined obligations to the other. The law recognizes a contract, when properly entered into, as legally binding and provides sanctions for its breach. Two elements are essential for the creation of a contract.

1. **Consideration**, which one party gives to the other to bind the other to the contract, consists of performing an act that the party is not otherwise bound to perform or refraining from an act that the party otherwise is entitled to do. The giving of consideration must be mutual for the contract to be binding.

2. An **offer** by one party and an **acceptance** by the other, which may occur formally or informally, is essential to the establishment of a consensual relationship.
   a. The offer and acceptance constitute a **bargained-for-exchange** through which the consideration given by one party is recognized as the agreed-upon price for the undertaking by the other party. This aspect of giving up something in return for action or forbearance by the other party is described by the term ***quid pro quo***, Latin for "this for that."
   b. The law consists of complex guidelines by which to determine whether an offer and acceptance have taken place—an issue that often is not clear-cut.

B. **Express or implied contracts**

1. **An express contract** is one that is stated in words, whether spoken or written.

2. **An implied contract** is one in which the agreement of a party is not expressly stated but may be inferred from the party's conduct. It is possible for the consent of *both* parties to be given by implication. For example, in the health care context, most contracts for care are implied. The patient registers his or her willingness to enter into a contract by presenting to the health care provider for care. The provider registers his or her willingness to enter into a contract by providing that care.
   a. When the parties agree upon a price, that price becomes a part of the contract regardless of whether or not others would consider it reasonable.
   b. When the parties do not agree on a price, the law presumes that a **reasonable price** was intended. A reasonable price is a factual matter, which may be determined by the court.

C. **Measure of damages.** The purpose of damages in a contract action is to place the aggrieved party (i.e., the one against whom a breach has been committed) as nearly as possible in the position he or she would have enjoyed had the contract been performed as agreed. This approach to compensatory damages attempts to give an aggrieved party the **benefit of the bargain** that was embodied in the contract.

1. In general, only economic losses are considered in awarding damages for a contract breach. Emotional distress and other intangible harms are not compensable, except in rare circumstances.

2. Similarly, punitive damages generally are not awarded against a breaching party, even though the breach may be deliberate (see section IV F for a possible exception).

D. Breach of warranty. An important application of contract law to the health care setting is illustrated by the suits brought by patients against health care providers for failure to obtain the positive results that the providers allegedly contracted to deliver—that is, for **breach of a warranty of cure**.

1. This approach, where allowed, may permit recovery of damages even though the provider has not been negligent in the provision of care. The patient's complaint is not that the provider failed to perform according to professional standards but that he or she failed to deliver the promised rèsult.
2. At least one court has held that the proper measure of damages in such a suit is the difference in value between the result promised by the provider and the result obtained—a **benefit of the bargain** approach, which is derived from classic contract actions outside the health care field (*Hawkins v. McGee*, New Hampshire, 1929).
3. Some courts have awarded damages following the rules of tort-based suits, allowing compensation only for deterioration of the patient's condition after care as compared to his or her condition before care was rendered (*Sullivan v. O'Connor*, Massachusetts, 1973).
4. Some courts restrict the use of contract theory in health care suits by imposing two important requirements.
   a. No breach of warranty is possible unless the provider makes a specific promise of cure.
      (1) Positive projections of the benefits of a planned treatment or promises that the provider will "do his or her best" do not constitute a warranty upon which a suit can be based.
      (2) Providers should choose their words of reassurance carefully to avoid crossing the line from a positive projection to a promise of positive outcome.
   b. Some courts insist that the alleged promise be expressly stated in a written document before it can serve as a basis for a breach of warranty suit.

E. Statute of limitations. One motivation for using a contract theory is that the statute of limitations for these actions may be longer than those for tort actions (see section II F).

F. Bad faith breach of contract. A curious hybrid of contract and tort reasoning has emerged in health care litigation, whereby a party who deliberately breaches a contract to provide health services may be held liable for the deliberate tort of **bad faith breach of contract**. This approach, which has been used in cases involving insurance companies:

1. Can arguably be used in the case of an HMO that fails to provide care specified in the subscriber's enrollment contract.
2. Makes it possible to award punitive damages for an unjustified, deliberate breach of contract.
3. Is controversial and has not had wide acceptance in the courts to date.

V. INFORMED CONSENT

A. Basic concepts. The law requires that diagnostic, medical, and surgical procedures must be authorized by a voluntary, knowledgeable consent of the patient or the patient's legal representative. This important aspect of patients' rights originates from the principles regarding battery.

1. Case law early in this century declared that "every human being of adult years and sound mind has a right to determine what shall be done with his own body" (*Schloendorff v. Society of New York Hospital*, New York, 1914). This is the **root premise** of the developing law of informed consent.
2. Since the late 1950s, courts have held that a patient's consent to treatment, even if formally obtained and documented in writing, is legally ineffective if the patient was not adequately informed about the treatment, including the inherent risks (*Salgo v. Stanford University Hospital*, California, 1957).

B. Informed consent obligations. Two approaches have evolved for defining the health care provider's informed consent obligations.

1. The older, **physician-based approach**, first adopted in the case of *Natanson v. Kline* (Kansas, 1960), requires that physicians disclose to patients all that is customary in the profession to disclose in similar situations. The law essentially adopts the **professional community standard**. Thus, in court the patient (plaintiff) is required to produce expert testimony as to what

physicians customarily tell their patients—obviously a difficult evidentiary burden. About half the states follow this approach.

2. The newer, **patient-based approach**, adopted in the landmark case of *Canterbury v. Spence* (U.S. Court of Appeals for the District of Columbia Circuit, 1972) requires that physicians disclose all that a reasonably prudent patient would consider **material** to the decision to accept or reject the proposed treatment. A factor is material if, either alone or in combination with other factors, it would significantly affect the patient's decision. Because expert testimony as to a "standard disclosure" is not needed, it is easier for patients to sue on informed consent grounds in states using this approach.

C. **Disclosure.** Under either the physician-based or the patient-based approach, the following elements must be disclosed in language that the patient can reasonably be expected to comprehend.

1. **Diagnosis.** The physician should also disclose any reservations he or she has about the diagnosis.
2. **Nature and purpose of the proposed treatment**
3. **Risks and consequences of the proposed treatment.** This includes only risks and consequences of which the physician has, or can be expected to have, knowledge.
4. **Feasible treatment alternatives.** This includes other treatment modalities that the medical community would consider using in this particular case, regardless of the personal recommendations of the physician making the disclosure.
5. **Prognosis without treatment.** If the patient elects not to have the recommended treatment, he or she must be informed of the implications of this choice.

D. **Causation.** To recover damages for a physician's failure to disclose information, a patient must convince the court that he or she would have made a different decision about the treatment had the information been known. Obviously, this is a difficult, speculative determination, which requires the court to determine, after a bad clinical result has occurred, what the patient would have chosen before the fact, not knowing the outcome.

1. Some courts base the causation analysis on an **objective standard**—that is, what an "average, reasonable patient" would have chosen.
2. Other courts use a **subjective standard**—that is, what "this particular patient" would have chosen.

E. **Therapeutic privilege.** Many courts have recognized that a physician may be justified under certain, limited circumstances, to withhold information in the patient's best interest.

1. This privilege applies *only* when a patient is unusually sensitive, anxious, or emotional. A general policy of not disclosing information because of the presumed hypersensitivity of patients is not an acceptable basis for this privilege.
2. A physician relying on therapeutic privilege should document carefully why a patient should have information withheld.
3. When the physician's use of therapeutic privilege is challenged, it must be determined whether the physician followed sound medical judgment in withholding information.

F. **Consent.** When the patient is adult and competent, the authority to give or withhold consent to treatment rests exclusively with the patient, unless he or she makes a valid delegation to someone else.

1. **A power of attorney** executed in writing by a competent adult (the patient) can delegate the responsibility for health care decisions to another person on the patient's behalf. The provider should take care to ascertain that the decision in question lies within the scope of the expressly authorized delegation, since the law interprets powers of attorney narrowly.
   a. Many states hold that a power of attorney becomes ineffective when the individual giving it becomes incompetent—that is, an **agent** can have no greater capacity than his or her **principal**.
   b. A **durable power of attorney**, which remains effective when the giver of the power becomes incompetent, is recognized in some states. This form of power is most useful in the health care setting.
2. **The legal age of majority** varies from state to state but is usually 18 or 19 years of age. Individ-

uals who have not attained this age cannot give legally effective consent except in the following situations.

a. Minors who are married, live away from their parents' home, or are financially independent are called **emancipated minors** and are regarded as having an adult capacity to consent to health care.

b. Some states, by statute, have fixed a **lower age of consent for health care**, especially regarding the diagnosis and treatment of sexual and reproductive problems (e.g., contraception, abortion, pregnancy, and venereal disease) and drug or alcohol abuse.

c. Some states, by case law, recognize a **mature minor** exception, allowing minors to give consent to health care under certain circumstances.

3. Next of kin. When a patient is incapable of giving consent because of age, incompetency, or incapacity, the law holds that the closest available relative has the power to authorize care on the patient's behalf.

a. The President's Commission for the Study of Ethical Problems in Medicine and Biomedical and Behavioral Research (1983) defined **competency** as "the patient's capability to understand information relevant to the decision and to reason about relevant alternatives against a background of reasonably stable personal values and life goals."

b. A health care provider who acts on the belief that a person is the patient's next of kin is legally protected if this turns out not to be the case. To assure protection, the provider should document the basis for believing that a person is the next of kin.

c. A difficult legal matter results when the next of kin refuses to authorize care that the provider believes is urgently needed. In such cases, a court order authorizing the treatment must be obtained. Where time or other circumstances do not permit this, the provider is not liable for action taken on sound medical judgment. However, this is a very risky situation, turning, as it would, on a court's after-the-fact determination of what the exigent circumstances required. Extreme caution is advised.

4. Emergency situations. The law recognizes an **exception to the requirement of consent** in cases where the patient is unconscious or otherwise unable to give consent and the need for care is so urgent that it is not feasible to contact the patient's next of kin.

a. The rationale for this emergency consent exception is that unless the health care provider has information to the contrary, he or she is entitled to presume that the patient would have chosen the care others have chosen in similar circumstances.

b. The exception does not extend beyond situations where immediate action must be taken to preserve life or, in some states, to prevent serious physical harm.

c. The circumstances justifying the emergency consent exception should be documented, including all efforts to contact next of kin before treatment is rendered.

d. Administrative authorization—that is, consent for treatment granted by the administration of a health care facility—helps merely to document the applicability of the emergency consent doctrine. Health care facility administrators have no inherent power to grant consent on behalf of patients.

VI. PATIENT'S RIGHTS

A. Refusal of treatment. A patient who is competent to give consent is also legally entitled to withhold it for whatever reasons he or she deems sufficient. This is true even if refusing treatment may result in serious harm or death to the patient.

1. When a patient refuses treatment, the provider should document all of the information given to the patient concerning the consequences of the refusal. Failure to provide such information or the inability to prove that it was provided could result in liability on informed consent grounds (*Truman v. Thomas*, California, 1980).

2. When the competence of the patient to make the treatment decision is questionable, the provider may rely on the principles of **emergency consent** and **consent by the next of kin**. Again, great care is advised, and a court order authorizing treatment should be obtained when feasible.

B. Treatment of terminally ill patients. Terminally ill patients whose death is imminent have a constitutionally protected **right of privacy**, which allows them to refuse life-support care that serves to prolong the process of dying.

1. Patients do not have an unrestricted "right to die." Courts and legislatures dealing with this matter have defined narrowly the cases in which patients can refuse life support.

2. Some courts distinguish between the use of ordinary and extraordinary life-support measures. **Ordinary measures** generally are held to include the provision of nutrition and water via a nasogastric tube; **extraordinary measures** encompass cardiopulmonary resuscitation and the use of a ventilator to maintain respiration.

a. In the much publicized *Karen Quinlan* case (New Jersey, 1976), the withdrawal of a respirator was held to be legally acceptable, even though its removal was likely to result in the immediate death of the irreversibly brain-damaged and comatose young patient.

b. In the case of *Claire Conroy* (New Jersey, 1985), the New Jersey Supreme Court extended the *Quinlan* ruling to allow the withdrawal of nasogastric feeding and hydration from a senile and semiconscious 84-year-old nursing home patient who was in failing condition but whose death was not thought to be imminent. The court established elaborate criteria and safeguards by which to determine as closely as possible what the patient would have chosen regarding the continuation of care had she been able to do so. This doctrine is known as **substituted judgment**.

3. Numerous states sanction the use of a **living will** or **natural death directive** by which a patient can direct what care should be rendered in a terminal illness when the patient is not competent to provide such direction. Even in states that do not recognize such devices, their use should help to protect those who act in response to sound medical judgment and the patient's wishes. Care should be taken to document the patient's wishes in such matters.

4. **No code** or **do not resuscitate** (DNR) orders generally are accepted legally in the treatment of terminally ill patients. If the patient is unconscious or incompetent, family members should be consulted about the decision not to resuscitate. Their concurrence with the provider's decision should be carefully documented. Extreme care should be taken when it is known that a relative opposes the entry of a DNR order.

VII. ACCESS TO CARE

A. **Duty to render care.** The law is struggling to balance the right of providers to choose who they will serve against the pressing needs of the community to have quality health care services readily available.

1. **Individual practitioners.** An individual health care practitioner has no common law duty to render care to anyone he or she has not accepted as a patient, even when a person is in need of immediate care. The physician who does not respond to such a call for aid has no liability for harm suffered by the patient.

a. **Moral duty.** There is a clearly recognized moral and professional duty, however, to render care to the best of the practitioner's ability under the circumstances.

b. **Abandonment.** Once a physician accepts a patient for care, the obligation to provide care within the scope of the agreed relationship continues until either the patient terminates the relationship or the physician terminates it with the patient's consent or with sufficient advance notice to allow the patient to secure an alternative source of care.

(1) The principle of abandonment is the source of the physician's legal obligation to arrange adequate coverage for a patient's care when the physician is not going to be available.

(2) Because of the possibility of an abandonment charge, the practitioner should document when a physician-patient relationship has terminated and provide the patient with unequivocal notice that this has occurred.

2. **Statutory imposition of duty to render care.** Vermont has adopted legislation requiring all citizens to do what they reasonably can to lend aid and assistance in emergency situations. The sanction for failing to obey the law's mandate is a minor criminal fine.

a. Although the law makes no specific mention of health care professionals, it applies to them as well.

b. Presumably, states could require health care professionals to aid in emergencies as a condition of licensure. No state has adopted such a requirement, however, and politically, if not constitutionally, it would be problematic.

3. **Good samaritan statutes.** These statutes have been passed in all states to encourage physicians to render care in emergencies.

a. Such statutes grant immunity from civil liability for injuries caused by a physician's good faith attempts to render care in emergency situations.

b. There is generally no immunity if the physician is grossly negligent—that is, if he or she acts with wanton or reckless disregard for the consequences of his or her actions—or expects to be compensated for the emergency care.

c. Some statutes cover health care professionals other than physicians, such as nurses, paramedics, and various emergency medical technicians. The immunity generally extends only to people who act within the scope of their properly certified abilities.

d. Even in the absence of good samaritan protection, persons attempting to assist in an emergency would run little risk of being held liable for harm suffered by the person they sought to aid. The standard by which a good-faith volunteer's actions is measured is what other persons similarly qualified would be expected to do under similar circumstances.

B. Health care facilities. Private hospitals are under no common law duty to accept patients or render care in emergencies. **Public hospitals**—those operated by federal, state, or local governments—have a broader obligation to provide care to the public. The law acts in various ways to encourage or require hospitals to expand access to their services.

1. Common law bases have been developed in case law to require admission—or at least initial treatment, advice, and referral—of patients by privately owned and operated health care institutions.

a. *Wilmington General Hospital v. Manlove* (Delaware, 1961) held that a private hospital that maintains an emergency department whose existence is known to the general public undertakes an obligation to provide emergency care to those presenting for treatment in an emergency situation. The rationale behind the decision was that the hospital led the public to rely on the availability of the emergency service.

b. The rendering of initial appraisal and advice may be held to constitute an acceptance of a patient for care. Failure to admit the patient after such initial steps have been taken could lead to a charge of abandonment (*O'Neill* v. *Montefiore Hospital*, New York, 1960).

2. Hospital licensure statutes in numerous states require general acute-care hospitals to maintain emergency facilities for the general public. (*Guerrero v. Copper Queen Hospital*, Arizona, 1972).

3. Some states have **statutes that require hospitals to provide emergency treatment** to the public without regard to health insurance coverage or other means of assuring payment for the care received.

4. Conditions for participation in the **Medicare and Medicaid programs** require that general acute-care hospitals must maintain emergency treatment facilities. In addition, these laws require hospitals to accept Medicare and Medicaid beneficiaries for treatment.

5. Rules for tax-exempt status under the federal tax laws (Internal Revenue Code section 501 C-3) contemplate the maintenance by hospitals of emergency facilities open to the general public. They do not, however, require tax-exempt hospitals to admit all patients regardless of their ability to pay for care.

6. Federal hospital financing laws (dating back to 1945) require that hospitals constructed or improved with federal funds must provide a reasonable volume of free or reduced-cost care to the general public. The so-called **Hill-Burton free-care obligation** helps to assure access to hospital care for persons who might not otherwise be admitted or treated. (*Cook v. Ochsner Foundation Hospital*, U.S. Court of Appeals for the Fifth Circuit, 1977).

7. The Joint Commission on Accreditation of Hospitals requires general acute care hospitals to maintain emergency facilities and staffing and to render initial appraisal and advice to individuals presenting for emergency treatment.

VIII. PUBLIC HEALTH AND GOVERNMENTAL POWER

A. Bases of governmental power. Under the United States constitution, the powers of the state (meaning the goverment at all levels: federal, state, and local) are limited. Much power and discretion are left to individuals to live as they wish and to control their own destinies. However, two important types of governmental power must be understood.

1. Police power. The state has an inherent authority, known as police power, to take necessary steps to **protect public health**, **welfare**, **safety**, **and morals**. Police power:

a. Can be exercised when the state has a legitimate interest in an activity and undertakes action reasonably related to the protection of that interest.

b. Must be balanced against the rights of the individual. When the individual right involved is a fundamental right, the state cannot take action unless it can demonstrate a **compelling interest**.

2. *Parens patriae*. When individuals cannot take adequate care of themselves, the state is both empowered and obliged to take protective action—that is, to assume a "parent" role.

B. Prohibition of dangerous activities. The prohibition of dangerous activities and other governmental interventions are justified under either police power or *parens patriae*, depending on who is at risk from the activity.

1. Activities that pose a threat to society, such as going to school with a communicable disease, are regulated under police power.
2. Activities that pose a threat only to the individual, such as riding a motorcycle without a helmet, are regulated under *parens patriae*.
3. Activities, such as driving an automobile while intoxicated, which pose a threat to both the individual and society, are regulated under both doctrines.
4. The nature and extent of the state intervention must be weighed against the seriousness of the harm to be avoided and the degree of interference with the rights of individuals. The following examples illustrate how such balancing may be done.
   a. Mandatory quarantine of individuals with contagious diseases like hepatitis A can be legally sustained because the disease is highly contagious through casual contact. Also, it has a finite, relatively brief period of contagion; thus, the quarantine would be for a limited time.
   b. Exclusion of a child with acquired immune deficiency syndrome (AIDS) from public school is legally questionable. The following factors favor the rights of the child and undercut the right of the state to restrict them.
      (1) Present knowledge of the disease indicates it cannot be spread by casual, nonsexual contact.
      (2) The period of contagion is indefinite, necessitating a restriction lasting perhaps for life.
      (3) The importance of education for children is widely recognized.

C. **Police tests.** In certain cases, physical tests of individuals may be necessary to obtain evidence of criminal activity. Determining the ability of law enforcement officials to order these tests against the will of the person being tested requires knowledge of the constitutional rights of the individual.

1. **Blood tests** can be ordered by the police when there is reasonable cause to believe a crime has been committed and necessary evidence can be obtained by a blood test.
   a. A search warrant must be obtained from a court if time and circumstances permit.
   b. If the time required to obtain a court order would result in the destruction of evidence, the need for a judicial warrant is obviated (*Schmerber v. California*, U.S. Supreme Court, 1966).
   c. Key factors in the law's recognition of the right to compel blood tests are that the degree and duration of bodily invasion are minor and the risk to the subject is minimal.
2. **Invasive tests** are less likely to be upheld as legal. In *Rochin v. California* (U.S. Supreme Court, 1951), the forcible pumping of a suspect's stomach to retrieve drug capsules allegedly swallowed was held to be a violation of the suspect's rights to due process.
3. **Breath analysis** (breathalyzer) to determine intoxication is routinely performed and upheld by the courts. It is a simple, noninvasive, painless, and risk-free test.
   a. In some states, consent to such tests is made a condition of obtaining a driver's license; in others, the use of highways is taken as implied consent.
   b. A suspect's refusal to allow breath analysis legally supports the presumption that the suspect is guilty of intoxication.
4. **Urinalysis** is treated like breath analysis from the standpoint of individual rights.
   a. The test is noninvasive, harmless, and poses no risk to the subject.
   b. The only possible issue would be the test's ability to prove what it purports to prove. Tests cannot be ordered if there is no demonstrable scientific basis for their use; some debate as to efficacy is tolerable.
5. **Skin and hair samples** may be removed for identification purposes.
6. **Semen samples** for rape and paternity identification pose a different and obvious problem. While removal of the samples poses no physicial threat to the subject, the cooperation of the subject is necessary. Thus, this test cannot be compelled without consideration of the legal rights of the subject.
7. **Removal of bullets** cannot be compelled without a court order since the time required for this step would not result in the loss of evidence.
   a. The judge must consider medical testimony as to the possible danger to the subject. Removal of a bullet cannot be authorized if it would jeopardize the life or safety of the subject.
   b. Problems are often avoided by the subject's desire to have the bullet removed.
8. **Health care personnel** cannot be compelled to perform tests whether on police request or court order.
   a. Even if police have a legal right to order a particular test, private individuals have no obligation to assist them.

b. Provided that the police appear to be within their rights in ordering a test, health care personnel are legally protected if they choose to participate.
c. Reasonable caution dictates that health care personnel should insist on documentation of the police order before performing the test.
d. If the subject consents to the test, a consent form signed by the subject should be obtained.

D. Reporting requirements for diseases and incidents

1. Confidentiality of information regarding patients' treatment must be scrupulously respected.
a. Both professional and legal requirements exist to protect against unauthorized disclosure of information related to patient treatment.
b. Health care personnel can be held liable for the violation of the right of privacy, defamation, breach of trust, or breach of implied contract if this results in harm to the patient.

2. Disregard of confidentiality. There are situations where revealing information about a patient's condition or treatment may be both ethically and legally required.
a. The American Medical Association's code of medical ethics recognizes and supports the disregard of patient confidentiality when there is a higher duty owed to the community or when the law requires the reporting of information. The following is an illustrative (not exhaustive) list of the types of information that must be reported in most states.
(1) Gunshot, knife, and other wounds indicative of a crime or other breach of peace
(2) Communicable diseases, including venereal diseases
(3) Evidence of use or abuse of, or addiction to, drugs or other substances prohibited by law
(4) Evidence of abuse or neglect of children, the elderly, animals, or other parties not capable of protecting themselves
(5) Epilepsy or other neurologic, visual, or motor control disorders, which make it dangerous to operate a motor vehicle or other device, thereby posing a threat to the individual and society
b. Health care personnel who reveal information without the patient's knowledge or against his or her objection should observe the following cautions.
(1) Disclosure of information should be made only to the proper authorities.
(2) Disclosure should not go beyond what is required by the situation and the law. Confidences should be preserved as far as possible.
(3) The reasons for and circumstances surrounding disclosure of confidential information should be carefully documented in a patient's record.
(4) Professional and personal ethics, as well as practical considerations, may dictate telling the patient that disclosures will be made to the proper authorities. In the absence of specific statutes, however, there is no legal duty to make such a disclosure to the patient.
c. Civil immunity (i.e., protection from a lawsuit charging defamation) is granted to health care providers who disclose patient confidences in good faith with reasonable justification. Disclosure is not protected if it is unnecessary or is motivated by malice or a desire to embarrass the patient.
d. A growing number of states requires, pursuant to case law, that mental health professionals (and presumably other health care providers) report reliable indications that a mentally disturbed individual intends to do harm to an identifiable individual or group.
(1) *Tarasoff v. Regents of University of California* (California, 1976) held that a psychotherapist had a duty to warn the intended murder victim of one of his patients.
(2) The *Tarasoff* decision, and others following its reasoning, is highly controversial because of the potential chilling effect it has on counselor-patient communications and because of the burden it puts on counselors to distinguish between patients' idle talk and real threats of harm.

BIBLIOGRAPHY

Danner D, Sagall E: Medicolegal causation: a source of professional misunderstanding. *Am J Law Med* 3:303–308, 1977

Eisenberg J, Rosoff A: Physician responsibility for the cost of unnecessary medical services. *N Engl J Med* 299:76, 1978

Roth M, Levin L: The dilemma of *Tarasoff*: should psychotherapists protect their patients or society? *Law Med Health Care* 11:104, 1983

Shoenberger A: Medical malpractice injury: causation and valuation of the loss of a chance to survive. *J Law Med* 6:51–84, 1985

COURT CASES

Canterbury v Spence, 464 F, 2d 772 (US Court of Appeals, DC Circuit, 1972)

Cook v Ochsner Foundation Hospital, 555 F, 2d 968 (US Court of Appeals, Fifth Circuit, 1977)

Gates v Jensen, 595 P, 2d 919 (Washington, 1979)

Guerrero v Copper Queen Hospital, 537 P, 2d 1329 (Arizona, 1972)

Hawkins v McGee, 146 A, 641 (New Hampshire, 1929)

Helling v Carey, 519 P, 2d 981 (Washington, 1974)

In the matter of Claire Conroy, 486 A, 2d 1209 (New Jersey, 1985)

In the matter of Karen Ann Quinlan, 355 A, 2d 647 (New Jersey, 1976)

Natanson v Kline, 350 P, 2d 1093 (Kansas, 1960)

O'Neill v Montefiore Hospital, 202 NYS, 2d 436 (New York, 1960)

Rochin v California, 342 US, 165 (US Supreme Court, 1951)

Salgo v Stanford University Hospital 317 P, 2d 170 (Ct App Cal, 1957)

Schloendorff v Society of New York Hospital, 105 NE, 92 (New York, 1914)

Schmerber v California, 384 US, 757 (US Supreme Court, 1966)

Shilkret v Annapolis Emergency Hospital, 349 A, 2d 245 (Maryland, 1975)

Sullivan v O'Connor, 296 NE, 2d 183 (Massachusetts, 1973)

Tarasoff v Regents of the University of California, 551 P, 2d 334 (California, 1976)

Truman v Thomas, 611 P, 2d 902 (California, 1980)

Wilmington General Hospital v Manlove, 174 A, 2d 135 (Delaware, 1961)

STUDY QUESTIONS

Directions: Each question below contains five suggested answers. Choose the **one best** response to each question.

1. The Anglo-American common law system places great emphasis on adherence to precedent. Which of the following Latin phrases is used to summarize this principle?

(A) *Res ipsa loquitur*
(B) *Stare decisis*
(C) *Parens patriae*
(D) *Quid pro quo*
(E) *Habeas corpus*

2. All of the following are elements that the plaintiff is required to prove in order to recover damages for a defendant's alleged negligence EXCEPT

(A) duty
(B) dereliction
(C) damage
(D) proximate cause
(E) deliberate wrongdoing

3. A physician has determined that a surgical procedure is needed to treat a condition suffered by a competent, adult patient. The physician is legally required to disclose to the patient in the course of obtaining the patient's informed consent to the procedure all of the following information EXCEPT for the

(A) nature and purpose of the proposed treatment
(B) physician's success rate in using the procedure
(C) risks and consequences of the proposed treatment
(D) reasonably feasible treatment alternatives
(E) prognosis if the proposed treatment is not implemented

4. Which of the following legal doctrines may be used, in appropriate circumstances, to relieve the plaintiff of the burden of introducing expert testimony to prove the defendant's negligence?

(A) Burden of proof
(B) Hearsay
(C) *Res ipsa loquitur*
(D) Conspiracy of silence
(E) Contributory negligence

Directions: Each question below contains four suggested answers of which **one or more** is correct. Choose the answer

A if **1, 2, and 3** are correct
B if **1 and 3** are correct
C if **2 and 4** are correct
D if **4** is correct
E if **1, 2, 3, and 4** are correct

5. Which of the following tests can the police order a criminal suspect to undergo without first obtaining a court order?

(1) Blood sample
(2) Urinalysis
(3) Breath analysis
(4) Removal of a bullet

6. Privately owned and operated hospitals may be required to render care to all individuals, including those they might otherwise choose not to serve by the

(1) reliance of the public on the hospital's custom of providing emergency services
(2) federal Hill-Burton program for financing of hospital capital expenditures
(3) Medicare and Medicaid, which require participating hospitals to maintain emergency facilities and treat eligible individuals under these programs
(4) federal tax laws governing the grant of tax-exempt status to nonprofit hospitals

7. A physician's duty to render care to a patient is described by which of the following statements?

(1) By accepting a license to practice medicine, a physician implicitly undertakes that he or she will serve all patients when they are in urgent need of care and none is procurable from another available source
(2) In general, a physician has no duty to accept someone as a patient, even in dire emergencies
(3) Good samaritan statutes in many states require physicians to come to the aid of persons threatened with serious and urgent medical problems
(4) A physician can be held liable for abandonment if he or she accepts a patient and later discontinues care without being discharged by the patient or giving the patient adequate notice

Directions: The groups of questions below consist of lettered choices followed by several numbered items. For each numbered item select the **one** lettered choice with which it is **most** closely associated. Each lettered choice may be used once, more than once, or not at all.

Questions 8–11

For each concept or doctrine listed below, select the legal term that most closely represents it.

(A) *Parens patriae*
(B) *Res ipsa loquitur*
(C) Substituted judgment
(D) Police power
(E) Therapeutic privilege

8. The government has the legal authority to take protective measures to safeguard individuals who are incompetent or otherwise unable to care for themselves.

9. When decisions are made on behalf of unconscious or incompetent patients, care must be taken to assure that the decision is what the patients would have chosen for themselves.

10. The plaintiff is relieved of the burden of introducing expert testimony to establish the defendant's negligence because a lay jury can discern the lack of care without expert guidance.

11. Physicians are generally required to disclose information to their patients concerning the diagnosis, treatment, risks, alternatives, and prognosis. However, this obligation is waived if the physician feels it is in the patient's best interest to withhold information.

Questions 12–15

In tort litigation, a number of different standards are used to determine various issues involving the provision of health services. For each of the issues listed below, select the standard that is most likely to be associated with it.

(A) Objective standard of causation
(B) Subjective standard of causation
(C) Court-imposed standard of care
(D) Physician-based standard of informed consent
(E) Patient-based standard of informed consent

12. The law can require a higher standard of medical practice than is currently observed in the medical profession under certain circumstances.

13. Physicians commonly tell their patients certain facts before undertaking a given medical, surgical, or diagnostic procedure.

14. A "particular" patient is entitled to damages for a physician's failure to disclose information about treatment.

15. An individual may consider certain things material to his or her decision to accept a proposed treatment.

ANSWERS AND EXPLANATIONS

1. The answer is B. (*II A 1–3*) *Stare decisis* means "let the decision stand." It is believed that justice is best served by equal treatment—that is, by having the law applied consistently in all similar cases. Existing precedents are generally followed by other courts at the same level or at lower levels in the same jurisdiction unless the case can be distinguished on its facts from the one that established the precedent or situations have changed in such a way as to make the precedent no longer appropriate.

2. The answer is E. (*III B 1 a–d*) Four conditions must be met if a plaintiff is to recover damages in a negligence claim. In addition to proving duty (an obligation recognized by the law and for the breach of which the law imposes sanctions), dereliction (that the defendent performed below the legally required standard of care), and damage (that the plaintiff was harmed), the plaintiff must also prove that the defendant's negligence was the proximate cause of the plaintiff's injuries. Deliberate wrongdoing, while it is an element in some tort suits, need not be proved in a negligence action, which charges that the defendant caused harm by careless or inattentive action.

3. The answer is B. (*V A–C*) While the physician's success rate for a given procedure might be important information for the patient to consider before authorizing the physician to perform the procedure, no court has yet required the physician to reveal this information. However, the physician would be bound to answer truthfully if the patient questioned his or her success rate.

The patient is entitled to be informed about the diagnosis; the nature, purpose, and risks of the proposed treatment; feasible treatment alternatives; and the prognosis if the treatment is not carried out. In courts that apply the "new rule" on informed consent, which requires that the patient be told all that a physician would reasonably anticipate a prudent patient would consider **material** to his decision, it is conceivable that a patient could convince the court that the physician's success rate was material to him. However, it appears that no case has yet so held this to be true.

4. The answer is C. (*III B 3 a*) *Res ipsa loquitur*, Latin for "the thing speaks for itself," applies when an occurrence is so unusual that a court can infer negligence from the mere fact of its happening. All courts hold that, at the least, when this doctrine is applicable, the plaintiff does not have to produce expert testimony to establish that there was negligence. Some courts hold that a rebuttable presumption of the defendant's negligence is established, shifting the burden of proof to the defendant.

5. The answer is A (1, 2, 3). (*VIII C 1–8*) In certain cases, physical tests may be necessary to obtain evidence of criminal activity. However, if a test is painful, invasive, or poses a significant risk to the patient, it must be authorized by a court order. Both breath analysis and urinalysis are painless, noninvasive tests that pose no risk to the subject and therefore can be ordered by the police without a warrant. The police would be justified in proceeding without a warrant to get a blood sample, if the information sought might be lost if the drawing of blood were delayed to obtain a court order. Removal of a bullet is subject to stringent safeguards to protect the health and inviolability of the suspect. A bullet may be removed without a court order only if the subject's life is in danger.

6. The answer is A (1, 2, 3). (*VII B 1–7*) Private hospitals, while under no inherent common law duty to accept patients or render care in emergencies, are encouraged under certain circumstances to render care to individuals they might otherwise choose not to serve. For example, a hospital that maintains an emergency department whose existence is known to the general public undertakes an obligation to provide emergency care to those individuals presenting for treatment in an emergency situation. Medicare and Medicaid programs have conditions for participation, including the requirement that general acute-care facilities maintain emergency treatment facilities and that these facilities accept Medicare and Medicaid beneficiaries for treatment. The Hill-Burton free-care obligation requires that hospitals constructed or improved with federal funds must provide a reasonable volume of free or reduced-cost care to those unable to pay. While rules governing tax-exempt status consider the maintenance by hospitals of emergency facilities open to the general public, they do not require tax-exempt hospitals to admit all patients regardless of their ability to pay for care.

7. The answer is C (2, 4). (*VII A 1–3*) Physicians have no inherent duty to take on any patients or render care except at their own choosing. Good samaritan statutes offer civil immunity to physicians who render care under difficult, emergency conditions, but they do not compel physicians to render such care. Once a physician has accepted a patient, he or she cannot unilaterally discontinue the relationship, unless the patient is given sufficient notice to allow the patient to secure needed assistance from another source.

8–11. The answers are: 8-A, 9-C, 10-B, 11-E. (*III B 2 a (2), 3 a (2); V E 1–3; VI B 2 b; VIII A 2*) *Parens patriae* ("the state as parent") is applied to individuals who are unable to care for themselves. Under these circumstances, the state is both empowered and obliged to take protective action—that is, to assume the role of parent.

The Supreme Court of New Jersey in the *Claire Conroy* case established elaborate criteria for determining the wishes of the patient. Thus, under the doctrine of substituted judgment, care must be taken to assure that any decisions that are made for unconscious or incompetent patients, particularly in regard to care, be as close as possible to those the patients would have chosen for themselves.

Under the doctrine of *res ipsa loquitur* ("the thing speaks for itself"), a judge or lay jury may infer the defendant's negligence even in the absence of expert testimony. Thus, the plaintiff is spared the burden of producing evidence of negligence, which can be difficult as a result of a conspiracy of silence among physicians.

The exercise of therapeutic privilege, the exception to the physician's duty to disclose information, must be related to properly documented concerns that the physician has about the mental or emotional status of the patient. A general policy of not disclosing information to patients because of a presumed hypersensitivity is not an acceptable basis for this privilege.

12–15. The answers are: 12-C, 13-D, 14-B, 15-E. (*III B 2 d (1)–(3); V B 1, 2, D 1, 2*) Generally, the standard of care required is that of the medical community—that is, a professional community standard. However, as in *Helling v. Carey* (Washington, 1974), it is possible for a court to hold that the standard of care observed by the profession is not adequate and that "reasonable care" requires a higher standard. While the *Helling* precedent has not been widely followed, it seems clear that a court *can*, where it seems appropriate, impose its own standards of required conduct.

The older rule on informed consent, still followed in roughly half of the states, concerns the adequacy of a physician's disclosure to his or her patient: It is measured by what other physicians commonly would disclose under a similar circumstance. Using such a physician-based standard supports professional autonomy with regard to the provision of information to patients. Practically, it means that patients cannot sue for lack of informed consent unless they can produce expert medical testimony as to what the prevailing standard of disclosure is for the procedure in question.

Under a subjective standard of causation—that is, one focused on the "particular patient" in question—the jury attempts to decide whether that person would have chosen differently with respect to treatment if the information had been disclosed. This approach is consistent with the concept of individual self-determination, which underlies the doctrine of informed consent. The problem with this approach is that it places great weight on what the patient says he or she would have done, since no one can really prove or disprove what a patient's response to particular information would have been.

The patient-based standard of informed consent focuses on patients' informational needs rather than on the standard practice of physicians, making it consistent with the "patient's rights" philosophy. Thus, a physician is expected to disclose all that a patient would consider material to the decision to accept or reject treatment. A factor is considered material if it is significantly likely to affect the patient's decision.

15
Medical Ethics

Thomas K. McElhinney

I. LANGUAGE OF ETHICS

A. Ethics is a discipline that includes the study of ideal human conduct and an understanding of the moral life in which actions are judged as right or wrong and persons and institutions are judged as praiseworthy or blameworthy.

B. Philosophy and theology. Ethics may be seen either as a subdivision of philosophy or of theology.

1. **Philosophical ethics** is concerned with ethical study and with analysis of our ethical judgments.

2. **Theological ethics** is the study of moral behavior, which provides judgments of proper conduct, drawing from specific religious sources.

C. Divisions of ethics. Like many disciplines, ethics has historical, theoretical, and practical dimensions (Fig. 15-1).

1. **Descriptive ethics** is concerned with analyses of facts obtained from anthropological, historical, psychological, or sociological studies. Such comparative studies and cross-cultural inquiries are conducted without judgments of the relative merits of the various systems.

2. **Normative ethics** concerns inquiry into actions and their worth.
   a. **General normative ethics** discusses principles of human conduct and how evaluations are to be effected.
   b. **Applied normative ethics** concerns the judgments of specific moral problems. It includes medical ethics, legal ethics, business ethics, and other professional ethics.

3. **Metaethics** is the study of the meaning and justification of ethical discourse and the nature of moral concepts.

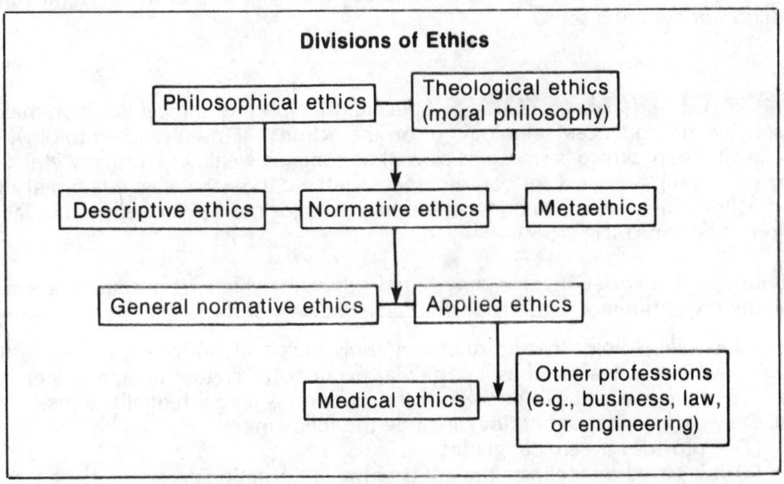

Figure 15-1

D. Moral and nonmoral values or goods. Both moral and nonmoral values are used in ethical analysis.

1. **Moral values or goods** are judgments of conduct, character, or actions of individuals or institutions (e.g., a saintly person or a despicable act).

2. **Nonmoral values or goods** are distinctions applied to estimates of the common worth of objects (e.g., a valuable painting or a good computer).

3. **Value levels** (adapted from Jurrit Bergsma and Raymond S. Duff) include personal values, group values, and society's values. Ethical conflict arises when any one value conficts with another.
   a. **Personal values** are the individual's unique interpretation of worth. While people may share values, even identical twins express different values.
   b. **Group values** are those of an individual's family, work unit, or organization, which an individual adopts.
   c. **Society's values** are general norms that are applicable to an individual or a group.

E. Virtues are desirable character traits—that is, virtues are a form of valuation about the moral worth of agents.

1. **Compassion** is a cardinal virtue of a health professional; it implies an ability to "suffer with" a patient.

2. **Integrity** of a health professional is expected by a patient; it is a virtue that demands honesty and allows the communication of personal matters that would not ordinarily be shared even with those closest to the patient.

F. Duties and rights

1. **Duties** are moral obligations owed by an individual, group, or institution to another individual, group, or institution.

2. **Rights** are generally correlative to duties and are claims by an individual, group, or institution on another individual, group, or institution.

G. Sources of morality. One or more sources may be drawn upon in any ethical situation. These sources operate as the basis for rights (and duties) and for the development of principles.

1. **Social contract** is the theory that specific rights may be drawn from implicit and explicit agreements by members of a society. This theory locates morality in human custom.

2. **Natural law** in morality may be regarded as the source of universal norms for human conduct. This theory holds that these norms can be discovered by reason and by an understanding of human nature.

3. **Divine command** is the belief that God reveals (directly or through inspired scripture) norms by which humans shall live.

4. **Individual insight** is the direct perception by the individual of what is right either through intuition or common sense.

II. NORMATIVE ETHICAL THEORIES. Specific principles for ethical decision-making center on judgments by consequences (teleology) or on the actions themselves (deontology). Because each major ethical theory provides strengths as well as contains weaknesses, many ethicists make decisions by combining a respect for consequences with a course that suggests moral rightness of the selected action. Such mixed theories attend to the major concerns of ethics but lack a center for validation of decisions (Fig. 15-2).

A. Deontological theories involve duty-based ethics in which right actions are determined independently of the moral goods or the consequences of those actions.

1. **Act deontology** holds that no rules can apply to specific judgments as each situation is unique. Each act is evaluated as a particular event according to its rightness or wrongness.
   a. When emphasized as "decision," this position is an existentialist ethics.
   b. Drawbacks of act deontology include the following:
      (1) It provides no ethical guides.
      (2) It is based on feelings; thus, it is emotive not rational.
      (3) It ignores the usefulness of rules.

Normative Ethical Theories

	Response	Theories		
		Particular	General	
Situation	Appeal to duty	1. Act deontology	2. Rule deontology	Action
	Appeal to consequences	1. Egoism 2. Act utilitarianism	3. Rule utilitarianism	

Figure 15-2

2. **Rule deontology** is the more popular deontological position; it holds that a rule or rules may be applied to decide ethical problems.
   a. **Monistic rule** deontology holds that one rule dominates all other rules; for example, Immanuel Kant's dictum: "Treat all persons as ends in themselves and never as means to an end."
   b. **Pluralistic rule** deontology holds that many moral rules exist (e.g., natural laws or the ten commandments) and that these rules must guide proper ethical decision-making.
   c. **Prima facie duties**—a modern modification of rule deontology—makes a distinction between those rules (duties) that seem appropriate for a certain situation and what may actually be best to do (the actual duty).
   d. Drawbacks of rule deontology include the following:
      (1) There is no agreement on one primary rule.
      (2) Judging conflicts among rules is difficult.

B. Consequentialist theories involve consequence-based ethics in which right actions are determined by the moral goods (results) produced without regard to the nature of the action.

1. **Egoism**
   a. Acts must be judged on the individual's best long-term interest.
   b. The good of the actor may be hedonistic (pleasure), but it may also be knowledge, power, or self-interest.
   c. Drawbacks to egoist theories include the following:
      (1) There are no guides or rules to settle conflicts.
      (2) There are no general principles to validate individual interest as primary human conduct.
      (3) There are no means by which to decide what is best.

2. **Act utilitarianism** is a consequentialist theory that promotes moral conduct that produces the greatest balance of good over evil.
   a. A balance of good and evil is applied to every action.
   b. The weaknesses of egoism are avoided by moving beyond self-interest.
   c. Drawbacks to act utilitarianism include the following:
      (1) It is difficult to assess consequences.
      (2) It ignores the usefulness of rules.
      (3) When two acts have equal consequences, they may still differ according to rightness of some principle.

3. **Rule utilitarianism.**
   a. The principle of balancing good and evil is used in conjunction with the application of rules to assess the balance; thus, there is a conformity of actions to valuable rules.
   b. Drawbacks to rule utilitarianism include the following:
      (1) There is no way to judge between contradictory rules with equal consequences.
      (2) The greatest good for the greatest number may be quite unjust to a minority.

III. MEDICAL ETHICS. Medical ethics is a branch of applied normative ethics supported by philosophical and theological presuppositions. It involves the study of general problems relating to health care, health care institutions, and biomedical research. While many issues are difficult to resolve because of conflicting social, political, legal, and economic pressures, there is considerable agreement about the general values that buttress the health profession. Moral disagreements are often amenable to rational discussion. The major issues have arisen from new technologies, increased respect for patient's rights, and financial restraints. Medical ethics will remain a strong interest in the medical profession as long as significant value differences remain and as long as ethics addresses the concrete concerns of patients and practitioners.

A. Background. The teaching of modern medical ethics began in the early 1960s. By 1985 virtually every medical school and several boards required courses in medical ethics, largely because:

1. New medical technologies challenged traditional patterns of care (e.g., genetic screening and life-support equipment).

2. Demands of public interest groups created new responses to rights questions from the professions.

3. Physicians and other health care professionals became concerned about the moral climate of their own fields.

B. Moral questions in medicine. Virtually every contact between a patient and a health professional contains moral dimensions, especially those that place demands upon the health professional. Most often the values of the patient, the health care worker, and the sponsoring institution conform, and there is no moral conflict. However, when values conflict, there is a need for medical ethical reasoning. The anatomy of moral conflict is best observed in an analysis of value levels.

1. Each physician has personal values, values formed at the level of practice partnership, service, or hospital, and values shared with other members of professional organizations and other general medical groups such as the County Medical Society (see section I D 3). At times demands from various levels may cause the physician internal conflict. When, for example, a physician who is opposed to abortion is a member of a medical group that is working for abortion rights, then the resultant pull of values between personal belief and professional loyalty is a subject for medical ethics.

2. Since patients also hold value claims at three levels similar to those of the physician, the possibilities for conflict are significantly increased. A physician opposed to abortion may argue for a woman's right to have an abortion against the wishes of her parents and spouse at the physician's hospital. Although not agreeing with the hospital policy nor the woman's choice, the physician may feel a moral duty to represent both value levels (the physician's group values and the patient's personal values) to a spouse and parents whose values coincide with the physician's personal values.

C. Professional codes of conduct. The Oath of Hippocrates, once widely subscribed to by graduating medical students, has been supplemented and revised by new interpretations of desirable medical behavior. The American Medical Association has produced a statement of professional principles, which is periodically revised. Medical specialties and other health professions have their own codes of conduct.

No code is able to foresee all possible moral situations or to provide exact behavior for particular situations. Virtues or desirable traits (see section I E) are often listed in codes of conduct and are often the core of a profession's sense of identity. To patients, high standards of behavior in a code are of no significance unless the character of the physician is beyond reproach.

IV. CLINICAL DECISION-MAKING.

Applied medical ethics seeks to relate general normative ethical theory to concrete decisions that must be made about specific situations. Standard decision-making procedures can be employed. The following is one method for clinical decision-making (Fig. 15-3).

A. Premise

1. Provide an action statement regarding conduct that should be initiated or discontinued because of a moral obligation of the physician to the patient or to an involved institution. Normally, it is phrased as "I ((We) ought (not) to do_______________."

2. Select the action statement that is positive as the original premise when opposite choices also appear attractive.

B. Ethical argument

1. List all reasons that support the premise.

2. Separate medical, legal, social, and personal reasons from moral ones.

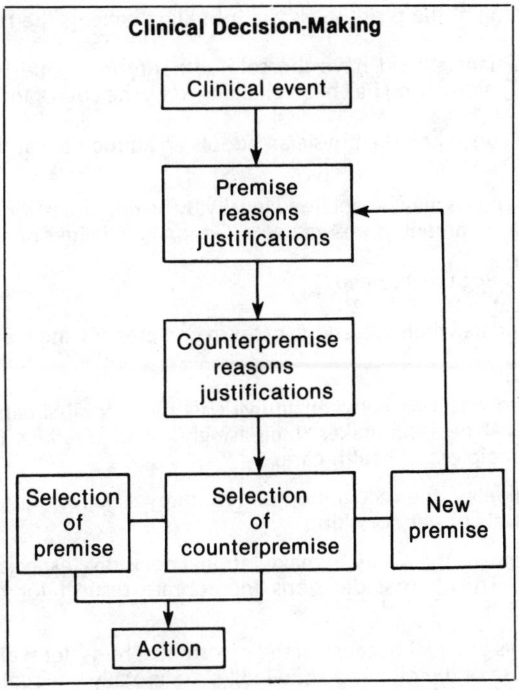

Figure 15-3

3. Provide justifications for all moral reasons listed. Justifications are "reasons for the reasons," and generally move to more abstract and general rules.
4. Hold objections until a later part of the argument.

C. **Counterpremise.** For each claim there will be one or more other moral claims.

1. List the first counterpremise.
2. List all reasons that support the counterpremise, including the objections noted earlier.
3. Sort the moral reasons from the other reasons.
4. Provide justifications for each moral reason.
5. List other counterpremises, if any, and complete steps 1–4.

D. **Evaluation.** Weighing alternatives is best done by concentrating on those reasons and their justifications that are the most appealing to the individual.

1. **General guidelines** include:
   a. **Consistency.** Be sure the decision is one that you would continue to support in similar cases.
   b. **Coherence.** Be sure the decision has internal logic and conforms to the general treatment plan for the patient unless there is an overriding reason for altering that plan.
2. **Alternatives** include:
   a. Accepting the original premise.
   b. Accepting a counterpremise.
   c. Developing a new premise as a modification of an earlier premise or counterpremise in which case the reasoning process should be repeated.

E. **Action.** Clinical medical-ethical decision-making is intended to culminate in the initiation of a particular action or procedure—one guided by moral insight.

V. MEDICAL-ETHICAL PRINCIPLES. Medical ethics may be divided into a consideration of some persistent general principles (this section) and into specific moral problems (see section VI).

A. **Fidelity.** By their professional standing, physicians and other health professionals make certain promises to society and thus to individual patients. Fidelity is the duty to observe the pledges made by the profession.

1. **Truthfulness.** One of the most troubling of the promises is that of telling patients the truth within the bounds of fidelity.
   a. The general assumption that physicians should have the sole authority to decide how much to tell their patients (directed paternalism) has been challenged by the courts and by physicians' organizations.
   b. A complete disregard for fidelity occurs when the physician adopts an attitude of careless truth-telling.

2. **Confidentiality.** Access to a patient's records may be obtained legally by health professionals, hospital personnel, and insurance or government representatives. General guidelines of confidentiality include:
   a. Limiting access to those who have a legitimate need.
   b. Avoiding idle conversation about patients.
   c. Using fake names and altering other data when presenting cases in conferences and teaching situations.

B. Autonomy. A basic understanding of the relations between individuals in a moral situation posits autonomy on the part of the moral decision-maker. Increasingly, medical ethics has stressed the autonomy of the patient or recipient of health care.

1. **Truth-telling.** In a manner similar to fidelity, the recognition of autonomy requires that the patient have access to the truth about his or her condition.

2. **Decision-making.** One mark of autonomy is the ability to make rational decisions, especially when considering one's own future. Truly moral decisions incorporate respect for the patient's own desires and needs.

3. **Respect for individuals.** Patients, always unequal because of their existential hurts (for which they have become patients) and because of their limited knowledge, are morally unequal to their caregivers and deserve respect as individuals.

C. Beneficence. The medical profession has a responsibility to do good for patients and the general public. This responsibility may be exercised through the care of individual patients or through efforts directed to preventing or ameliorating health problems in a community. Beneficence includes all efforts to increase the health of a community.

D. Nonmaleficence. The duty to "do no harm" is one of the oldest guiding principles of the medical profession.

1. **Deliberate acts to harm.** Only under limited concepts of self-defense is it permissible to harm another person.

2. **Calculated risk**
   a. When possible harm may occur, then there must be a compensating and compelling possibility of benefits in order to justify the action.
   b. For health care professionals, standards of "due care" include knowledge, craft (skill), and perseverance.

E. Justice. Equitable distribution of benefits and burdens constitute the subject matter of the principle of justice.

1. **Procedural justice.** One means of just distribution is the establishment of rules. To be fair, exceptions to rules should be clearly built into the procedures. The distribution of services on the basis of "first come, first served" is an example of a procedural rule.

2. **Distributive justice.** Equal sharing may not always be the most just way to distribute benefits or burdens; additional claims may be involved. Claims requiring decisions based on distributive justice arise when resources are limited; thus, reductions on spending for health care generate the questions of who shall have health care and who shall not (see section VI B).

3. **Compensatory justice.** Punishment as retribution is one form of compensatory justice. The more positive aspect is the attempt to reward victims for losses not the consequences of their own action—for example, quotas to combat discrimination.

4. **Individual and society.** Often issues of justice rest upon claims of the rights of individuals against claims of the society in which the individual lives. Decisions made for the "good of society" are particularly painful when they discriminate against an individual patient. The physician is often caught between primary duty to the patient and obligations to society.

VI. SELECTED MORAL PROBLEMS. Ethical consideration may be developed through principles (see section IV) or through review of specific problem areas (see below). Each problem represents a question of limits and of the moral stress arising from boundaries.

A. Limiting technology. New pharmacologic agents and sophisticated diagnostic and therapeutic machines have given physicians access to procedures that alter the traditional relations between physician and patient. Problems include:

1. Initiating life-support treatment. Legal and moral uncertainties surrounding the *removal* of life-support systems have in turn raised issues about initiating treatment at the onset of a medical crisis.

a. To not initiate treatment means the loss of a life that might be saved.

b. To begin treatment means the possibility of sustaining individuals who have no prospect for recovery, which can be costly in terms of patient, staff, and family suffering as well as in the use of resources that might be applied to other health problems.

2. Control and autonomy. Many of the new technologies promise methods of mind and behavior control, which have beneficial effects for some patients but which are subject to abuse by repressive governments, or even by well-meaning but overbearing health professionals. It is difficult to establish limits between the beneficial applications of technology and uses that may debase individuals and populations.

B. Limiting resources. The availability and types of medical care are restricted by the choices of individual physicians about their practices and through the process of congressional budget setting. Choices of **microallocation** (decisions affecting individuals) and **macroallocation** (decisions about which goods are available) produce many ethical questions.

1. The right to treatment. Ideal moral consensus expects that individuals be treated equally with respect to health care. However, the complexity of treatment systems and the diversity of illnesses make such an ideal impossible to maintain. Decisions by society determine which diseases and patients receive support, resources, and access to treatment. For example, the decision to fund renal dialysis changed a limited resource to a more readily available therapy but at significant economic expenditure. The right to treatment as decided by society determines:

a. What diseases get funded.

b. Which patients receive support for catastrophic illnesses.

c. Which theory of justice can best serve the decisions about the right to treatment.

2. Individual physician decisions. Although some government intervention has attempted to redistribute physicians by requiring certain locations for practice to repay educational assistance, physicians remain relatively free to choose where they practice and in what specialty. They also choose whom they will serve and, to a great extent, how much time they will spend with each patient. Those physicians working within prepaid plans report pressures to meet quotas. Physicians as a group, with some help from society, still determine:

a. How many physicians are needed.

b. The eligibility of physicians to pursue certain medical specialties and subspecialties.

c. The time that physicians should spend with patients.

3. Medicine and other social needs. The total expenditure on health care by society is balanced against other needs of that society—for example, defense, education, and measures against crime.

a. If it is determined that American expenditures on health care need to be changed, then responsible parties to determine the directions and amount must be assigned.

b. It is also important to determine how much money and resources go into prevention and into maintenance of good health habits and how much into treatment of existing illnesses, especially those affecting small numbers of people or those having high individual cost.

C. Limiting research. The new technologies are the result of the burgeoning research that occurred during and after World War II. The problems associated with research, although generally present throughout history, were highlighted by the medical experiments performed on humans in Nazi concentration camps. Articles written in the past 20 years continue to direct attention to unethical behavior by experimenters.

1. Deception. It should be determined when, if ever, deception is necessary in research. The investigator must ask if an altered design or a different protocol could obtain the necessary information; if not, under limited and controlled circumstances where the risk of harm seems minimal, it may be possible ethically to use deception.

2. Informed consent. The rights of individuals to choose risks has led to the move for informed consent in research. At one end of the spectrum, this doctrine means freedom to reject participation; at the other end, it requires a thorough evaluation of the individual's role in the experiment.

a. **Children.** Children cannot grant informed consent because of their limited capacity to assess risks and benefits. Nontherapeutic research in children is generally proscribed even where limited risk exists.

b. **Prisoners.** Prisoners once served as a major source of research subjects. As the doctrine of informed consent was strengthened, it became apparent to some that consent by those held in special restraint may be impossible to obtain. Critics of prisoner research argue that consent that offers good financial rewards to generally poorly paid convicts, that allows relaxation from otherwise strenuous and tedious duties, or that promises consideration for early parole or favorable attention when parole comes up is not comparable to the consent of nonprisoners. Additionally, since the concept of consent includes the right to refuse, prisoners who may be judged "uncooperative" for not volunteering to be research subjects do not have the same right of nonparticipation as do other potential subjects. Those advocating prisoner research refer to elevated prisoner morale from a sense of contributing to society, the chance to earn extra money, and relief from the monotony of prison life, as positive factors that promote freely informed consent from prisoners.

c. **Proxy consent.** For small children, the mentally retarded, and comatose patients, consent must be obtained from a legal guardian. Great restraints have been placed on proxy consent except in cases of possible therapeutic benefit for the patient or, in fatal illnesses, for others with the same disease.

3. **Privacy.** One constraint on researchers is the need to maintain patient confidentiality. However, with the general use of computerized records the problem of access to private information has increased.

4. **Reporting unethical research.** Journal editors have disagreed about the editorial responsibility for ensuring that published papers adhere both to high standards of research and to ethical means of obtaining data. The pressure of the news media for information as well as the fame and fortune to be gained by being "first" exacerbate this problem.

D. **Limiting risk of disease.** The continuing problem of the health profession to weigh the risks of the increased incidence of a disease against other public and private goods, such as the invasion of privacy, the rise of unneccessary panic, and confidence in health care has been illuminated recently by the health problems generated by the acquired immune deficiency syndrome (AIDS).

1. **General ethical concerns** involving infectious diseases, such as AIDS, venereal disease, and the common cold raise some very interesting questions. For example, attempts to limit the spread of a disease may place unnecessary restrictions on individuals not affected by the illness. General ethical concerns include:
   a. Caring for infected individuals.
   b. Reducing the spread of the disease.
   c. Finding treatments and eventually cures.

2. **Public health issues**, such as smoking, the use of alcohol or other drugs, or the possession of firearms, also raise issues of control and judgment concerning who shall be limited and in what ways. These items also balance the cost of measures to reduce ill effects while still permitting freedom to choose life-styles.

BIBLIOGRAPHY

Beauchamp TL, Childress JF: *Principles of Biomedical Ethics*. New York, Oxford University Press, 1979

Bergsma J, Duff RS: A model for examining values and decision-making in the patient-doctor relationship. *The Pharos*, 1980, pp 7-12

Institute of Science, Ethics and the Life Sciences: *Hastings Center Report*, Hastings, NY

Kennedy Institute of Ethics: *Bioethicsline*, National Library of Medicine, Washington, DC

Kennedy Institute of Ethics: *Encyclopedia of Bioethics*, 4 vols. New York, Free Press, 1978

Society for Health and Human Values: *Newsletter*, McLean, Va

STUDY QUESTIONS

Directions: Each question below contains four suggested answers of which **one or more** is correct. Choose the answer

- **A** if **1, 2, and 3** are correct
- **B** if **1 and 3** are correct
- **C** if **2 and 4** are correct
- **D** if **4** is correct
- **E** if **1, 2, 3, and 4** are correct

1. Moral limits on research include the

(1) need for informed consent
(2) high cost of equipment
(3) need for ethical means of conducting research
(4) scarcity of researchers

2. The general guidelines for observing the principle of confidentiality are

(1) limit access to patient information
(2) avoid idle conversation about patients
(3) use false names and alter data when teaching
(4) do not lie to patients

3. Factors that can be expected to continue the importance of medical ethics include

(1) the rise of new technologies
(2) the demands of the public
(3) physician concern
(4) new moral discoveries

Directions: The group of questions below consists of lettered choices followed by several numbered items. For each numbered item select the **one** lettered choice with which it is **most** closely associated. Each lettered choice may be used once, more than once, or not at all.

Questions 4–9

For each comment about a correct action to be taken, identify the probable moral theory from which the comment is drawn.

(A) Act deontology
(B) Rule deontology
(C) Egoism
(D) Rule utilitarianism
(E) None of the above

4. This action is likely to help me learn more about the disease and complete my project.

5. Telling the truth will maintain the patient's confidence.

6. It is clearly our duty to do this.

7. The law says to do it this way.

8. It must be done this way because the alternatives are too costly.

9. It is God's will.

ANSWERS AND EXPLANATIONS

1. The answer is B (1, 3). (*VI C 2, 4*) Informed consent is one doctrine that has arisen in response to a concern about unethical practices. Informed consent not only means freedom to reject participation but also requires a thorough evaluation of an individual's role in an experiment. For example, prisoners once served as a major source of research subjects, but it has been argued that perhaps incarcerated populations can never really be "free" to give their consent. Unethical research practices may lead to publishing restrictions and general rejection by the scientific community. The high cost of equipment and the scarcity of researchers may limit the ability to conduct research, but they are not *moral* limits. It may be a moral problem of the *allocation of resources* to not fund expensive equipment or the training of researchers.

2. The answer is A (1, 2, 3). (*V A 1, 2 a–c, B 1*) While truthfulness is a desirable moral behavior, it is related to the principles of fidelity and autonomy rather than to confidentiality. Limiting access to information, avoiding idle conversation about patients, and using simple means to change patient information when teaching are general guidelines for observing the principle of confidentiality. It is important to note, however, that access to a patient's record may be obtained *legally* in certain situations.

3. The answer is A (1, 2, 3). (*III A 1–3*) Basic moral theory has changed little since Socrates, Plato, and Aristotle made contributions that formally established the field 2500 years ago; it is, therefore, unlikely that medical ethics will be important because of new moral discoveries. However, changing technology, public demand, and physician concern have prompted the current interest in medical ethics and will be significant in the future of medicine and of medical ethics.

4–9. The answers are: 4-C, 5-D, 6-A, 7-E, 8-E, 9-B. (*II A 1, 2, B 1 a, b, 3 a*) The claim for carrying out the particular action based on the agent's needs and ultimate own best interest is called egoism. Even though the object is knowledge (and perhaps ultimately power) and not simply hedonism, the consideration is basically self-centered.

The principle of considering the good and evil consequences of an action and appealing to the general rule of telling the truth is rule utilitarianism. The specific consequence, undoubtedly worthwhile, is maintaining the patient's confidence.

The flat claim to authority without recourse to any specific rule or regulation or regard to consequence is the principle of act deontology. Each act is evaluated according to its rightness or wrongness. It is not simply enough to do one's duty, but it is necessary to understand "clearly" the proper action.

Knowing the law does not satisify a moral claim. There may be a presupposition that obedience to law is required if an act is to be moral. More sophisticated moral reasoning recognizes the place of law but also recognizes the exceptions that a moral claim may make. Thus, none of the answers apply.

Economic considerations may have moral impact, but they must be specifically identified. The claim may be consequentialist, but it does not explain the best nonmoral good. It may also be duty referenced toward accountability for expenditures. Both possibilities still need reference to some moral theory. Thus, none of the answers apply.

The principle that rules may be applied to decide ethical problems is the principle of rule deontology. Consequences are not considered: The only reference is to religious duty or "following God's will."

16 Health Care Manpower

Brett J. Cassens

I. INTRODUCTION. Health care manpower comprises those individuals employed in personal and public health. One in ten individuals in the work force are employed in medically related occupations. Because of the large number of health care professionals and the costs of their education, training, wages, and salaries, manpower issues are a major priority. This chapter describes the major categories of medical care personnel, their numbers, and their educational and licensure requirements.

A. Health care providers. Adequate numbers of personnel to provide health care has always been a concern of society. This is especially true of physicians whose costly training takes 7 years or more.

1. Shortages. A perceived shortage of physicians received widespread publicity in the 1960s as society struggled to improve access to medical care through Medicare and Medicaid. Many areas also reported shortages of nurses despite the large number of registered nurses in the United States.

2. Expansion of facilities. During the 1960s and early 1970s, federal funding supported the construction of new health professional schools and expansion of classes through the 1963 Health Professions Education Assistance Act. Between 1964 and 1975:

a. The number of medical schools mushroomed from 88 to 114, a 30% increase.

b. The total enrollment of medical students rose from 32,428 to 54,074, a 67% increase (Table 16-1).

3. Maldistribution. Despite this astounding increase in physicians, underserved areas persist as a result of maldistribution. Physicians tend to cluster near urban areas, avoiding rural and economically depressed communities. Even in physician-dense cities, physicians' services are not accessible to everyone. Table 16-2 demonstrates the geographic variations in the density of several medical professions. Health care planners continue to grapple with this issue.

4. The Graduate Medical Education National Advisory Committee (GMENAC) was chartered in 1976 by the Department of Health, Education, and Welfare (now Health and Human Services).

a. The task of GMENAC was to project physician manpower requirements for the year 1990 and for each specialty. The report predicted that an excess of 70,000 physicians can be expected by 1990, particularly in the surgical specialties.

b. The physician surplus projected by GMENAC will give a physician: population ratio of 215 physicians per 100,000 population. Experts have suggested that a ratio of 141 per 100,000 is adequate.

B. Costs. The costs of medical education and salaries for health care personnel are major components of medical care costs today. For example, 1 year of medical school costs $40,000 or more.

1. Medical school expenditures. Medical school and graduate medical education expenses are increasing by 12% per year.

a. Medical school expenditures for 1984–1985 exceeded $9.8 billion.

(1) Approximately 33% of revenues came from patient care.

(2) Approximately 25% came from federal funds, a steadily decreasing portion.

b. Rising medical school costs are reflected in increasing medical student debt. In 1985, the average graduating senior owed $30,256; however, 10% of graduates owed over $50,000.

Table 16-1. Graduates of Health Professional Schools and Number of Schools, According to Profession in the United States: Selected 1950–1983 estimates and 1990 and 2000 projections

Year	Medicine	Osteopathy	Nursing*	Dentistry
		Graduates		
1950	5553	373	25,790	2565
1960	7081	427	29,895	3253
1970	8367	432	43,103	3749
1975	12,714	702	73,915	4969
1978	14,393	963	77,874	5324
1979	14,966	1004	77,132	5424
1980	15,135	1059	75,523	5256
1981	15,667	1151	73,985	5550
1982	15,985	1017	74,052	5371
1983	15,824	1317	77,408	5756
1990	16,240	1480	68,400	4390
2000	16,080	1460	57,800	4080
		Schools		
1950	79	6	1304	42
1960	86	6	1128	47
1970	103	7	1340	53
1975	114	9	1362	59
1978	122	12	1358	59
1979	125	14	1374	60
1980	126	14	1385	60
1981	126	15	1401	60
1982	127	15	1432	60
1983	127	15	1466	60

Note.—Data are based on reporting by health professional schools. (Reprinted from Bureau of Health Professions: *Report to the President and Congress on the Status of Health Personnel in the United States*. Health Resources and Services Administration. DHHS Pub. No. HRS-P-OD 84-4, Rockville, Md., 1984; unpublished data; and American Chiropractic Association: unpublished data.)

*Some nursing schools offer more than one type of program. Numbers shown for nursing are the number of nursing programs.

c. A physician surplus means unnecessary educational costs absorbed by the medical care system or the taxpayer and increasing competition among physicians for available revenue.

2. Wages and salaries. Medical care is labor intense, and wages and salaries comprise a major percentage of the costs.

a. An average of 418 people were employed in community hospitals for every 100 patients in 1983. The figure was 226 employees for every 100 patients in 1960.

b. Labor costs for these personnel in 1983 comprised 56.5% ($208) of the adjusted average cost per patient per day ($368).

II. PHYSICIANS control the majority of medical care expenditures and are, with rare exception, the only practitioners licensed to diagnose and treat medical problems. Two philosophies of medicine dominate today: allopathic medicine and osteopathic medicine.

A. Allopathic physicians. Of the 443,285 physicians practicing in 1983, 96% possessed the Doctor of Medicine (MD) degree. They are called allopathic physicians (see Table 16-2).

1. Allopathic, or conventional medicine, originated in the heroic therapies of bloodletting and purging. The term allopathic refers to the concept that heroic medical treatments bore little relationship to the diseases to which they were applied.*

*The terms allopathic and homeopathic were coined by Samuel Hahnemann, founder of the latter philosophy of medicine. This eighteenth century German physician felt illnesses could be treated best by dilute solutions of elements thought to be related etiologically to a given symptom—thus, the concept of homeopathy, employing treatments "like the disease." In retrospect, Hahnemann's therapeutic conservatism doubtlessly saved many who would have died from the heroic methods of the day.

Table 16-2. Active Health Personnel and Number per 100,000 Population, According to Occupation and Geographic Region in the United States in 1983

Occupation	No. Active Health Personnel	United States	Geographic Region: Northeast	North Central	South	West
Physicians*	443,285	192.6	242.9	177.7	165.0	205.2
Doctors of medicine†	425,795	185.0	233.6	164.9	160.5	200.7
Doctors of osteopathy	17,490	7.6	9.3	12.8	4.5	4.5
Dentists*	129,920	55.7	67.5	56.5	44.7	60.9
Optometrists	23,770	10.1	10.2	11.5	8.0	11.9
Pharmacists†	152,600	65.0	66.3	72.7	65.7	52.5
Podiatrists	10,400	4.4	7.6	4.6	2.6	4.1
Registered nurses	1,404,200	600.0	772.2	648.5	477.4	564.7

Note.—Ratios for physicians and dentists are based on civilian population; ratios for all other health occupations are based on resident population. (Reprinted from Division of Health Professions Analysis, Bureau of Health Professions: *Supply and Characteristics of Selected Health Personnel*. DHHS Pub. No. (HRA) 81-20. Health Resources Administration. Hyattsville, Md., June 1981; Bureau of Health Professions: *Report to the President and Congress on the Status of Health Personnel in the United States*. Health Resources and Services Administration. DHHS Pub. No. HRS-P-OD 84-4, Rockville, Md., 1984; and unpublished data.)

*Excludes doctors of medicine in federal service; excludes dentists in military service. Data for 1982.

†Excludes United States possessions.

2. Medical education

a. Study leading to the MD degree requires 4 years of education beyond the baccalaureate degree, including 2 years of the basic sciences—anatomy, biochemistry, microbiology, pathology, physiology, and pharmacology—followed by 2 years of clinical rotations in the medical specialties.

b. In 1986, 66,604 students were enrolled in the 127 accredited medical schools in the United States. This is 1500 fewer students than in 1985.

(1) Enrollment in medical schools declined in 1985 as in the 2 prior years. This decline is expected to continue.

(2) A total of 32,893 students applied for first-year positions in medical school in 1986, down from 35,944 students who applied in 1985. The trend downward continues.

(3) Approximately 17,000 first-year students were accepted. About 1.9 times as many students apply as there are positions available.

(4) Approximately 17% of new enrollees were categorized as minority group members, including:

(a) Blacks: 5.3%

(b) Puerto Ricans: 2%

(c) Asians: 5.8%

(5) Women comprise 32% of all students, and their numbers are growing.

(a) In 1974, only 8% of medical students were women.

(b) In 1986, 4960 women graduated from medical school.

(6) The number of Americans studying in foreign medical schools is increasing, but no accurate means exist to estimate their numbers. In 1984, 247 Americans studying abroad transferred to schools in the United States with advanced standing, while 340 transferred in 1985.

(7) The Fifth Pathway is a program for Americans who have graduated from foreign medical schools to complete their graduate medical education in the United States.

(a) These programs usually provide lectures and clinical rotations to prepare students for residency positions in the United States.

(b) In 1985, 208 students entered the Fifth Pathway program.

3. Graduate medical education—that is, training programs beyond medical school—is accredited by the Accreditation Council for Graduate Medical Education (ACGME) of the American Medical Association (AMA).

a. Most specialty programs now include the first year after medical school (formerly known as the internship) as the first postgraduate year (PGY-I), which is followed by 2 postgraduate years (PGY-II and PGY-III) in the specialty residency program.

(1) In 1986, 20,997 PGY-I positions were available for the 16,291 graduates of the United States medical schools.

(2) The number of residents in all specialties declined in 1985. For example, 75,100 residents were on duty in 1984, but 74,500 residents were working in 1985.

(3) While the primary care specialties of family medicine, pediatrics, and internal medicine have been promoted in recent years, only 42% of students enter such programs.
(4) Surgery, which is generally over represented, showed a decrease in PGY-1 positions as did family practice and internal medicine.

b. The term "fellow" denotes a resident in a subspecialty program. Subspecialty training, or fellowship programs, follow residency programs in a general specialty. For example, residents complete 3 years of general internal medicine before entering a 2-year fellowship program in infectious diseases.

c. The number of graduates of foreign medical schools in American residency programs has been steadily declining. Since the mid-1970s, foreign medical graduates decreased from 25% to 16.89% of all residents in 1985. A total of 6868 American foreign medical graduates worked in residency programs in this country from 7400 in 1984.

d. Board certification or eligibility for certification is the end-point of specialty training. Each of the 24 specialties has its own board or in two cases, a conjoint board formed by representatives of two or more other boards. While board certification has no legal significance like licensure, it does establish a practitioner as a specialist. Some forms of insurance compensate specialists at higher rates.

4. Licensure. Regulation of medical practice is a function held by the states and territories. Texas passed the first modern licensure and medical practice act 100 years ago.

a. Eligibility for licensure requires:
(1) Graduation from a medical school accredited by the Association of American Medical Colleges (AAMC).
(2) Successful completion of an objective examination—either Parts I, II, and III of the National Board of Medical Examiners examinations or the Federal Licensing examination (FLEX).
(3) Completion of 1 year of postgraduate medical training.

b. While medical graduates are licensed as "physicians and surgeons" and thus not legally restricted to practice in a specialty, liability coverage and hospital privileges act to limit the scope of practice.

c. Reciprocity of licensure permits a physician licensed in one state to seek similar privileges elsewhere in the United States. Licensure is usually limited to a fixed number of years after completion of the aforementioned examinations; thereafter, an applicant may be required to take a state licensing examination.

d. Although states do not currently require re-examination to maintain licensure, many seek evidence of 50 credit hours of continuing medical education (CME) per year.

B. Osteopathic physicians graduate with the Doctor of Osteopathy (DO) degree. In 1983, 17,490 osteopathic physicians were in practice, comprising 4% of practicing physicians in the United States (Table 16-2).

1. Osteopathic medicine (literally "bone treatment") was developed by Andrew Tayler Still in the 1870s. Still was informally educated in allopathic medicine but was wary of the poisonous compounds used in the therapies of the day. Through a chance discovery, he learned to alleviate his own headaches by tension on the cervical spine. Based on his theories of musculoskeletal manipulation, he abandoned medications for this new osteopathic manipulative therapy.

2. Osteopathic education

a. Study leading to the DO degree requires 4 years of education beyond the baccalaureate degree. Curriculum content closely parallels that required for the allopathic education with the addition of training in manipulation therapy. Manipulation is now largely used as an adjunct to more traditional medical treatments.

b. In 1985, a total of 5600 students were enrolled in osteopathic schools.
(1) There are currently 15 schools of osteopathy. Michigan and New Jersey have parallel medical and osteopathic schools.
(2) Approximately 1400 students graduated in 1985.
(3) Although Still's original school pioneered the admission of both blacks and women, ironically the percentages of blacks and women in osteopathy schools in the 1983–1984 school year were smaller than those in medical programs (e.g., 2% to 5.5% blacks and 22.6% to 30.6% women, respectively).

3. Graduate medical education for osteopathic physicians has been limited until recently.

a. Traditionally, osteopathic physicians have followed a primary care path. After completing the obligatory osteopathic internship, most entered general practice.

b. Recently, graduates of osteopathic schools have increasingly sought positions in residency programs.

(1) Such programs could be either allopathic programs approved by the ACGME of the AMA or programs approved by the American Osteopathic Association (AOA).
(2) In 1985, 1277 osteopathic residents participated in ACGME-approved programs.
(3) Of these graduates, 50% were in the primary care specialties of family medicine, internal medicine, or pediatrics.

4. **Licensure.** All states license graduates of medical and osteopathic schools, permitting them similar privileges, although some states have separate licensing boards. Requirements for licensure are analogous to those described previously for medical physicians (see section II A 4).

III. NURSES.

Nursing services have traditionally focused on the needs of hospitalized or institutionalized individuals with most nurses employed in hospitals. In 1983, there were 1,404,000 registered nurses (RNs) and 549,000 licensed practical nurses (LPNs) in the United States. However, despite large numbers, many areas experience shortages.

A. **Registered nurses** constitute 70% of the nurses in the United States.

1. **Qualifications and training**
   a. A variety of degrees can qualify a registered nurse (Table 16-3).
   (1) **Diploma programs** graduate nurses after 3 years in a program that includes didactic work and extensive practical experience. However, diploma programs are being phased out in favor of college and university programs.
   (2) **Associate degrees** in nursing are granted after 2 years of study, usually at a junior college. Associate degree students acquire limited practical experience. Students with associate degrees comprise the largest number of graduates.
   (3) **Bachelor of Science degrees** in nursing (BSN) are granted by 4-year colleges or universities and require more extensive class work. The emphasis is now being placed on earning the BSN (Fig. 16-1).
   b. Registered nurses must pass a licensing examination to be registered in any state.

2. **Specialization**
   a. **Hospital-based nurses** often elect to practice in one specialty, such as pediatrics, operating room, medical/surgical, or intensive care nursing, for prolonged periods. The technical complexity of care, including more complex monitoring and drug regimens, is the principle force behind this specialization.

Table 16-3. Educational Requirements for Nurses

Educational Level	Training Required beyond High School	Curriculum	Training Site
Registered nurse PhD and DNS (Doctor of Nursing Science)	3–5 years post-baccalaureate	Academic program integrated with practical work throughout the years	University
Master's degree	5–6 academic years	1- to 2-year academic program integrated with practical work	University, hospital, and community health agencies
Baccalaureate degree	4 years and summer sessions	4-year academic program integrated with practical experience	University, hospital, and community health agencies
Diploma	27–36 months	1-year academic program and 2 years of practical experience with clinical courses	Hospital
Associate degree	2 years	2-year academic program integrated with practical experience	Junior college
Licensed practical nurse	1 year	1-year academic program integrated with practical experience	Vocational technical school and hospital

Reprinted with permission from Snook DI: *Hospitals: What They Are and How They Work*. Rockville, MD, Aspen Publishers, 1981, p. 81.

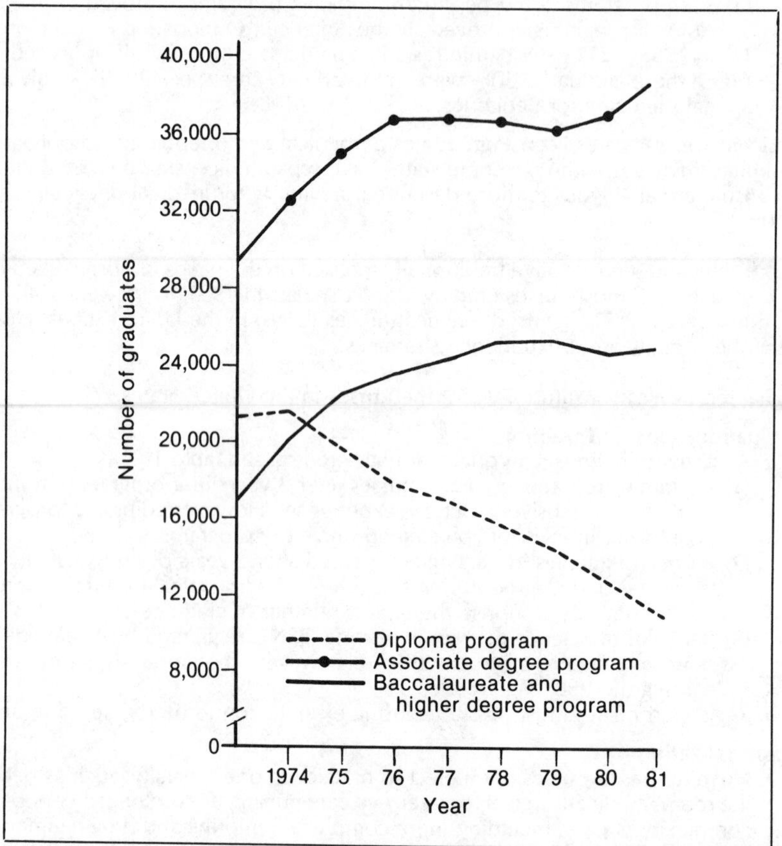

Figure 16-1. Registered nursing students graduated from initial programs of nursing education, 1973-74 to 1980-81. (Reprinted with permission from *Facts About Nursing*. Kansas City, MO, American Nurses' Association, Inc., 1983, p. 130. Based on information in *State-Approved Schools of Nursing—R.N. 1982*. New York, National League for Nursing, 1980.)

b. **Public health nursing**, or community nursing, is a field that focuses on the health care needs of large segments of the population.
   (1) Working in state or local health departments, public health nurses develop and implement programs in such fields as:
      (a) Immunization.
      (b) Maternal and infant health care.
      (c) Control of infectious diseases.
   (2) There are currently 72,600 public health nurses or 33 per 100,000 population.

c. **Home health care services**, provided by such groups as the Visiting Nurses Association, are playing a growing role in providing nursing and therapy in the patient's home. Medicare and Medicaid legislation, which provide payment for home services, spurred the establishment of these agencies. Home health care planning for hospital patients eases the transition from hospital to home. Discharge planning uses home nursing extensively to allow early discharge. Prospective payment systems emphasize early discharge (see Chapter 18).

3. **Licensure.** Registered nurse licensure is handled by state boards of nursing. Each state administers a licensing examination. All nurses must be licensed to provide patient care. Additional licenses must be obtained for each state in which a nurse wishes to practice.

B. Licensed practical nurses

1. **Qualifications and training.** Licensed practical nurses (LPNs) or licensed vocational nurses (LVNs) are certified health care workers trained in basic manual skills and techniques for assisting the registered nurse in the care of patients. They must train for 1 year. A major limitation of licensed practical nurses is their inability to administer medication.

2. **Salaries** for licensed practical nurses are lower than those of registered nurses; thus, a hospital

ward is usually staffed with one or two registered nurses who are assisted by several practical nurses.

3. **Licensure** for licensed practical nurses is similar to that of registered nurses (see section III A 3).

IV. DENTISTS. Dentistry is generally confined to care of the teeth and oral cavity.

A. Education

1. In 1983, 60 dental schools operated in the United States, granting Doctor of Dental Surgery (DDS) or Doctor of Medical Dentistry (DMD) degrees to students after 4 years of study. DDS and DMD degrees are equivalent.

2. Dental and medical students study similar subjects (e.g., pharmacology, anatomy, and physiology); however, dental students focus on the clinical and technical aspects of oral and tooth diseases.

3. In 1983, 5756 students graduated from dental school.

B. Licensure. Each state has a board of dentistry and laws regulating the practice of dental medicine. Licensing examinations are required, and a practitioner must obtain a license for each state in which he or she wishes to work.

C. Practice. In 1983, 130,000 nonfederal dentists were in active practice in the United States. There is an average of 55 dentists per 100,000 civilian population. A surplus of dentists exists.

1. **Solo practice** of dentistry has dominated the profession historically. However, dentists are currently working in small groups or as employees of hospitals, municipalities, or chains of dental offices managed by a central administration in increasing numbers.

2. **Dental assistants or hygienists** are technicians employed in virtually all practices. Patient preparation, including history review, radiographs, and teeth cleaning, is performed by these specialized personnel who also focus on preventive oral health.

3. **Specialization** in dentistry is expanding. It includes:
   - **a.** Orthodontics.
   - **b.** Periodontics.
   - **c.** Pediatric dentistry.
   - **d.** Endodontics.
   - **e.** Cosmetic dentistry.
   - **f.** Oral surgery.
   - **g.** Facial reconstructive surgery.

V. MIDLEVEL PRACTITIONERS are health care providers such as nurse midwives, nurse practitioners, and physician's assistants. These professionals usually work with and are supervised by physicians in teams. They are seen as physician extenders—that is, they increase a physician's productivity—although their skills in areas such as health education and prevention may exceed those of a physician. In a few states, midlevel practitioners are licensed to practice independently. Most midlevel practitioners are either licensed or regulated by state nursing or medical boards. The quality of care provided by midlevel practitioners compares favorably with that provided by physicians treating similar problems.

A. Nurse practitioners are registered nurses who have completed additional study in a specific area such as pediatrics. There are approximately 26,000 active nurse practitioners.

1. **Education.** Most programs, which grant a Master of Nursing (MSN) degree, last 1 to 2 years and prepare candidates for diagnosing and treating patients within their areas of expertise.

2. **Certification.** Candidates must pass a certifying examination and then are generally registered or licensed through state nursing boards.

B. Nurse midwives are registered nurses with special training in managing uncomplicated pregnancies, childbirth, postpartum and gynecologic phases of the reproductive cycle, and normal newborns. There are an estimated 2500 certified midwives currently living in the United States, 70% of whom are practicing.

1. **Education.** University programs for nurses with bachelor's degrees grant master's degrees after 1 to 2 years of midwifery study and experience. Additional 9- to 12-month programs are available to registered nurses with diplomas and associate degrees.

2. **Certification.** The American College of Nurse Midwives (ACNM) is a professional organization of midwives founded in 1955. ACNM administers a national certifying examination. Successful completion of this examination plus evidence of sufficient clinical experience leads to certification and the title certified nurse midwife (CNM).

3. **Licensure.** Most states require licensure that is specific to nurse midwives and require close cooperation with and supervision by an obstetrician.

C. **Physician's assistants (PAs)** are described by their professional organization, the American Academy of Physician's Assistants (AAPAs) as "skilled members of the health care team. . . working under the supervision of licensed physicians, providing a broad range of medical services." Physician's assistants working in surgical practices are known as surgeon's assistants. About one-third of physician's assistants are women. In 1985, 19,000 physician's assistants were in practice.

1. **Education.** The first educational program for physician's assistants was based on former military corpsmen—that is, military medics returning to civilian life were given additional medical education to provide them with an official status in civilian medical care. Since 1965, over 50 programs have been accredited by the Committee on Allied Health Education and Accreditation (CAHEA). Programs last 18 to 24 months and cover the basic medical sciences and clinical skills. Certificates or degrees are awarded upon completion of the program.

2. **Certification** is achieved on examination by the National Commission on Certification of Physician's Assistants. A certified physician's assistant must pass an examination every 6 years.

3. **Licensure or registration** varies by state, but the Board of Medical Examiners usually oversees licensure.

4. **The scope of practice** depends on the tasks delegated by the physicians with whom the physician's assistants work as well as the state laws or regulations. Generally, physician's assistants take medical histories, perform physicals, order diagnostic studies, and initiate treatment. Medications are usually prescribed by physicians.

5. **Practice patterns** of the 19,000 physician's assistants active in the United States in 1985 are rapidly changing. Ten years ago, most physician's assistants worked in a physician's office; today 64% are based in institutions and are replacing housestaff on some services. Physician's assistants are viewed as economically attractive alternatives to physician's services.

VI. ALLIED HEALTH PERSONNEL include professionals and workers in the fields of patient care, public health, and health research who assist independent practitioners in providing health services. They are defined as individuals working under the general supervision of a physician in providing medical services to members of the public while exercising independent judgment within their areas of competence. Over 8 million allied health personnel were active in 1984. Table 16-4 lists 24 CAHEA accredited allied health occupations.

A. **Education.** A high school diploma or equivalent is necessary for admission to all programs. The programs may also require college level work or a baccalaureate degree. The program itself may be as short as 6 months for an electroencephalogram technician to 4 years for a radiographic technologist. The educational programs discussed here are those accredited by the CAHEA, a voluntary organization established by the AMA in 1976, which is composed of 14 members representing the government, the public, and numerous health organizations.

B. **Certification** of allied health professionals is carried out by individual professional organizations. For example, a respiratory therapist must take the test administered by the National Board of Respiratory Therapy. Upon successful completion, he or she would be a registered respiratory therapist (RRT). Some allied health professions do not have certification processes, but some states may require registration or licensure.

C. **Licensure** of allied health personnel is not uniform and because of the cumbersomeness of establishing individual state examinations for the many allied professions, certification by a national organization has been proposed. By contrast, physical therapists are not nationally certified, but must apply for registration or licensure in each state in which they wish to practice. Diagnostic radiographic technicians may be required to pass a state licensing examination, even though they might be registered or certified.

Table 16-4. Enrollments, Graduates (Academic Year 1982–1983), and Programs by Occupational Type (1983) for Allied Health Professionals

Occupation	Enrollments	1982-1983 Graduates	1983 Programs
Cytotechnologist	310	256	66
Diagnostic medical sonographer	113	79	10
Electroencephalographic technologist	255	102	19
Emergency medical technician-paramedic	782	505	13
Histologic technician technologist	272	135	49
Medical assistant	12,382	5777	165
Medical assistant in pediatrics	10	3	1
Medical laboratory technician (associate degree)	7129	2231	206
Medical laboratory technician (certificate)	2302	1627	66
Medical record administrator	1759	621	54
Medical record technician	3028	851	83
Medical technologist	9283	5199	638
Nuclear medicine technologist	1464	772	141
Occupational therapist	6571	2044	55
Ophthalmic medical assistant	60	37	7
Perfusionist	76	26	8
Physician's assistant	2695	1294	53
Radiation therapy technologist	872	413	97
Radiographer	19027	7007	768
Respiratory therapist	9684	3627	213
Respiratory therapy technician	6920	3813	187
Specialist in blood bank technology	146	169	66
Surgeon's assistant	81	23	3
Surgical technologist	2049	1416	102
Totals	87,270	38,027	3,070

Note.—Totals reflect only one level of program per occupation offered by a sponsoring institution. (Reprinted with permission from *Allied Health Education Directory*, 13th ed. Chicago, Department of Allied Health Education and Accreditation, American Medical Association, 1986.)

VII. PHARMACISTS, OPTOMETRISTS, AND PODIATRISTS

A. Pharmacists. There were 153,000 pharmacists in the United States in 1983. They provide a range of services from retail pharmacy to clinical pharmacology. Pharmacy education usually requires 5 years of a combination of undergraduate work and pharmacy experience. Registered pharmacists have completed the required educational program and passed appropriate examinations. All states register or license pharmacists.

B. Optometrists are trained to diagnose eye disorders and fit corrective lenses. The educational program leads to a Doctor of Optometry (OD). In 1983, 1040 optometrists graduated, and 24,000 were in practice in the United States.

C. Podiatrists are health care professionals trained in the diagnosis, treatment, and prevention of diseases of the foot and ankle. Podiatrists complete a 4-year doctoral level curriculum to receive the Doctor of Podiatric Medicine (DPM) degree. Because of conflicting philosophies, podiatrists are usually excluded from allopathic and osteopathic hospitals, where orthopedic surgeons practice. There are separate podiatric hospitals in most large cities. In 1983, 2600 podiatric students were enrolled, and 10,400 podiatrists were in practice—that is, 4.4 podiatrists practice per 100,000 population.

STUDY QUESTIONS

Directions: Each question below contains five suggested answers. Choose the **one best** response to each question.

1. Which of the following statements bests describes allopathic physicians graduating this year?

(A) Upon completion of medical school, they may complete a Fifth Pathway program permitting residency training in a foreign country
(B) They are likely to have accumulated over $30,000 in student loans and debt
(C) They are more likely to enter a primary care specialty than their osteopathic counterparts
(D) They will graduate in a class with a nearly equal number of men and women
(E) When originally applying for medical school, they had a 1 in 5 chance of being accepted.

Directions: Each question below contains four suggested answers of which **one or more** is correct. Choose the answer

A if **1, 2, and 3** are correct
B if **1 and 3** are correct
C if **2 and 4** are correct
D if **4** is correct
E if **1, 2, 3, and 4** are correct

2. To assure their citizens that medical personnel have met minimum educational requirements, all states

(1) require licensure of all physicians and nurses
(2) accredit their own medical schools
(3) require certification or licensure, depending on the type of position
(4) require continuing medical education hours for physician license renewal

3. The Graduate Medical Education National Advisory Committee report

(1) was sponsored by the American Medical Association
(2) was chartered to project physician manpower requirements
(3) found that both physicians and populations were increasing proportionately
(4) projected continued heavy physician specialization in the surgical fields

4. There were approximately 549,000 licensed practical nurses in the United States in 1983. Accurate statements about licensed practical nurses include which of the following?

(1) Their salaries are lower than those of registered nurses
(2) They assist patients with personal care
(3) They are referred to as licensed vocational nurses' in some states
(4) They usually dispense routine medications

5. Statements that accurately describe nursing in the United States include

(1) licensed practical nurses outnumber registered nurses 2:1
(2) nursing education emphasizes obtaining the Bachelor of Science degree in nursing
(3) diploma nursing programs are university based
(4) a high level of specialization has evolved in nursing practice

Directions: The group of questions below consists of lettered choices followed by several numbered items. For each numbered item select the **one** lettered choice with which it is **most** closely associated. Each lettered choice may be used once, more than once, or not at all.

Questions 6–10

For each description listed below, select the professional that most closely fits it.

(A) All practicing physicians
(B) Registered nurses
(C) Diploma program registered nurses
(D) Public health nurses
(E) Osteopathic physicians

6. Although these professionals are only a small percentage of all medical personnel, they are strongly oriented to primary care.

7. Predicted to be in surplus by 1990, the number of these professionals continues to expand, consuming considerable economic resources.

8. Relatively few in number, these professionals have traditionally focused on preventive health care and health education.

9. Among the most numerous of all health professionals, shortages of these professionals are still common.

10. Educational programs for these professionals emphasize practical hospital-based experience but such programs are rapidly disappearing.

ANSWERS AND EXPLANATIONS

1. The answer is B. (*I B 1 b*) The rapidly rising cost of medical education as well as the perceived complexity of medical practice may contribute to the decline in medical school applicants and medical students. Projections of a sizeable surplus of physicians in 1990 have led to shrinking medical school classes. Student loans are an average of $30,000 at graduation with some debt exceeding $50,000. Osteopathic physicians predominately enter primary care, while 42% of allopathic physicians currently enter pediatrics, internal medicine, or family medicine. Twice as many applicants apply for available medical school positions as there are first-year openings.

2. The answer is B (1, 3). (*II A 4 a, d*) The process by which an individual practitioner acquires credentials is complex but involves the individual states only at the point of licensure or registration. Accreditation, the process of approving institutions, is carried out by independent nongovernmental groups. The Association of American Medical Colleges alone accredits American and Canadian medical schools. All states license nurses and physicians, but the sheer number of different allied medical personnel has led many states to accept national certification of allied personnel. Continuing medical education (CME) hours were adopted by many states in the late 1970s as a means of ensuring that physicians kept up-to-date. Experience over several years has yielded mixed results, and less than half of the states still require proof of adequate CME for re-licensure.

3. The answer is C (2, 4). (*I A 4 a–b*) Chartered by the Department of Health, Education, and Welfare, the Graduate Medical Education National Advisory Committee (GMENAC) is considered a landmark attempt to project needs for health care providers in the United States by 1990. The report suggested that current numbers of physicians were excessive overall. A total physician excess of 70,000 was projected with especially heavy excesses in the surgical specialties.

4. The answer is A (1, 2, 3). (*III B 1, 2*) Licensed practical nurses provide much of the hands-on care of patients, but they are prohibited from dispensing drugs. Because licensed practical nurses earn less than registered nurses, it is common for a hospital to employ fewer registered nurses but several licensed practical nurses to assist them. Licensed practical nurses are known as licensed vocational nurses in some states.

5. The answer is C (2, 4). (*III A 1 a, b, 2*) As nursing has become increasingly specialized and technical, the education of nurses has become more demanding, emphasizing the 4-year program required for a Bachelor of Science degree in nursing (BSN). Diploma nursing programs are primarily those established by hospitals and lack the university or college affiliation to grant a BSN degree. There are more than twice as many registered nurses as licensed practical nurses.

6–10. The answers are: 6-E, 7-A, 8-D, 9-B, 10-C. (*I A 4 a; II B 3 a; III A 1 a (1), 2 b*) While the number of osteopathic physicians is small, the numbers continue to grow, with 28,000 practitioners projected for 1990. Osteopaths traditionally have been more strongly oriented toward primary care. Relatively few specialize, though more are taking that route.

The number of physicians, both MDs and DOs, continues to increase yearly. Since 1965 there has been a greater than 40% increase in practicing physicians. The projection for 1990 is a total of 595,000 practicing physicians.

It is estimated that 72,600 registered nurses were employed as public health nurses in state and local agencies in 1979. These numbers have doubled since 1966 but still reflect a small number of nurses who are available for community medicine.

From 1965 to 1980, there was a 75% increase in the number of registered nurses in practice. While nursing personnel nearly doubled in this period, many areas still felt acute shortages of registered nurses.

Virtually all diploma programs are administered by hospitals and require 3 years of training. Recent trends have shown a steady decline in the number of graduates from these programs with larger numbers receiving associate and bachelor degrees.

17
Health Care Services

Brett J. Cassens

I. INTRODUCTION. This chapter describes institutions and organizations that focus on the health of 230 million Americans who spend over $400 billion annually in the pursuit of health. Health care services focus on maintaining, restoring, and improving a state of physical and mental well-being that is free from illness or infirmity. The American Medical Association (AMA) points out that "both mental and physical health are influenced by many factors, including environment, education, housing, civil rights, and to a very great degree by economic status." The concept of social well-being is generally excluded from the responsibilities of health care providers, though health and social well-being are arguably inseparable. The success of these services is measured in terms of the longevity, survival, and prevalence of disease in a given population. Health care services encompass individuals and institutions that provide both personal and public health services.

A. Personal health care refers to services provided to an individual by a health professional to preserve or restore health. A patient visit to a physician for treatment is personal health care in its simplest form. There are several categories of personal health care.

1. **Ambulatory care**, or outpatient services, refers to services provided for nonhospitalized patients in medical offices, clinics, emergency departments, urgent care centers, and physical therapy offices.
2. **Hospital care**, or inpatient services, are institutional services that include bed and board. Physicians, nurses, and ancillary personnel work together to provide intensive, sophisticated care in the hospital environment.
3. **Long-term care** refers to health services provided in nursing homes or by home health care specialists who provide personal and medical care for patients who are dependent but not sick enough to remain hospitalized.

B. Public health is defined as the combination of sciences, skills, and beliefs that is directed to the maintenance and improvement of the health of an entire population. Public health typically is in the domain of government. The World Health Organization (WHO) states that "governments have a responsiblity for the health of their peoples which can be fulfilled only by the provision of adequate health and social services." In the United States, federal, state, and local governments provide health services.

1. **Federal government** involvement in health care is a function of the Department of Health and Human Services (DHHS), which was established in 1953 as the Department of Health, Education and Welfare (DHEW) and renamed DHHS in 1979.
   a. Figure 17-1 shows the organization of DHHS. The Secretary, a cabinet level position, "advises the President on health, welfare, and income security plans, policies, and programs of the Federal government."
   b. The Public Health Service (PHS) is the division of DHHS that is responsible for public health services research, and to a limited extent, personal health care (e.g., Indian Health Service). The Assistant Secretary for Health and the Surgeon General head the PHS, which has its origins in the Marine Hospital Act of 1798. The seven major divisions of the PHS are listed in Figure 17-2.
2. **State and local governments** fund 85% of all public health activities, usually through cooperative programs. Control of infectious diseases; medical laboratory services; environmental health, including air, food, and water quality; maternal and children's health; health education; immunizations; and vital statistics are major responsibilities of state and local health departments. Federal agencies, especially the Centers for Disease Control (CDC), regularly

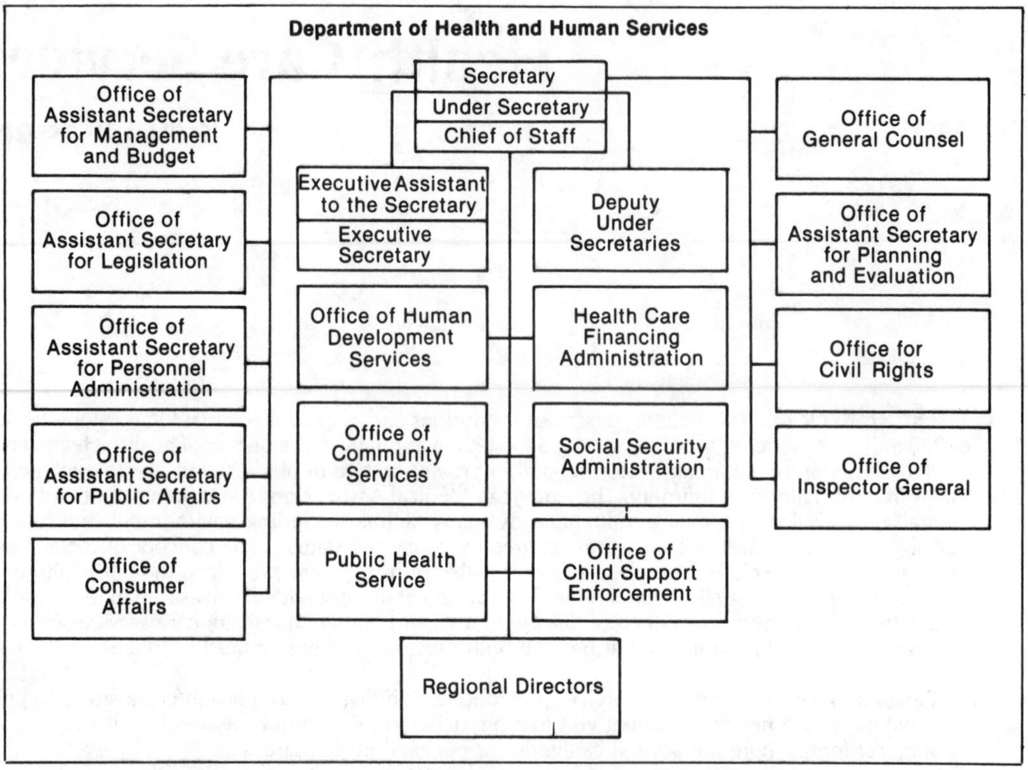

Figure 17-1. Organization of the Department of Health and Human Services.

provide funding, technical assistance, and frequently personnel to support local health departments. Teams of CDC specialists or members of the CDC Epidemic Intelligence Service (EIS) often work with local health departments on unusual or complex public health problems, such as the acquired immune deficiency syndrome or rubella outbreaks.

a. State health departments are headed by boards of health or by a secretary or commissioner of health. In the latter case, governors appoint their health officers and exercise significant political control over the appointees. The state department of health sets minimum standards for hospitals, nursing homes, and laboratories and licenses institutions and many health care professionals. In rural and unincorporated areas, the state has responsibility for immunizations, rabies control, and water and air quality.

b. Cities, large municipalities, and counties may also have boards of health, health commissioners, or directors of public health. While the local responsibilities parallel those of the states, local services may exceed those of the state. Most local health departments operate with boards of health composed of community members. Such boards advise on health matters and formulate codes of health, which govern the community. Many cities provide free community health centers, but few still support large municipal hospitals, such as Cook County Hospital in Chicago and Bellevue Hospital in New York City.

II. CHARACTERISTICS OF MEDICAL PRACTICE.

Numbering nearly 500,000, physicians (MDs and DOs) control and direct the activities of the 8 million other health care workers. In the past, physicians were either general practitioners or specialists, depending on whether or not they completed a residency program beyond the obligatory internship. However, all medical students today enter residency programs in either family medicine or one of the other specialties.

A. Primary care is a fundamental concept in the organization of medical practice because it involves the point of entry into the medical world. Efforts to streamline and economize medical practice have placed increasing importance on the role of the primary care physician.

1. Primary care physician. According to the AMA, the primary care physician is "one whom the public generally contacts directly, and whose practice is characterized by a broad scope of medical services, including the management of slowly progressive and chronic illnesses, preventive and emergency services, and personal and family counselling .... The primary care physician is often the one to whom a patient turns for counselling on personal life situations as well as with concerns about illness or injury."

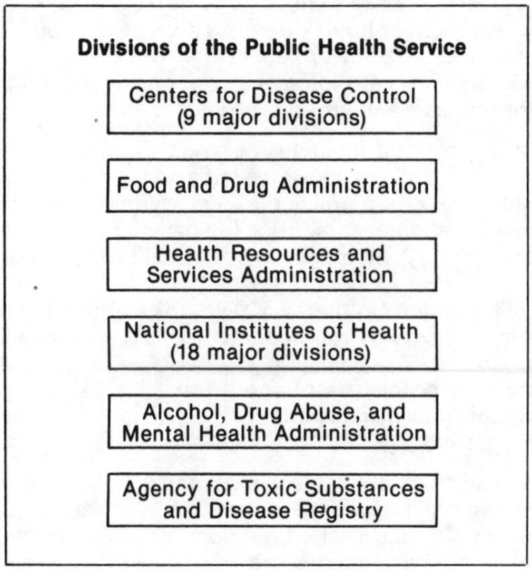

Divisions of the Public Health Service
Centers for Disease Control (9 major divisions)
Food and Drug Administration
Health Resources and Services Administration
National Institutes of Health (18 major divisions)
Alcohol, Drug Abuse, and Mental Health Administration
Agency for Toxic Substances and Disease Registry

Figure 17-2. Organization of the United States Public Health Service—a division of the Department of Health and Human Services.

2. **Primary care specialties** include family medicine, internal medicine, pediatrics, and rarely obstetrics and gynecology. Approximately 49% of residents are trained in primary care; however, only 33% of practicing physicians are in these primary specialties.

3. **Role of the primary care physician** has alternately been described as a keystone or a gatekeeper. The difference is significant.
   a. **The keystone role** of the primary care physician holds that primary care physicians coordinate the care provided by an increasing number of disparate specialists and technicians, each of whom is concerned with only a single aspect of an individual's overall medical condition. As a keystone, the primary care physician oversees these interactions and ties them together in a most effective manner, just as a keystone unites and stabilizes the sides of an arch.
   b. **The gatekeeper role** of the primary care physician, by contrast, coordinates care but also controls access to other specialists. For example, primary care physicians in Health Maintenance Organizations (HMOs) are encouraged to provide "a broad scope of medical services," thus avoiding expensive referrals to specialists for elementary problems. Family practitioners, for example, competently treat acne, usually without dermatologic consultation.
   c. **Pros and cons** of these two conceptual models focus on the issues of a patient's freedom of choice of providers, the economic ramifications of these choices, and the quality of care.
      (1) Advocates of the keystone concept argue that patients should be free to select whomever they wish for a given service, and the specialist, though potentially more expensive, may actually be more efficient by virtue of his or her expertise and a superior level of care. Nonprimary care specialists in particular may favor patient freedom to exercise preference for one specialist over another.
      (2) Advocates of the gatekeeper function accept the restrictions of patient choice, but believe that this loss of freedom is justified because better care results when it is provided by one physician rather than numerous consultants, and savings accrue when expensive consultations are avoided. Critics charge that HMOs reward primary care providers for not referring, thus providing incentives for not making referrals, even when they are medically indicated. The expanding influence of alternative delivery systems, like HMOs, predicts a greater role for primary care gatekeepers.

B. Organization of physician practice gains greater importance each year as physicians participate in complex practice arrangements and office visits continue to be a major portion of physician/patient contacts each year. In 1983, there were 1.5 billion patient visits, 956 million of which were office visits with the remainder consisting of hospital rounds and emergency room and outpatient department visits. (Although total visits increased over the last decade, they decreased by 2% from 1982–1983; visits per physician decreased by 5%.) The choice between solo and group practice and between self-employment and employee status are important issues that confront physicians today.

1. **Solo practice.** Two-thirds of physicians practice alone. As entrepreneurs, they are at risk for all aspects of the business. They tend to work longer hours—that is, 52 versus 50 hours per week for physicians in group practice. They see 10% fewer patients per week—that is, 115 versus 123 for physicians in group practice, and they earn somewhat lower net incomes—that is, $104,000 versus $112,000 per year for physicians in group practice.

2. **Group practice** has been viewed with suspicion, and members of groups have been sanctioned by local medical societies in the belief that groups foster impersonal, "corporate" medical practice. While offering less autonomy, group practice fosters sharing of expertise and, in multispecialty groups, ease of referral without fear of losing the patient to the consultant. Advocates of group practice argue that groups on average provide better care because of the sharing of cases among partners.
   a. Group practices in 1984 offered 140,000 positions in the 15,500 groups registered in the AMA census. In 1965, by contrast, only 4300 groups were counted. This is an annual increase of 7% for the past 20 years.
   b. Most groups are small, numbering only three or four practitioners, usually in a single specialty. However, the average size of groups has increased to nine physicians per group; thus, 160 groups had over 100 practice positions.

3. **Self-employed and salaried physicians.** The traditional solo entrepreneur is becoming a thing of the past as young physicians opt for more limited time commitments and early guarantees of a stable income. As recently as 10 years ago, salaried positions for physicians were limited. Now as hospitals and large health care corporations provide patient care through clinics, HMOs, and urgent care centers, the number of salaried positions is growing. Fully 45% of physicians under the age of 35 years are now working as employees.
   a. **Work patterns** of self-employed and salaried physicians differ significantly. Although both groups worked an average of 47 weeks per year in 1984, AMA statistics reveal a shorter work week for salaried doctors—that is, 53 hours versus 58 hours for self-employed physicians. Similarly, salaried physicians had fewer patient visits but longer patient hospital stays—that is, 9 days versus 6 days for patients of self-employed physicians.
   b. **The economics of practice**
      (1) Salaried physicians carry no overhead. Rent, insurance, office staff, and supplies are all paid by the employer. Fringe benefits, such as health, disability, life insurance, and retirement accounts, are also paid by the employer. In 1984, the average total professional expenses for self-employed doctors was $92,600.
      (2) Average annual net income is the total amount of money earned in the practice per year less expenses (overhead). Net income is taxable income. For salaried physicians, salary is net income. Average net income for self-employed physicians in 1984 was $118,000 versus $80,000 for salaried physicians. The greater financial risk and longer hours of self-employed physicians translates into 50% higher earnings.

4. **Midlevel practitioners** include physician's assistants, nurse midwives, and nurse practitioners. These physician extenders totaled 46,000 in 1985, providing many of the services of the primary care physicians. Although most midlevel practitioners work under the supervision of physicians, a small number practice independently in some states. With salaries in the range of $20,000 to $30,000 annually, they are attractive alternatives to more expensive physician manpower. Although the scope of practice of midlevel practitioners is more limited than physicians, they have replaced house physicians in some hospitals and nursing homes, and physicians in some rural and city clinics. These providers increasingly compete with physicians for the growing number of salaried positions in health care organizations.

C. **Practice economics** is an area with which medical students and residents have limited training and expertise. Yet the ability of a physician to achieve a target salary is essential to job satisfaction.

1. **Physician numbers** are large. A ratio of 150 physicians per 100,000 population is thought to be ideal. In 1985, 220 physicians were available per 100,000 population, and the ratio is projected to be even higher in the future. Physician extenders are also more numerous each year, and increasing numbers are accepting salaried positions in institutions rather than in physicians' practices. The combination of the efforts to contain health care expenditures and physicians' fees and the rapidly rising office overhead will assuredly make physicians' practices less lucrative than previously.

2. **Average annual net income** of physicians in 1984 was $108,400, including pensions and retirement plan contributions. As a 2% increase over 1983, this represented a net loss of 2% when inflation is considered. Small increases in physicians' salaries will be the rule in the near future.

Table 17-1. Average Physician Net Income after Expenses and before Taxes (1983 and 1984)

Specialties	1983	1984	Percent Change
All physicians	$106,300	$108,400	2.0
Specialty			
General/family practice	68,500	71,100	3.8
Internal medicine	93,300	103,200	10.6
Surgery	145,500	151,800	4.3
Pediatrics	70,700	74,500	5.4
Obstetrics/gynecology	119,900	116,200	−3.1
Radiology	148,000	139,800	−5.5
Psychiatry	80,000	85,500	6.9
Anesthesiology	144,700	145,400	4.8

Reprinted with permission from Reynold RA, Duann DJ (eds): *Socioeconomic Characteristics of Medical Practice*. Chicago, American Medical Association Center for Health Policy Research, 1985.

a. **Specialty differences.** Physicians are among the highest paid professionals in this country, though not worldwide. Variation among specialties, however, is great. Table 17-1 demonstrates a range of incomes from $151,000 for surgeons to a low of $71,000 for family medicine. This disparity of 114% demonstrates the difference in compensation for procedure-oriented care such as surgery, as compared to the cognitive services of pediatricians, internists, and family physicians.

b. **Regional differences** in net income are shown in Table 17-2. Physicians in New England experienced the lowest net incomes of $87,000 in 1984, while those in the South averaged $120,000. Income in the Rocky Mountain states increased 12%, six times greater than the national average.

D. **Alternative delivery systems**, such as HMOs, contrast to the traditional fee-for-service practice where the physician established a fee schedule, and the patient paid for each service. Either through prepayments or carefully negotiated service discounts, newer systems of providing medical service have been established in an attempt to minimize costs.

1. **Definitions**

a. **Health Maintenance Organizations (HMOs)** provide prepaid comprehensive health care, and providers are placed at financial risk for excessive use of services. Preventive, diagnostic, and therapeutic services are provided.

b. **Independent Practice Associations (IPAs)** are a form of HMO where physicians are in private practice but agree to accept either a reduced fee or a capitation fee for services rendered.

c. **Preferred Provider Organizations (PPOs)** are fee-for-service plans where insured individuals are given financial incentives to use "preferred providers." Other than the agreed upon discount from their charges, physicians are not at risk, and patients may use any physican, though nonmember physicians' services require copayments or deductibles.

d. **Exclusive Provider Organizations (EPOs)** are a rare form of fee-for-service plan where an

Table 17-2. Average Physician Net Income after Expenses and before Taxes (1983 and 1984)

Census Division	1983	1984	Percent Change
New England	84,500	87,300	3.3
Middle Atlantic	98,600	98,400	−0.2
East North Central	114,300	109,400	−4.3
West North Central	110,500	110,700	0.2
South Atlantic	106,700	114,500	7.3
East South Central	114,900	122,200	6.4
West South Central	124,400	119,100	−4.3
Mountain	91,400	102,300	11.9
Pacific	103,100	109,400	6.1

Reprinted with permission from Reynold RA, Duann DJ (eds): *Socioeconomic Characteristics of Medical Practice*. Chicago, American Medical Association Center for Health Policy Research, 1985.

employer selects hospitals and physicians with favorable charges and rates. Patients within such plans are required to use the physicians and hospitals felt to be most cost-effective. Providers are at no financial risk.

e. Capitation is the typical prepayment form of reimbursement. A provider receives a fixed payment per month to provide a specified set of services to an enrollee or arrange for such services. Capitation fees usually take age and sex into consideration. The physician does not bill either the patient or the plan.

f. Copay is a plan whereby the patient pays a percentage of the bill for medical services or a fixed amount per service. All forms of health insurance require that employees copay to reduce premiums and to constrain the use of services. If an insurance policy or HMO has a 20% copayment plan, then a complete physical costing $100 would cost the patient $20 and the insurance company $80, and an HMO requiring a $3 copayment would collect this amount whenever the patient saw a provider.

g. Deductible is the amount an enrollee must pay each year before the insurance plan begins to pay. A typical deductible is $200. If a patient incurred $800 of medical expenses in 1987, the patient would pay the first $200, and the plan would pay the remainder. Insurance plans and HMOs may employ deductibles and copayments together.

h. Enrollees are individuals who have paid premiums and are on the membership roster for an insurance company or health plan. In an HMO, a physician group would be capitated per enrollee.

i. Plan refers to insurance companies and HMOs. Within an IPA, however, the plan would be the central administrative services collecting premiums, establishing benefits, and paying capitation with which the IPA or physician group would negotiate a contract for services.

j. Provider describes anyone rendering health care within a health plan. Physicians, mid-level practitioners, and a variety of therapists are all providers who serve enrollees.

k. Prepaid medical care refers to the concept that hospitals or providers are paid in advance a predetermined amount for services that enrollees are entitled to receive. Implicit in prepayment is risk. A skillful provider with healthy patients might earn a handsome sum, whereas a less efficient physician or one with sicker enrollees, might receive a meager reimbursement relative to services rendered—that is, payment is independent of the health status of the patient or the efficiency of the provider.

2. History of prepaid health care

a. The earliest prepaid health plans date back to the Depression. In 1929, the Ross-Loss Clinic contracted with the city of Los Angeles to provide prepaid health care to city employees. In 1934, consumers in Elk City, Oklahoma organized a health cooperative, hired physicians, and provided services on a prepaid basis.

b. Despite the staunch resistance of organized medicine to the concept of "contract" medicine, prepaid health care slowly spread in the 1940s and 1950s. It was during this period that the Kaiser Health Plans gained a strong foothold on the West Coast.

c. The Medicare and Medicaid programs established in the 1960s have had a decisive effect on prepayment. These two programs rapidly inflated federal health care expenditures to such an extent that reform was desperately sought by 1969.

d. The concept of prepaid care emphasizing health maintenance over expensive hospital care was the proposal of Paul Elwood, the Executive Director of the American Rehabilitation Foundation. He coined the term Health Maintenance Organization. His proposals were eagerly adopted by the Nixon administration, but strong resistance from organized medicine and liberals alike postponed passage of the HMO Act (P.L. 93-222) until 1973. This Act funded only limited demonstration projects and precluded state laws, which might prohibit HMOs. Amendments to the HMO Act in 1976 and 1978 finally spurred a true federal commitment to prepaid health care.

3. Prepaid health care today

a. Although the 1971 projection of 1700 HMOs by 1977 proved wildly optimistic, recent growth has been impressive (see Fig. 17-1). Currently over 17 million Americans are covered by HMOs, and these numbers are increasing by 20% per year.

b. Ironically, though prepayment was seen as the means by which to reduce federal health care expenditures under Medicare and Medicaid, it was not until 1984, a decade later, that these programs were promoted within HMOs.

c. The basic form of an HMO, which is illustrated in Figure 17-3, consists of the plan, a group of physicians, and a hospital. Enclosures in the circles indicate ownership by the plan, while straight line linkages are contractual relationships.

(1) Staff model HMOs. In these HMOs, physicians are employed by the plan, while the hospitals may be plan-owned or independent.

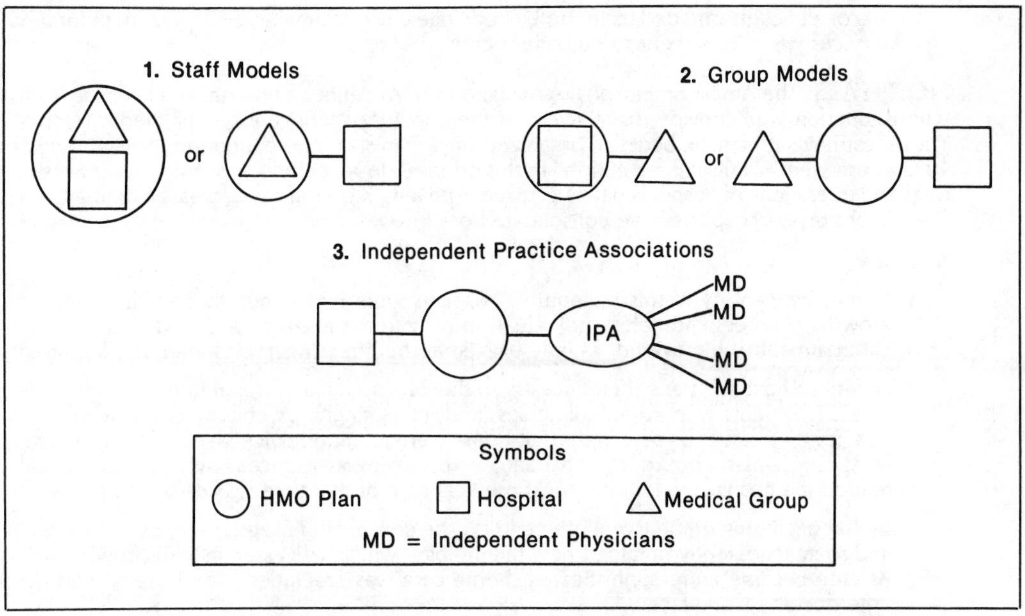

Figure 17-3. Health Maintenance Organization models.

(2) **Group model HMOs.** In these HMOs, physician groups contract with the plan, but the physicians remain employees of the group.

(3) **IPAs** differ from staff and group model HMOs because the physicians are private practitioners who agree to see prepaid enrollees. Physicians band together in an IPA, and then this entity contracts with the HMO. Because of the independent position of the practitioner, IPAs are more palatable to organized medicine.

d. An HMO is operated in the following manner.

(1) A group of investors, usually physicians and hospitals, formulates a plan for an HMO.

(2) After licensure by the state insurance authority, the plan, which is actually an insurance company, formalizes contracts with hospitals and either hires physicians or contracts with a group.

(3) The plan then attempts to convince employers in the area to offer the HMO health insurance to their employees for a premium, depending on whether the employee is single, married, or has a family.

(4) The plan collects premiums, and the new enrollee selects a physician.

(5) In a staff model HMO, the plan pays a salary to the physician, who then provides care, but does not bill. Hospitals are usually paid a negotiated rate, often 15% to 20% less than their standard charges.

(6) All routine and emergency care is provided at little, if any, charge to the enrollee.

(7) If the HMO has an average number of sick patients, it will break even or perhaps make a small profit. If patients are quite ill, a debt is incurred. The distribution of financial risk is ideally dispersed among providers, hospitals, and the plan. The appropriate sharing of risk is fundamental to HMO management.

e. Continued HMO development is inevitable as insurance companies start HMOs of their own to compete with independent prepaid plans. So called triple-option plans are the wave of the future. Under these arrangements, an insurance company offers its own indemnity (traditional) plan, an HMO, and preferred provider option. This is designed to enable one insurance company to offer these three different products to an employer.

D. Veterans Administration services. The Veterans Administration provides extensive health services to eligible veterans. Medical care is provided without charge for any service-related illness or disability. Veterans with nonservice-related problems may receive care based on financial need. Hospital care, nursing home care, and outpatient medical and dental care are offered.

1. Facilities. Veterans Administration facilities include 173 medical centers, 16 domiciliary facilities, 225 clinics, and 105 nursing homes. Most of these are affiliated with teaching programs.

2. Costs. Health care expenditures within the Veterans Administration totaled $8.3 billion or

2% of all health care dollars in the United States. Approximately 61% was spent for inpatient services while 19% went to outpatient care.

III. HOSPITALS.
The American Hospital Association (AHA) defines a hospital as a licensed institution whose function is to provide diagnostic and therapeutic patient services for medical conditions. They must have at least six beds, an organized physician staff, and continuous nursing services. In 1983, there were 6700 such institutions in this country. In recent years, substantial changes in the roles and operations of hospitals have occurred. The length of stay has decreased dramatically, and financially pressed hospitals have consolidated or closed.

A. History

1. In the first century of this millenium, hospitals were established to provide shelter for the growing number of homeless individuals moving from the countryside to the cities. No medical treatment was provided, as little existed at the time. Incurables were not admitted.
2. American hospitals trace their ancestry to the Pennsylvania Hospital founded in Philadelphia in 1751. Patients with curable illnesses (and interestingly, psychiatric cases) who could not care for themselves or be cared for at home were admitted twice weekly at a specified time. Most care was simply room and board with nursing assistance. Physicians periodically attended the hospitalized ill, but most medical care of that time was delivered in the home.
3. By the beginning of the twentieth century, the concepts of asepsis, surgery with anesthesia, and roentgenography heralded new technology, which was essentially institutionally based. As care became more sophisticated, home care was precluded. The hospital had become "the doctor's workplace."

B. Definitions

1. **Admissions** include the total number of patients, excluding newborns, accepted for care.
2. **Average length of stay** is the total number of patient days counting the day of admission but not the day of discharge, divided by the total number of patients discharged during that time period.
3. **Hospital discharge** is the completion of any continuous period of stay of 1 night or more in a hospital as an inpatient. Deaths, transfers to other hospitals or nursing homes, and patients returning home are all considered discharges. The stay of a well newborn is excluded. The number of discharges does not equal the number of admissions because of the minimum length of stay requirement and the inclusion of sick newborns.

C. Types of hospitals.
Hospitals are classified according to the average length of stay, the type of ownership, and the focus of care.

1. **Short- and long-stay hospitals.** Short-stay hospitals are those in which the average length of stay is less than 30 days. Long-stay hospitals usually involve psychiatric problems, rehabilitation, or chronic illness, such as tuberculosis and drug dependency. In 1983, there were 6148 short-stay and 528 long-stay hospitals in the United States.
2. **Community and noncommunity hospitals.** Community hospitals are defined as nonfederal short-stay general hospitals whose facilities are open to the public. Noncommunity hospitals include federal hospitals, such as military, Veterans Administration medical centers, and the Indian Health Service hospitals, as well as the long-stay hospitals listed above.
3. **Voluntary, proprietary and government hospitals**
   a. **Voluntary hospitals** are established by community members rather than the government. They are not-for-profit organizations operated by churches, fraternal groups, and other community or charitable institutions. Voluntary hospitals can, of course, have revenue in excess of expenses, but this is then termed a "surplus." Not-for-profit organizations do not pay income or property tax.
   b. **Proprietary hospitals** are operated for profit by individuals or corporations explicitly to make a profit, which is then returned to the investors.
   c. **Government hospitals** may be federally funded (e.g., the Veterans Administration system), state funded (e.g., state university hospitals or facilities for the mentally retarded), or supported by city and county funds (e.g., Cook County Hospital or Boston City Hospital for indigent individuals). Government hospitals are often large institutions with over 1000 beds. In 1983, there were 6148 government, voluntary, and proprietary short-stay hospitals (Table 17-3).
4. **General and specialty hospitals.** General hospitals provide both diagnostic and treatment services for patients with a variety of medical conditions, both surgical and nonsurgical. Spe-

Table 17-3. Short-stay Hospitals, According to Type of Ownership in the United States (1981–1983)

Type of Ownership	1981	1982	1983
Hospitals			
All ownerships	6190	6173	6148
Federal	311	310	305
Nonfederal	5879	5863	5843
Nonprofit	3356	3354	3363
Proprietary	729	748	757
State-local government	1794	1761	1723

Reprinted with permission from *Hospital Statistics,* 1982–1984 editions. Chicago, American Hospital Association.

cialty hospitals provide a particular type of service. Common specialty hospitals are listed in Table 17-4.

E. Hospital operations. Voluntary community general hospitals provide most of the medical services in this country.

1. **Hospital governance** consists of an appointed hospital board of community members, physicians, or members of the sponsoring organization, such as a religious order. The Board delegates the day-to-day responsibilities of running the hospital to a hospital director who is the chief executive officer. This person then manages other administrators and personnel who operate the various departments of the hospital.

2. **The medical staff** is a formal organization of practitioners who have been accepted by the Board to practice in the hospital. These physicians elect a set of officers and representatives who meet with the Board to advise on medical matters.

3. **Hospital services** include medicine, surgery, obstetrics and gynecology, and pediatrics. Hospitals may also have rehabilitation and psychiatric units. As hospitals have become more sophisticated, highly specialized units have been established; thus, oncology, stroke, and metabolic units are now common. In addition, most hospitals have a constellation of intensive care units, such as neonatal intensive care, surgical and medical intensive care, coronary care, respiratory intensive care, and neurologic intensive care.

4. **Ancillary services** encompass all of the departments that assist physicians in diagnosing and treating patients. The principal ancillary service departments, which are staffed by various allied health professionals are listed in Table 17-5.

5. **Hospital licensure and accreditation**
   a. **Hospital licensure** is a legal function carried out by the individual states. All states license hospitals and have standards for the construction and operation of hospitals. All nonfederal hospitals must be licensed to operate.

Table 17-4. Types of Specialty Hospitals

Children's
Maternity
Ear, nose, and throat
Eye
Rehabilitation
Tuberculosis
Psychiatry
Drug and alcohol dependency

Table 17-5. Hospital Ancillary Services

Anesthesia
Clinical laboratories
Radiology
Respiratory care
Pharmacy
Physical medicine

b. Hospital accreditation is, in theory, voluntary though over 95% of allopathic hospitals are accredited. The Joint Commission on Accreditation of Hospitals (JCAH) is comprised of representatives of the AMA, American Dental Association (ADA), AHA, the American College of Physicians (ACP), and the American College of Surgeons (ACS). Detailed hospital standards are established and updated by JCAH, which does on-site surveys every 3 years, if a hospital is fully accredited.

(1) Hospitals must be accredited to receive federal funds for patient care under Medicare.

(2) Osteopathic hospitals are accredited by the American Osteopathic Association (AOA).

F. Dimensions of hospital care. A number of statistics reflect hospital activity.

1. Admissions. Both admissions and discharges (see section III B) are used to tabulate the number of patients who have received care. Steadily increasing until 1983, total admissions to community hospitals dropped by 0.6% to 36,000,000 in that year.

2. Average length of stay of 7.6 days per admission has remained stable for several years. The implementation of Diagnosis Related Groups (DRGs) in 1984, has steadily decreased length of stays. Nearly a full day reduction has been effected.

3. Average occupancy rate. For the 1,018,000 community hospital beds available in 1983, there was an average daily census of 750,000 individuals for an average occupancy rate of 73.5%. Occupancy rates of 73% are similar to those of the last 25 years. This is an important factor economically, as it reflects the average number of revenue-producing beds. Obviously, hospitals cannot easily control the number of admissions at all times. Sometimes a large bed capacity is needed to accommodate the ill, while at other times there is less demand. Low occupancy, however, is bad financially for any hospital.

4. Labor intensity. Hospitals are labor intense. In 1983, an average of 418 employees were needed for every 100 patient days. However, hospital statistics reflect wide regional variations. For example, the Pacific coast hospitals employed 497 people per 100 daily patients, while Kentucky, Tennessee, and Alabama hired only 361—a 38% difference. These differences are important because 48% of community hospital expenditures are payroll expenses. Staffing is both an important patient care and financial issue.

5. Hospital costs constituted 39% of total health care dollars in 1985 or $166 billion. This was a 7% increase over the prior year and was nearly twice the general rate of inflation of 3.8%. In 1983, the average community hospital spent $370 per inpatient day. Today that figure is over $475.

G. Trends in hospital care. Health care has become big business in the last 10 years. Major health care corporations have developed with national networks of institutions to earn a share of the 10.7% of gross national product spent on health. Between 1980 and 1983, these for-profit hospitals increased by 4% (i.e., 730 to 757), while voluntary institutions increased by 1% (i.e., 3339 to 3363). Similarly, hospital closures and consolidations have increased, because of tougher competition.

1. Costs. Hospital care is expensive, and costs continue to rise. In 1983, the average community hospital spent $370 per inpatient day compared with $20 in 1950. Three factors have contributed to this trend.

a. As the population ages, there is an increasing demand for medical services, the costs of which are concentrated among the elderly.

b. As the technical quality of care increases, so does cost. CT scanners, which cost $2 million, are now being replaced by magnetic resonance imagers, which cost two to three times as much as CT scanners.

c. The cost of labor and supplies always increases. Inflation in health care continues to outstrip inflation in other sectors of the economy.

2. Outpatient care. Costly hospital care has lead to an increased emphasis on outpatient care, thereby decreasing admissions and length of stays. More care is given at home, in nursing homes, and on an outpatient basis.

IV. LONG-TERM CARE INSTITUTIONS. Long-term care is the delivery of ongoing medical, rehabilitative, and maintenance care to chronically impaired individuals. The AHA defines long-term institutions as facilities where the average length of stay is greater than 30 days. In contrast, the Commission on Chronic Illness considers care long-term when it extends beyond 90 days. Regardless of the definition, the concept conveys the need for services for months at a time.

A. Need for long-term care

1. **Decreased length of stays at acute care hospitals** has lead to an increased need for institutions where inexpensive, low-intensity care can continue until the patient is ready to return home. Between 1979 and 1983, short-stay hospital use measured in days of care per 1000 population declined by 10%. Some of this was accomplished by early discharge to nursing homes.

2. **Increased care for the elderly**, who comprise only 10% of the population, accounts for 75% of the utilization of long-term care facilities. Only 5% of individuals over 65 years of age are in nursing homes at one time. Yet over their lifetimes, 20% of the elderly will use such institutions. However, the elderly over 85 years old (i.e., the "old old") will number over 1.4 million more in the year 2000 than in 1980. Elderly over 65 needing institutionalization will increase from 1,541,000 in 1985 to 2,367,000 in the year 2000.

3. **Home care agencies**, such as the Visiting Nurse Association (VNA), are growing to meet the demands of the elderly and younger individuals discharged home but still needing assistance. About one-third of the elderly require support in their homes.

B. Funding long-term care

1. **Out-of-pocket costs.** In 1985, long-term care costs totaled $35.2 billion, the third greatest expense in health care after hospital and physicians' services. During this period, there was greater out-of-pocket payment for these services than in the past. The percent of costs paid by various payers includes:
   a. Medicare—2%.
   b. Medicaid (state and federal)—45%.
   c. Out-of-pocket by patients—51.4%.

2. **Insurance.** Of the elderly, 59% have private nursing home insurance, but this covers only skilled care, which is similar to the Medicare coverage.

C. Types of long-term care facilities. In 1980, over 24,000 nursing homes were licensed. Of these, 8% were government owned, 17% were not-for-profit, and 75% were proprietary. The National Nursing Home Survey of 1977 listed four categories of nursing homes based on the nursing care provided. For the purpose of this survey, nursing care was defined as the provision of any of a number of different services (Table 17-6).

1. **Nursing homes** must provide full-time nursing care by registered nurses or licensed practical (vocational) nurses. Skilled nursing facilities and intermediate care facilities belong to this category. Skilled nursing and intermediate care facilities are defined by each individual state, which in turn has the responsibility for licensing such nursing homes. Often part of a facility will provide different levels of care on different floors. In the 1977 National Nursing Home Survey, 24% of certified facilities provided both skilled nursing and intermediate care.
   a. Skilled nursing facilities provide the most intensive care. These services are covered by Medicare and Medicaid. Medicare Part A pays for care up to 100 days per episode of illness. A spell of illness begins on the day the patient is provided skilled nursing services and ends when the patient has not been a skilled nursing patient for 60 days. In the 1977 survey, 43% of nursing homes provided skilled nursing services. Medicare Part A eligibility requirements for skilled nursing care include:
   (1) Hospitalization in an acute care hospital for at least 3 days.
   (2) Admission to the skilled nursing facility within 30 days of discharge.
   b. Intermediate care facilities provide health-related services that are less sophisticated than

Table 17-6. Nursing Care Services

Application of bandages
Bowel and bladder retraining
Bladder catheterization
Enemas
Full bed bath
Hypodermics
Intramuscular or intravenous injections
Irrigation
Nasal feeding
Oxygen therapy
Monitoring of vital signs

skilled nursing but more comprehensive than simply room and board. Medicaid covers such care in appropriately certified homes. Medicare does not cover such services. In 1977, 56% of certified homes provided intermediate services.

2. **Personal care homes** *with nursing* employ registered nurses or licensed practical nurses but provide nursing services only to a limited number of clients. They administer medication and provide personal services, such as assistance with daily activities like eating, bathing, dressing and ambulation. Personal care homes *without nursing* typically provide only administration of medication and assistance with personal care.

3. **Domiciliary care homes** provide room and board and limited assistance with personal services. Such homes are appropriate for persons who are not entirely self-sufficient but require no nursing care.

D. Comprehensive long-term care. Approximately one-third of the elderly population require some type of assistance though not institutionalization. For some, these needs can be met by home health care services. There has been growing interest in the concept of long-term care insurance and facilities that can meet the needs of the elderly who may need only minor assistance to live independently. These have been termed lifecare centers or Social Health Maintenance Organizations.

1. **Lifecare centers** provide a wide range of health and personal services up to and sometimes including skilled nursing care.
   - **a.** Payment for these organizations may be out-of-pocket by the client or may be covered by private insurers. Premiums or monthly payments regularly cover the cost of room and board and nursing care when needed.
   - **b.** The number of lifecare centers is growing. In 1983, not-for-profit centers grew 14%, while multihospital systems developed 11 new centers, a 26% increase over 1982. Table 17-7 lists lifecare centers by type of ownership.

2. **Home health care** is an important and growing segment of long-term care. Home care provides health services to individuals at home, after a hospital stay or even in lieu of hospital services. These services promote, maintain, and restore health while maximizing patient independence.
   - **a. Types of services** provided largely follow Medicare reimbursement guidelines.
     - **(1)** Skilled nursing services
     - **(2)** Physical and occupational therapy
     - **(3)** Medical social services
     - **(4)** Home health aid
   - **b. Reimbursement for home health services** may be private or governmental. Home health care services, are, however, less than 2% of total Medicare/Medicaid expenditures.
     - **(1)** In 1982, for example, Medicare spent about $1 billion on home health care out of a budget of $51 billion, while Medicaid spent $310 million out of a budget of $31 billion.
     - **(2)** Nursing home care, consumed $12.4 billion, 40% of the 1982 Medicaid budget. Other types of health insurance, Blue Cross, and indemnity carriers cover services similar to those provided by Medicare.
   - **c. Ownership of the 3500 Medicare certified home health agencies** is diverse. The original not-for-profit home nursing services were operated by VNAs. Today, over 85% of home health care services are operated by hospitals, nursing homes, public health departments, and private, for-profit and not-for-profit organizations.
   - **d.** Emphasis on early discharge under prospective reimbursement plans like DRGs have made home health care units important parts of all acute care hospitals.

V. AMBULATORY CARE FACILITIES.

Ambulatory care refers to health services provided for nonhospitalized patients. Physicians' offices, outpatient departments, emergency rooms, and community health centers are examples of ambulatory care. Table 17-8 lists several types of outpatient facilities. This section describes three new developments in ambulatory care.

Table 17-7. Lifecare Centers in 1983

Type of Ownership	No.
Investor owned	40
Not-for-profit	194
Multihospital systems	54

Table 17-8. Types of Ambulatory Care Facilities

Birthing centers
Drug and alcohol treatment centers
Surgery centers
Urgent care centers
Occupational health centers
Diagnostic centers
Rehabilitation centers
Psychiatric clinics

A. **Birthing centers** specialize in the delivery of uncomplicated pregnancies. In the late 1960s and early 1970s interest arose in returning childbirth to a home-like environment rather than a hospital. Forces mitigated against home deliveries, however, and groups began developing out-of-hospital sites for childbirth. Some hospitals have since developed birthing rooms adjacent to the delivery suites.

1. Birthing centers are often operated by not-for-profit women's groups. In 1984, only three centers were run by hospital systems. The deliveries are usually performed by certified nurse midwives.
2. Since the first birthing center opened in 1975, proponents have argued that the centers provide a more intimate personal experience surrounding the delivery than the barren hospital delivery room. Costs have also been lower, approximately 50% of hospital charges.
3. Critics cite the limited knowledge of the nurse midwife and the lack of medical backup if the mother or infant develop complications. To counter these concerns, all patients are screened by an obstetrician for any potential risks, and then only low-risk pregnancies are followed. Virtually all centers have physician and hospital backup.
4. Although nurse midwives have a favorably low incidence of malpractice suits, several insurance carriers have refused to renew their liability insurance. Limited access to low-cost insurance constrains the availability of nonhospital-based birthing centers.

B. **Urgent care centers** are freestanding emergency care centers.

1. The first urgent care center opened in Newark, New Jersey in 1973. There are currently 2000 such facilities. Growth has been rapid, averaging 70% per year.
2. The purpose of most of these centers is to compete with hospital emergency departments for acute, ambulatory medical visits. Estimates suggest that over 80% of emergency room visits are nonemergencies, requiring low-intensity care.
3. Proponents of urgent care centers see them as an efficient, cost-effective means of providing basic ambulatory care. Not only do such centers expand the service area (and potentially revenue) for the hospitals, but they can increase access to care in underserved areas.
4. Critics charge that urgent care centers are often not equipped to handle serious injuries or medical problems. The issue of intensity of care offered is of critical importance to the economic viability of these centers. As the seriousness of the medical problem to be handled increases, so do the costs of operating the center.

C. **Freestanding outpatient surgery centers**, are independent facilities designed to provide same-day surgery for selected problems.

1. The first surgery center was opened in Phoenix, Arizona in 1970; this facility was unique in that it was a nonhospital outpatient surgery facility.
2. Freestanding surgery centers offer a cost-competitive alternative to hospital surgery. While most surgeons perform some surgery in their offices, the availability of anesthesia and recovery rooms limit the type of procedures that can be performed. Table 17-9 lists several catagories of surgery commonly performed in freestanding centers.
3. In 1984, there were 330 freestanding outpatient surgery centers in the United States. Twice that number is expected in the next 4 years. It has been estimated that 9 million procedures each year (or 40% of all surgery) are appropriate for these surgery centers.
4. Ownership of surgery centers is independent (local entrepreneurs, 61%), corporate chains (33%), or hospital affiliated (6%).

Table 17-9. Common Surgery Center Procedures

Dilation and curettage
Laparoscopy
Orthopedic procedures
Myringotomy
Excision of skin lesions
Arthroscopy
Tonsillectomy/adenoidectomy
Dental procedures
Plastic surgery
Cystoscopy

5. Licensure and accreditation of surgery centers are not uniform. In 1983, 22 states required licensure while a growing number require accreditation. JCAH and the Accrediation Association for Ambulatory Health Care (AAAHC) both accredit surgery centers.

VI. QUALITY AND COST OF CARE

A. Introduction. Quality of care reflects the adequacy of the services provided. While desirability of quality is universally accepted, the realities of health policy and health care financing have often dressed cost-containment in the guise of quality assurance. For practical purposes, cost-effectiveness is an essential component of effective, quality care.

1. **Cost-effectiveness** attempts to relate the quantity of resources expended in the pursuit of a given outcome with the desirability of the outcome. Cost-effective medical care implies that the outcome of a medical intervention, polio immunization for example, is less costly than treating the complications of polio. Such decisions, of course, have ethical and economic consequences.

2. **Dimensions of quality assessment** are threefold.
   a. **Structure** refers to the characteristics of medical manpower, the organizational setting, and physical resources. For example, JCAH has established requirements for the physical layout of a hospital to inhibit nosocomial (hospital acquired) infections.
   b. **Process.** The manner in which health care professionals diagnose disease and implement treatment is known as the process of care.
   c. **Outcome.** Outcome assessment is an essential and expanding area of health care research because it is the bottom line. The complex series of factors that affect outcome make the evaluation of outcomes difficult. Socioeconomic status, level of education, compliance, and health beliefs all have an impact on the outcome of a course of treatment.

3. **Definitions**
   a. **Medical audit**, which is synonymous with quality assessment or appraisal, is a technique of evaluating care based on review of the medical record. Charts may be audited by non-expert personnel, using explicit criteria (i.e., written guidelines) or by experts, using personal criteria that may apply to the review.
   b. **Quality assurance** is a program that evaluates care and then institutes programs to improve care where needed.
   c. **Utilization review** assesses the necessity of medical services—that is, the appropriateness of admissions and length of stays. Specific procedures include:
      (1) **Certification**—a statement by the physician or reviewer confirming the need for admission.
      (2) **Concurrent review**—the process of monitoring the duration of hospitalization while the patient is actually in the hospital.
      (3) **Retrospective review**—the process of reviewing the charts after discharge. Such a review could lead to retrospective denial of an admission, placing the hospital or admitting physician at financial risk for the costs incurred.

B. Assessing quality of care. The goal of quality inputs is approached through the processes of accreditation, certification, and licensure.

1. **Accreditation** is a process carried out by nongovernmental organizations whereby an institution or educational program is recognized as voluntarily meeting a set of quality standards. These standards are established from within the profession to assure adequate programs of education or care. Medical schools are accredited and regularly reviewed by the American Association of Medical Colleges (AAMC). JCAH accredits hospitals.

2. **Certification** is a process applied to individuals. Again, a nongovernmental agency establishes standards of achievement and recognizes individuals who attain these standards by certification. Certification is carried out by examination. For example, a physician's assistant may become certified by successful completion of the examination of the National Commission on Certification of Physician's Assistants. Internists are "board certified" by the American Board of Internal Medicine. While certification has no legal status, virtually all specialists seek board certification to compete effectively for positions in teaching institutions.

3. **Licensure** is the legal process government agencies use to grant permission to individuals or institutions to practice or provide services. Licensure is a function of the individual states, and a practitioner must be licensed by the jurisdiction in which he or she wishes to practice. Disciplinary actions may lead to suspension or permanent revocation of a professional's license; however, it does not necessarily prevent that individual from working in another state.

C. Cost assessment. Medicare and Medicaid rapidly increased the percentage of the federal budget that is spent on health care and spurred congressional interest in the quality of care provided. As the Medicare budget mushroomed, however, quality control yielded to cost-containment. Two federal programs focus on the cost implications of the process of care.

1. **Professional Standards Review Organizations (PSROs)**
   - **a.** The Bennett Amendment to the Social Security Act (P.L.92-603) established the PSRO program in 1972. The intent of the program was to assess the quality of medical care that Medicare, (Title XVIII) and Medicaid (Title XIX) recipients were receiving. It sought to curb cost escalation in these programs by utilization review.
   - **b.** Associations of physicians, usually from within a hospital, constituted the utilization review committee. These committees were charged with approving the appropriateness of admissions of Medicare and Medicaid patients and monitoring length of stays.
   - **c.** By 1981, 182 federally funded PSROs existed. The outcome of care provided, and hence quality assessment, was not carried out. PSROs were expensive themselves and appear to have had little impact on the cost of medical care. After 10 years of lackluster performance, PSROs were replaced by Peer Review Organizations.

2. **Peer Review Organizations (PROs)**
   - **a.** The Tax Equity and Fiscal Responsibility Act of 1982 (P.L. 97-248) mandated the formation of PROs to accompany the implementation of prospective payment systems, legislation for which was passed in 1983. One year later, the Health Care Financing Administration, (HCFA) issued a request for proposals for the first PROs.
   - **b.** The 54 PROs are to monitor hospital use and quality of care for Medicare patients. Both admissions and procedure objectives and quality objectives were established (Fig. 17-4). Quality of care has become a major issue because legislators fear that the financial incentives of the prospective payment systems lead to inadequate care. Under prospective payment, a hospital is paid a fixed amount per admitting diagnosis. Intensive care and long stays may actually cost the hospital more than it receives; however, less care for short stays means a profit. Congress feared care could suffer from profiteering. Cost-containment is still the overriding concern.
   - **c.** Organizationally, most PROs are reformed PSROs. To receive a HCFA contract, a PRO must demonstrate either physician sponsorship, or broad-based representation of a least 17 different medical specialties. They should not be associated with hospitals or insurance companies.
   - **d.** PRO contracts include lengthy lists of specific goals for reducing hospital use and monitoring quality. For example, a PRO might set an admission objective of eliminating all hospitalizations for cataract surgery. A quality objective might be a 60% reduction in urinary tract infections caused by Foley catheters.
   - **e.** To maintain their contracts, PROs have had to demonstrate effectiveness in achieving their selected goals. While the PRO programs are still too new to assess effectiveness overall, close government scrutiny of medical practice has become a fact of life.

VII. HEALTH CARE PLANNING.

The purpose of health care planning is the coordinated and comprehensive provision of medical treatment, prevention of disease, and promotion of health. Only in the last 20 years have serious attempts at national health care planning been initiated. The impact of these efforts remains unclear.

A. The Comprehensive Health Planning and Public Service Amendment of 1966 (P.L. 89-749) was the first federal effort at planning and coordinating services. It established health planning as a priority and funded training for health planners. Tangible results of this legislation resulted from federal funding of regional comprehensive health planning agencies.

Admission and Procedure Objectives and Required Review Activities

One or more objectives are required in each of the following areas:

1. Reduce admissions for procedures that could be performed effectively and with adequate assurance of patient safety in an ambulatory surgical setting or on an outpatient basis.
2. Reduce the number of inappropriate or unnecessary admissions or invasive procedures for specific diagnosis-related groups (DRGs).
3. Reduce the number of inappropriate or unnecessary admissions or invasive procedures by specific practitioners or in specific hospitals.

Quality Objectives

At least one objective is required in each of the following five areas:

1. Reduce unnecessary hospital readmissions resulting from substandard care provided during the prior admission.
2. Assure the provision of medical services which, when not performed, have significant potential for causing serious patient complications.
3. Reduce avoidable deaths.
4. Reduce unnecessary surgery or other invasive procedures.
5. Reduce avoidable postoperative or other complications.

Figure 17-4. Federal performance requirements for peer review organizations (PROs).

B. **The National Health Planning and Development Act** of 1974 (P.L. 93-641) superceded the 1966 law by legislating 203 health service areas, each to be covered by a health systems agency.

1. The purpose of health systems agencies was strongly influenced by cost-containment pressures. The principle function of these organizations was to help hold the purse strings on health care spending.
2. Health systems agencies monitored health care costs by approving local requests for federal health care grants, particularly in certificate of need determinations (see section VII C).
3. The future of health systems agencies is uncertain. Recent federal policy has emphasized local planning and has stopped funding health systems agencies. While some states continue to support these agencies, most have dissolved these vestiges of federal health planning.

C. **Certificate of need statutes** are state laws enacted to review major capital health care expenditures.

1. The original certificate of need laws were developed by several states in the 1960s. Federal legislation led all states to pass certificate of need laws by 1981.
2. These laws required health systems agency approval for new hospital or nursing home construction or renovations. Expensive equipment and ambulatory services were also subject to review. By 1982, certificate of need laws in 11 states applied to equipment in physicians' offices. One of the most celebrated confrontations of the certificate of need process was the

then newly developed CT scanner. Each CT scanner in theory required health systems agency approval or risked denial of federal reimbursement for services.

3. Generally, certificate of need applies to expensive technology or buildings. Items costing over $100,000 to $200,000, depending on the individual state, are subject to review. At the heart of this legislation is the awareness that new technology contributes substantially to higher health care costs. Unfortunately, it is doubtful that certificate of need has significantly inhibited the spiral of health care costs.

STUDY QUESTIONS

Directions: Each question below contains five suggested answers. Choose the **one best** response to each question.

1. An important decision for physicians entering practice is whether or not to practice alone or in a group. A solo practice is best characterized by which of the following statements?

(A) Two-thirds of physicians practice this way
(B) Approximately 10% more patients are seen by solo practitioners
(C) Physicians who work alone often work fewer hours by choice
(D) Physicians who have their own practice have higher incomes than those who are employed by a group
(E) Solo practice offers less autonomy without partners with whom to share the work load

Directions: Each question below contains four suggested answers of which **one or more** is correct. Choose the answer

A if **1, 2, and 3** are correct
B if **1 and 3** are correct
C if **2 and 4** are correct
D if **4** is correct
E if **1, 2, 3, and 4** are correct

2. Certificate of need legislation is characterized by

(1) the need for health systems agency approval of major health care expenditures
(2) a review of hospital or nursing home expenditures over $100,000
(3) a review of equipment purchases by hospitals and private physicians
(4) the refusal of several states to implement such laws

3. Which of the following are major components of the United States Department of Health and Human Services?

(1) Veterans Administration medical centers
(2) Public Health Service
(3) Department of Housing and Urban Development
(4) Health Care Financing Administration

4. A primary care practitioner is generally contacted directly by the public and has a practice that is characterized by a broad range of medical services. Which of the following may be considered primary care specialities?

(1) Pediatrics
(2) Internal medicine
(3) Family medicine
(4) Obstetrics and gynecology

Directions: The group of questions below consists of lettered choices followed by several numbered items. For each numbered item select the **one** lettered choice with which it is **most** closely associated. Each lettered choice may be used once, more than once, or not at all.

Questions 5–8

Match the following definitions with the appropriate terms.

(A) Preferred Provider Organizations
(B) Independent Practice Associations
(C) Group model Health Maintenance Organizations
(D) Staff model Health Maintenance Organizations
(E) Exclusive Provider Oragnizations

5. A medical care plan where the physicians are employed directly by the plan

6. A medical care plan that provides financial incentives for the patient to see selected doctors but also pays for care outside of the plan, though at greater cost to the patient

7. A medical care plan where individual physicians contract to see prepaid patients at an agreed rate or capitation but generally are occupied seeing fee-for-service patients

8. A medical care plan that contracts with a physicians' group to provide care to the prepaid patients

Directions: The group of questions below consists of lettered choices followed by several numbered items. For each numbered item, select the one lettered choice with which it is most closely associated. Each lettered choice may be used once, more than once, or not at all. Choose the answer

A if the item is associated with **(A) only**
B if the item is associated with **(B) only**
C if the item is associated with **both (A) and (B)**
D if the item is associated with **neither (A) nor (B)**

Questions 9–12

Match the following.

(A) Gatekeeper role
(B) Keystone role
(C) Both
(D) Neither

9. A primary care physician who makes decisions about when and to whom to refer a patient for additional evaluation

10. A primary care physician who assists the patient with referrals as the patient chooses

11. A primary care physician who coordinates care provided by an increasing number of disparate specialists

12. A primary care physician who provides a broad scope of medical services

ANSWERS AND EXPLANATIONS

1. The answer is A. (*II B 1, 2*) Two-thirds of all practicing physicians currently practice alone. However, young physicians seem to be preferring group practice over solo practice. While offering less autonomy, group practice fosters a sharing of expertise and often an ease of referral without the fear of losing the patient to a consultant. In addition, solo practitioners see approximately 10% fewer patients, make less money, and work longer hours than group practitioners.

2. The answer is A (1, 2, 3). (*VII C 1–3*) Certificate of need legislation was first implemented by several states in the 1960s. However, federal legislation eventually required all states to pass certificate of need laws by 1981. These laws required health systems agencies to review expensive equipment purchases and hospital building programs. While such review was targeted primarily at hospitals and nursing homes, 11 states extended it to physicians' offices as well.

3. The answer is C (2, 4). (*I B 1 a, b; Figure 17-1*) The federal government involvement in health care is a function of the Department of Health and Human Services (DHHS). The Public Health Service (PHS) and the Health Care Financing Administration (HCFA) are two major divisions of DHHS. The PHS includes the Centers for Disease Control, the National Institutes of Health, and the Food and Drug Administration. HCFA is responsible for Medicare and Medicaid. The Veterans Administration (VA) hospitals are part of the VA, and the Department of Housing and Urban Development is a department that is parallel to DHHS.

4. The answer is E (all). (*II A 2*) The primary care specialties include family medicine, internal medicine, pediatrics, and general practice. In addition, obstetrics and gynecology is considered a primary care specialty for women in some health plans. The primary care physician is often the patient's first contact with the medical care system, for counseling as well as general diagnosis and treatment.

5–8. The answers are: 5-D, 6-A, 7-B, 8-C. [*II D 1 a–d, 3 c (1)–(3)*] Alternative delivery systems, which contrast with the traditional fee-for-service practices, have been established in an attempt to minimize costs.

Health Maintenance Organizations (HMOs) provide prepaid comprehensive health care, and providers are placed at financial risk for excessive use of services. Staff model HMOs have physicians who are employed directly by the plan, while hospitals may be plan-owned or independent. Group model HMOs have physicians' groups who contract individually with the plan but the physicians remain employees of the group not the plan.

Preferred Provider Organizations (PROs) are fee-for-service plans where insured individuals are given financial incentives to use the panel of preferred providers. Patients may choose their own physicians, though nonmember physicians require copayments or deductibles.

Independent Practice Associations are plans where physicians are in private practice but agree to accept a capitation fee for any patients referred by the plan.

Exclusive Provider Organizations are a rare form of fee-for-service plans where an employer selects hospitals and physicians with favorable charges and rates. Thus, patients are required to use the most cost-effective providers and hospitals. Providers are at no financial risk.

9–12. The answers are: 9-A, 10-B, 11-C, 12-C. (*II A 3 a, b*) The role of the primary care physician has been alternately described as a keystone or a gatekeeper. The difference is noteworthy.

The gatekeeper role of the primary care physician holds that the primary care provider controls access to other specialists and subspecialists. The patient sacrifices freedom of choice, to some extent, but the more efficient use of consultants provides better coordinated care at a lower cost.

The keystone role of the primary care physician holds that the primary care provider assists patients with referrals and then oversees these interactions. However, the patient freely chooses consultants and makes the decision of choosing a primary care physician or other specialist.

The primary care physician in both the keystone and gatekeeper roles coordinates the care provided by an increasing number of disparate specialists, each of whom is concerned with only a single aspect of an individual's overall medical condition. All primary care physicians, too, are encouraged to provide a broad range of medical services.

18
Health Care Financing

Anthony J. Buividas
Mark L. Richards

I. OVERVIEW OF HEALTH CARE EXPENDITURES

A. Health care expenditures in the United States are estimated at $439 billion for 1986, a 14% increase over 1984. In 1985, health care expenditures equaled almost 10.6% of the gross national product (GNP) or $413.4 billion, which amounts to approximately $1773 per capita annually. The percentage distribution of the 1984 health expenditures is given in Figure 18-1. Hospital care accounted for 42.4% of the total 1984 health expenditures.

B. Government funding. The growth in health care expenditures from 5.3% of the GNP in 1960 to 10.6% in 1985 has resulted from:

1. Increased government funding through Medicare and Medicaid.
2. Growth in private insurance coverage.
3. New technologies.
4. Greater access and availability of care and facilities.
5. Shifting demographics resulting in an older population.

C. Employer contributions. Between 1960 and 1982, total employer contributions for health insurance, expressed as a percentage of corporate profits, increased from 7.6% to 57.4%. Between 1970 and 1982, employers' health benefits expenditures have increased 700%, which is three times the rate of growth of the GNP during that period.

II. FUNDING SOURCES FOR HEALTH CARE EXPENDITURES.

Health services are either paid by an insurer or government agency (third-party payer) or directly by the consumer (out-of-pocket expenditure). The percentage of total health services paid by third-party payers has increased dramatically while the percentage paid directly by consumers has declined. Economists believe that this growth in third-party payments has resulted in excessive inflation in health costs since the con-

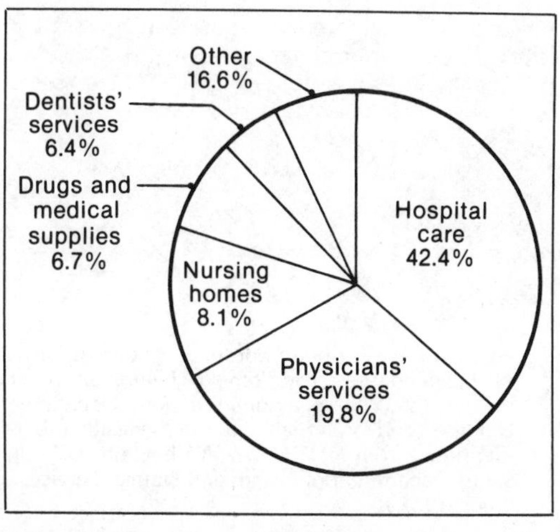

Figure 18-1. Distribution of health care expenditures. The "other" category includes: other professional and health services, eyeglasses and appliances, program administration and insurance costs, public health expenses, construction, and research. (Reprinted from *Health Care Financing Review*. Baltimore, HCFA, United States Department of Health and Human Services, Fall, 1985.)

sumer has little incentive to be cost-effective in purchasing services. The distribution of funding sources is presented in Figure 18-2.

A. Third-party payers. Typically, third-party payers tend to provide more coverage for inpatient and hospital diagnostic services and less for outpatient services, such as office visits, immunizations, or prescription drugs.

1. Government pays for approximately 42% of all personal health care expenditures in the United States. Government programs include the:

a. Veterans Administration.
b. Department of Defense.
c. Maternal and Child Health Programs.
d. Medicare and Medicaid.

2. Private health insurance. As health insurance costs are tax deductible for businesses and health insurance coverage is included within the scope of collective bargaining items under the Taft-Hartley Act, it is not surprising that nearly 85% of Americans have some type of health insurance coverage. Private health insurance, which pays for 58% of all personal health care costs, includes:

a. Over 100 not-for-profit Blue Cross and Blue Shield insurance organizations, which pay providers directly according to agreed upon fee schedules.
b. Indemnity coverage offered by for-profit commercial insurers. Indemnity insurers pay the insured person after submission of a claim form.
c. Employer "self-insurance." Under self-insurance programs, the company that provides employee benefits assumes the financial responsibility for the benefits rather than passing the risk to an external insurer. These programs have become popular due to:
(1) Cash flow advantages whereby the benefit payments are made as incurred rather than prepaid as premium.
(2) Lack of regulation as self-insurance plans are not subject to the extensive state regulations governing group health insurance.
(3) Flexibility in benefit design and administration as a result of the lack of regulations.
(4) Ability to manage health care utilization efficiently by:
(a) Utilization review programs.
(b) Employee incentives to use low-cost providers.
(c) Direct contractual arrangements with health care providers.
d. Health Maintenance Organizations (HMOs), which usually pay providers (physicians and hospitals) directly and maintain participation agreements with providers that specify payment terms (see section IV A).

B. Out-of-pocket expenditures refer to health benefit costs incurred directly by consumers that are not covered under health insurance plans. These expenditures result either because a particular health service is not covered (e.g., cosmetic surgery) or because the benefit plan requires patients to pay a portion of the benefit.

C. Uncompensated care. A 1983 Census Bureau study found that approximately 15% of Americans (35 million people) lacked any type of health insurance coverage. As health care providers

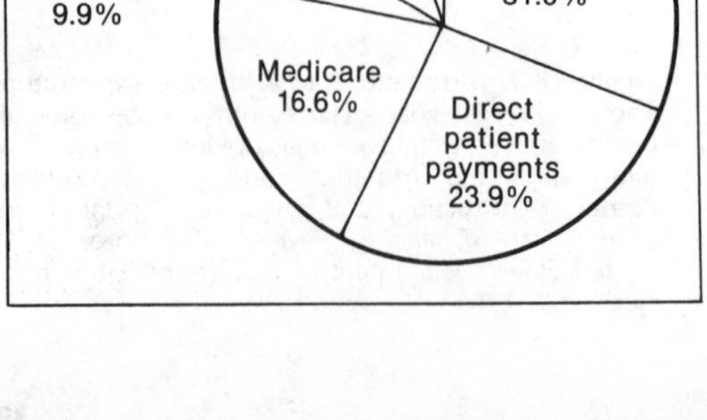

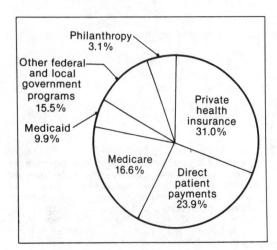

Figure 18-2. Distribution of funding sources for health care expenditures. The "other" government programs include the Veterans Administration, Department of Defense, and Maternal and Child Health programs. (Reprinted from *HHS News*. Washington, DC, United States Department of Health and Human Services, October, 1984.)

respond to changing political and health financing structures, which reward cost-efficient hospitals, the provision of care to the uninsured and medically indigent (i.e., those not poor enough to qualify for Medicaid benefits but whose medical expenses when subtracted from income would lower their financial means below the poverty line) has become a more pressing societal problem. The uncompensated care issue has the following three dimensions:

1. **Change in hospitals' historic mission.** As hospitals move from a mission orientation to a profit motivation in a newly competitive health services marketplace, they have cut back on uncompensated care.
2. **Inequity by hospital.** Although uncompensated care, or charity cases, account for only 5.4% of gross hospital patient revenues, the burden is not shared equally.
3. **An unresolved flaw in the competition model.** The inequity in providing uncompensated care mars the competition model that Congress has tried to establish via the Diagnosis Related Group (DRG) payment system used by Medicare (see section III D).

III. METHODS OF PAYMENT

A. Defintions

1. **Contractual allowance.** Although hospitals and physicians generally bill on a fee-for-service or itemized charge basis, they often accept less than the billed amount. This discount, or contractual allowance, is based on the provider's contract or participation agreement with the particular third-party payer. For example, a physician who participates in the Medicare program:
   a. Agrees to accept the maximum "allowed" fee, determined by the regional Medicare administrative organization, or "carrier."
   b. Writes off the difference between the usual fee and Medicare's allowed amount. This difference is called the "Medicare contractual allowance."
   c. May bill the individual patient for any deductibles or copayments included in the Medicare program. The payment from the Medicare carrier will reflect a subtraction for applicable deductibles and copayments, which are the patient's personal responsibility.
2. **A deductible** is a threshold amount incurred directly by the patient before the third-party payer picks up coverage. For example, the first $75 per year in covered outpatient expenses under the Medicare program is the patient's personal responsiblity.
3. **Copayment** refers to a sharing of financial responsibility for the health service cost by the patient and the third-party payer. For example, under the Medicare program, the patient is responsible for 20% of the amount "allowed" by Medicare for outpatient services once the $75 annual deductible has been satisfied. Many Medicare recipients purchase individual supplemental insurance policies to cover deductibles and copayments not included within Medicare's coverage.

B. **Four payment methodologies** employed by third-party payers to reimburse providers are listed below.

1. **Fee-for-service** charges are billed on an itemized invoice.
2. **Per diem** is an all inclusive flat rate for each day of hospital care provided.
   a. Per diems usually include all ancillary services, supplies, and other services billed by the hospital.
   b. Per diems for different clinical services can be arranged (e.g., obstetrics, surgery, medical, intensive care, or pediatrics) to take account of the differences in the intensity of care provided.
3. **Per admission** is an all inclusive flat rate for each hospital admission. The admission reimbursement can be further refined to encompass different rates by admitting service or diagnosis.
4. **Capitation** is a fee that the provider agrees to accept per patient per month for each patient enrolled in the practice in exchange for providing all specified health services to such enrolled patients. The reimbursement is fixed and paid regardless of the actual number or types of services provided.
   a. **Example of capitation used by HMOs.** HMOs increasingly employ the capitation payment method for both hospitals and physicians. Under a capitation payment method, the health care provider receives a fixed monthly amount for each patient who relates to that provider. A hospital might receive a per capita amount to provide all required inpatient

services, a general surgeon might receive a per capita amount to provide all general surgery services, or a multispecialty group might receive a per capita amount to provide all outpatient physician and diagnostic services.

b. Adjustments to capitation.

(1) Usually, the capitation amount is adjusted for the age and sex of the patient.

(2) Often "stop loss" limits are used to protect the provider from atypical, catastrophic expenses.

(3) Under a "risk corridor" adjustment, additional payments to, or refunds from, the provider would occur if the variance between actual, itemized costs and the capitation amount exceeded a certain threshold percentage (e.g., 5% or 10%).

C. DRG payments. The DRG payment system, begun in 1983, is based on a fixed hospital payment rate for each of 470 treatment classifications called Diagnosis Related Groups. A weighted average of each hospital's historic, cost-based per admission payment rate and the national DRG rates will be used for several years to gradually phase in fixed national DRG rates by 1988.

1. In fiscal 1986, 50% of payments were based on a hospital-specific cost-allocation amount per admission and 50% on regional DRG rates.
2. Teaching hospitals presently receive a percentage adjustment to the DRG rates to compensate them for direct and indirect costs of graduate medical education (residency programs).
3. The DRG rates have excluded capital costs, which include depreciation, interest, and financing expenses for buildings and equipment.
4. Medicare has used an allocation formula to determine what part of each hospital's capital costs it will pay by comparing Medicare service volume to total patient service volume. In the future, it is likely that capital costs will be capped at a fixed percentage of the DRG payment rate rather than based on a year-end cost allocation.
5. Other third-party payers, like some state Medicaid programs and some Blue Cross plans, have adopted a DRG payment system.
6. Presently, the DRG payment system applies only to the hospital: Physicians' services are excluded. HCFA is studying the feasibility of including all physician and hospital services in one payment.

D. Retrospective versus prospective payment

1. **Prospective payment.** In October 1983, the Health Care Financing Administration (HCFA), which administers Medicare and the federal portion of Medicaid, introduced a new "prospective" payment system to reimburse hospitals for inpatient expenses of Medicare patients. The new payment method, based on fixed prices for 470 DRGs ended nearly 20 years of retrospective, cost-based reimbursement to hospitals.
2. **Retrospective payment.** Under the cost-based system, each hospital's payment for Medicare patients was determined by employing complex cost-allocation formulas designed to apportion total hospital expenditures to Medicare and other third-party payers. Although each hospital received interim payments from the Medicare program for each Medicare admission, the final payment was not determined until year-end settlement, when the cost-allocation formulas were employed to assess Medicare for its share of the hospital's total allowed costs. Medicare used detailed definitions to differentiate allowed from disallowed costs, which it refused to pay.

IV. NEW HEALTH INSURANCE ARRANGEMENTS.

To manage health benefit costs better, new arrangements that relate the beneficiary's coverage to the use of selected health care providers have emerged. These arrangements include: Health Maintenance Organizations (HMOs), Preferred Provider Arrangements (PPAs), and Health Insuring Organizations (HIOs).

A. Health Maintenance Organizations (HMOs)

1. **Definition.** HMOs are medical care organizations that accept responsibility for the provision and delivery of a predetermined set of comprehensive health services to insureds who voluntarily choose an HMO for health insurance coverage. The HMO differs from a health insurance company because it arranges a health delivery network and conditions benefit payments on the use of this network and the observance of certain referral and authorization procedures.
2. **Models.** There are four models of HMOs: medical group HMO, staff model HMO, indepen-

dent practice association (IPA), and network model HMO. Some HMOs are combinations of these different models.

a. Group model HMO. In this model, the HMO contracts with an organized medical group practice, which provides all medical services to the enrolled population in the HMO. The group is usually paid on a capitation basis. If a service is not available within the group practice, a physician in the group must authorize the referral. The Kaiser Health Plan is a well known group model HMO.

b. Staff model HMO. The staff model HMO is similar to the group HMO except that physicians are hired directly by the HMO and paid a fixed salary. The Group Health Association in Washington, D.C. is a staff model HMO.

c. Independent practice association (IPA). Under this model, an HMO contracts with an association of individual practitioners, called an IPA. The IPA, in turn, contracts with private practice physicians, who see HMO and non-HMO patients in private offices. An example is HMO-Pennsylvania.

d. Network model HMO. The network model HMO is similar to the IPA except that the HMO contracts directly with several group practices and individual physicians. There is no physician association involved in the transaction.

3. History

a. Government role. Although HMOs have been operating in the United States for half a century, HMO enrollment grew slowly for many years because of opposition from organized medicine, restrictive state laws, and lack of adequate capital. In response to rapidly escalating health care costs, Congress enacted the Health Maintenance Organization Act of 1973 to promote the establishment and growth of HMOs. This Act:

(1) Authorized loans and grants to community organizations to establish HMOs.

(2) Required employers with more than 25 employees to offer federally qualified HMOs as an alternative health care delivery system to their employees.

(3) Preempted various restrictive state laws.

b. HMO coverage for Medicare recipients. In January 1985, the federal government issued final regulations, which permit eligible HMOs to enroll Medicare recipients under a "risk-based" capitation contract with HCFA, whereby the HMO retains the profit or loss if the actual cost of delivering defined health benefits to Medicare recipients varies from the fixed capitation payment.

c. Enrollment trends. From 1970 to 1984, the number of HMOs in the United States increased from 26 to approximately 380. During this period, HMO enrollment increased at a compound rate of 13%, from approximately 2.9 million members to approximately 17 million members. In 1984, the growth rate was 22.6%. This growth in HMO membership is a result of:

(1) Increased consumer acceptance.

(2) Employer support.

(3) Physician interest as a result of increased competition for patients.

(4) Growth in private sector investment.

(5) Premium advantages over traditional group health insurance.

4. Management of health care. HMOs can provide more health benefits per premium dollar for a given population than traditional group health insurance by:

a. Emphasizing low cost alternatives to inpatient care, such as outpatient services.

b. Restricting patient referrals to participating providers who agree in advance to certain fee schedules and utilization review programs.

c. Requiring that each HMO member select a primary care physician who coordinates the member's total health care needs.

d. Employing maximum fee schedules for participating providers to control the unit cost of health benefits.

e. Implementing profit- and deficit-sharing arrangements with providers whereby they share in variances from expected health benefit costs.

f. Operating concurrent and retrospective peer review and utilization review programs.

g. Negotiating volume discounts with tertiary hospitals and other suppliers, such as home health agencies, medical equipment companies, laboratories, and pharmacies.

B. Preferred Provider Arrangements (PPAs)

1. Definition. PPAs are agreements between a network of health providers (i.e., physicians, hospitals, and other health suppliers) and a health benefit purchaser (i.e., insurance company or self-insured employer). Typically, the agreement includes:

a. A discounted provider fee schedule.

b. Peer and utilization review programs.

c. Representations as to the potential insured population covered under the agreement.
d. Incentives for the insured to use the preferred providers, usually in the form of a lower deductible or copayment.

2. Characteristics
a. Provider panel
b. Fee schedule accepted by the provider panel
c. Utilization or claims review
d. Free choice of providers, including those outside the network of participating providers on every occasion a health service is sought

3. Differences between PPAs and HMOs are listed in Table 18-1.

4. Organizing PPAs. Preferred Provider Organizations (PPOs) organize and market PPAs. Sponsoring entities include: insurance companies; third-party administrators, which administer claims systems; self-insured companies; health care providers; and independent consultants or brokers.

5. Evaluating PPAs. Historically, PPAs have focused on fee schedules (price control) to win benefit purchasers' support. However, as health benefit costs are a function of price (fee schedule) *and* volume (utilization), it is very difficult to evaluate the effectiveness of PPAs in controlling health benefit costs. Specific evaluation difficulties include:
a. There is no patient "lock-in." The insured population can opt into or out of the preferred network every time a health service is obtained.
b. The population served by the PPA is constantly changing because there is no "lock-in." Evaluation, therefore, would require a controlled study, where two *matched* populations had the same benefit plan except for the PPA. Such a study is unfeasible.

C. Health Insuring Organizations (HIOs)

1. Definition. HIOs are risk-bearing entities that arrange and provide a health benefit program for an enrolled, defined population. HIOs are paid a fixed amount per capita for each enrollee and assume the risk that the payment is adequate to provide a specified set of benefits. The HIO arrangement is a new concept that has been employed by Medicaid programs in Kentucky and Pennsylvania. It provides the purchaser (in these cases, the state Medicaid programs) a means to cap benefit expenditures, since the risk is passed to another entity.

2. HIOs versus HMOs. Unlike the HMO enrollment process, the HIO enrollee has no choice in selecting this insurance coverage. The benefit purchaser mandates that the beneficiary accept the HIO benefits plan, including all restrictions on provider choice, as well as referral and prior authorization procedures. The mandatory enrollment feature makes the HIO system very controversial. The HIO typically employs the same features to manage patient care that were discussed under section IV A.

V. MEDICARE

A. Origin

1. Medicare began on July 1, 1966 under Title XVIII of the Social Security Act to provide health insurance coverage to patients 65 years of age and over.

2. Subsequently, the program was expanded to cover the disabled under 65 and individuals suffering from chronic renal disease.

Table 18-1. Differences between HMOs and PPAs

Characteristics	PPA	HMO
Insured's "lock-in" to providers under contract	No	Yes
Primary physician gatekeeper	Sometimes, but not binding	Generally, yes
Provider incentives	Possible	Generally, yes
Provider risk-sharing for deficits	Usually capped if present	Often unlimited
Peer review and utilization review	Usually	Yes

B. Overview

1. Part A coverage, which is for inpatient hospital services, skilled nursing facility care, and home care, is funded by the Social Security payroll tax paid by employers and employees.
2. Part B, which helps pay for physician services, outpatient services, and medical supplies outside the hospital, is funded by monthly insurance premiums paid by the beneficiary and from general tax revenues.
3. **Benefit limitations.** Due to the exclusions and limitations of the benefits, Medicare covers less than one-half of the consumer health expenditures for the covered population. Thus, many Medicare recipients buy supplementary or "wrap-around" policies from private insurers to fill in the gaps in Medicare coverage.
   - **a.** While Medicare covers many basic health services, there are patient deductibles and coinsurance payments for both inpatient and outpatient services.
   - **b.** There are also day or dollar limitations on inpatient hospital, skilled nursing facility, and psychiatric coverage.
   - **c.** Medicare does not pay for:
     - **(1)** Routine dental care.
     - **(2)** Outpatient prescription drugs.
     - **(3)** Hearing aids.
     - **(4)** Eyeglasses.
     - **(5)** Routine physical examinations.

C. Administration

1. The Medicare program is administered by HCFA, which is part of the Department of Health and Human Services.
2. HCFA has regional offices that contract with intermediaries to oversee benefit payments under Part A (mainly inpatient care) and with carriers, which oversee payments under Part B (mainly physicians' services).

D. Benefit payments

1. **Part A: inpatient hospital.** In 1983, HCFA introduced a new payment system based on diagnostic categories called DRGs. After, a phase-in period of several years, HCFA intends to use a uniform payment rate for each DRG. Presently, there are "pass through" adjustments to the DRG payment rates for items such as graduate medical education and capital budget items.
2. **Part B: outpatient services.** Under Part B, Medicare usually pays 80% of reasonable costs or charges for covered services, subject to a $75 per year deductible. This general rule is subject to many exceptions or limitations.
   - **a. Definition of reasonable.** In determining the reasonable charge under Part B, Medicare historically paid the lower of either the individual physician's median charge for the procedure or the prevailing charge for the procedure (defined as the 75th percentile charge for that specialty and geographic location). In the 1970s Medicare began to limit the increase in prevailing charges to the medical price inflator index, rather than reassessing the 75th percentile charge.
   - **b. Payment methods.** There are two ways in which Medicare Part B pays its share of the bills of physicians or medical suppliers:
     - **(1) Directly to the physician** if the patient and physician both agree to this assignment method. If the physician accepts Medicare's determination of the reasonable charge as his full charge, he can only charge the patient for any deductible or the 20% coinsurance.
     - **(2) Directly to the patient** after the patient submits an itemized bill to Medicare. Medicare pays the patient the reasonable charge for the procedure or service. It is the patient's responsibility to pay the physician, including any difference between the billed fee and Medicare's reasonable charge.

VI. MEDICAID

A. Origin

1. Medical Assistance, commonly called Medicaid, was established in 1965 under Title XIX of the Social Security Act.
2. The federal government shares in 50%–83% of state assistance to the medically indigent. The

percentage varies according to per capita income of the state and therefore the state's ability to share costs.

3. Originally, state participation was voluntary. By 1970, states had to participate or lose aid for ongoing, federal programs targeted for the blind, crippled, and aged.

4. Beyond the mandated services—that is, inpatient and outpatient hospital services, laboratory and radiology, basic physician medical services, and skilled nursing facility coverage for patients over 21—tremendous variation in scope of benefits by state exists, particularly with respect to dentistry, drug prescriptions, physical therapy, prosthetic devices (including dentures), and ambulance coverage. New York and California have the most extensive benefits.

B. Program administration

1. Eligibility for Medicaid benefits, based on income and means criteria, is determined by county welfare boards. Medicaid applications and claims generally come under the state's Public Welfare or Health Department. Many states subcontract administrative functions to private, third-party administrators.

2. Formulas and methods for provider payment vary by state. Increasingly, state Medicaid programs have moved from cost-based reimbursement to prospective payment, such as per diem or DRG rates.

3. Medicaid is a state-directed program, with eligibility and benefit limits set within a framework established by federal law. Each state must have an advisory committee comprised of provider and health professional representatives, which oversees policy decisions, quality assurance, and payment methods and levels, within the state-approved budget.

4. A federal advisory council advises on policy for both Medicare and Medicaid.

5. In order to control the rapid increase in Medicaid costs, states have instituted several measures, including:
   a. Copayment or deductibles.
   b. Enrollment in HMOs and HIOs.
   c. Preadmission authorization procedures.
   d. Restricted provider network.
   e. Primary care "gatekeepers" (see Chapter 17, section II A 3 b).
   f. Bulk purchasing for medical supplies, eyeglasses, hearing aids, and laboratory equipment.
   g. Prospective reimbursement plans, including capitation and DRG rates.

C. Benefits information

1. Medicaid spending between 1981 and 1983 grew by 22.3% compared to 14.2% for state tax revenues. Medicaid is the fastest growing portion of state budgets.

2. The number of individuals covered by Medicaid doubled between 1969 and 1984, from 12.1 to 22.7 million.

3. The single largest Medicaid expenditure is for nursing home care, which represents approximately one-third of expenditures.

4. States use Medicaid funds to pay deductibles and coinsurance under Medicare Part A (hospital insurance) and the monthly premium for Part B (outpatient and physician services).

5. Medicaid has reduced significantly bad debt levels for hospitals.

D. Medically indigent programs

1. Due to the variability and timing of income for Medicaid eligibility, Medicaid covers only about half of the people whose income falls below the poverty line. To deal with this problem, 33 states have joined the federal-state medically needy program.

2. States have the option of participating in federal government programs for the "categorically needy"—that is, Aid to Families with Dependent Children (AFDC), Aid to the Aged (AA), Blind (AB), and Disabled (AD). These recipients surpass income limits but qualify for medical assistance because of their condition.

STUDY QUESTIONS

Directions: Each question below contains five suggested answers. Choose the **one best** response to each question.

1. After hospital services expenditures, the category that accounts for the next highest percentage of total health expenditures is

(A) drugs and medical supplies
(B) nursing homes
(C) physicians' services
(D) dentists' services
(E) research

2. The population served by the Medicaid program includes individuals who are

(A) over 65 years of age
(B) unemployed
(C) disabled
(D) poor
(E) chronically ill

Directions: Each question below contains four suggested answers of which **one or more** is correct. Choose the answer

A if **1, 2, and 3** are correct
B if **1 and 3** are correct
C if **2 and 4** are correct
D if **4** is correct
E if **1, 2, 3, and 4** are correct

3. Health services not covered by Medicare include

(1) routine dental care
(2) eyeglasses
(3) outpatient prescription drugs
(4) routine physical examinations

4. Characteristics of Medicare coverage include

(1) deductibles and coinsurance for inpatient and outpatient services
(2) inpatient hospital services and skilled nursing care
(3) physicians' services and outpatient services
(4) monthly insurance premiums for Part B coverage

ANSWERS AND EXPLANATIONS

1. The answer is C. (*I A; Figure 18-1*) Health care expenditures in the United States are estimated at $439 billion for 1986, a 14% increase over 1984. Hospital services account for approximately 42.4% of the total expenditures—the largest category by far. Physicians' services account for 19.8%, followed by nursing homes at 8.1%, and drugs and medical supplies at 8.1%.

2. The answer is D. (*VI A 2, B*) Medicaid, or Medical Assistance, was established in 1965 under Title XIX of the Social Security Act. The federal government shares 50%–83% of the state's assistance to the medically indigent. Eligibility for Medicaid benefits is based on income, which must be below a certain level set by each state. Medicaid claims generally come under the state's Public Welfare or Health Department.

3. The answer is E (all). (*V B 3 c*) Medicare pays less than one-half of the average beneficiary's total health care costs. Many Medicare recipients purchase private supplemental insurance to fill the gaps in Medicare coverage. Medicare does not pay for routine dental care, outpatient prescription drugs, hearing aids, eyeglasses, and routine physical examinations.

4. The answer is E (all). (*V B 1–3*) The Medicare system has deductible and coinsurance amounts for both inpatient and outpatient services. Part A coverage, funded through the Social Security payroll tax, is primarily for inpatient hospital services and skilled nursing care. Part B coverage, funded by monthly premiums from beneficiaries and through tax revenues, covers physicians' services and outpatient services.

Post-test

QUESTIONS

Directions: Each question below contains five suggested answers. Choose the **one best** response to each question.

1. Cerebromacular degeneration involves a group of disorders in which there is progressive deterioration and loss of mental function for which there is no treatment. The different types, which are distinguished by age of onset, include all of the following EXCEPT

(A) Tay-Sachs disease
(B) Gaucher's disease
(C) Kuf's disease
(D) Jansky-Bielschowsky disease
(E) Spielmeyer-Stock-Vogt-Koyanagi disease

2. Which of the following statements regarding the plaintiff's burden of proof in a medical malpractice suit is true?

(A) The plaintiff is required to prove the material elements of his or her case beyond a reasonable doubt
(B) The plaintiff is allowed to present proof to a jury only if the defendant agrees; otherwise, the case is heard by a judge
(C) Once the plaintiff demonstrates injury in the course of receiving medical care, the burden of proof shifts to the defendant to show lack of negligence
(D) The plaintiff cannot recover damages, even though the defendant's negligence is clear, unless it is proved that the defendant's negligence was the proximate cause of the plaintiff's injury
(E) The plaintiff is relieved of the burden of proof if the court feels the defendant's acts are sufficiently offensive to deserve public censure

3. A case series report is useful for addressing all of the following clinical problems EXCEPT

(A) the natural history of a specific disease
(B) the clinical characteristics of disease
(C) the outcomes from two different treatments
(D) unusual or unexpected findings resulting from a new treatment
(E) comparing two or more treatments

4. The critical ratio or z score is applicable to which type of distribution?

(A) t
(B) Normal
(C) Chi-square
(D) Binomial
(E) Skewed

5. Which of the following statements concerning the epidemiology of alcohol use in the United States is true?

(A) Nearly 100 million people can be considered heavy drinkers
(B) Between 8% and 10% of adult men and between 3% and 5% of adult women are alcoholic
(C) American Indians have a low rate of alcoholism because of an enzyme deficiency
(D) Heavy drinkers are most likely to be 55–59 years of age and belong to high socioeconomic groups
(E) Alcoholic individuals are associated with 15,000 homicides and suicides annually

6. All of the following statements are true concerning homicide in the United States EXCEPT

(A) Current homicide rates for most age groups of both sexes are as high or higher than any previously recorded in the United States
(B) Homicide is the leading cause of death for black American men between the ages of 15 and 24
(C) Hispanic men are 8 to 15 times more likely to be victims of homicide than white men
(D) Use of alcohol and other drugs has been documented in 45% of all homicides
(E) Men are four times as likely to be victims of homicide than women

7. According to the American Association on Mental Deficiency, mental retardation refers to below average intellectual functioning that is further characterized by which of the following?

(A) Overwhelming brain disease caused by infection
(B) Occurrence at birth in 50% of cases
(C) Nonadaptive behavior during the developmental period
(D) Normal development until 5 years of age in 50% of cases
(E) Masked by illness or emotional or epileptic syndromes in 30% of cases

8. All of the following statements about screening tests are true EXCEPT

(A) they are used as a basis for therapy
(B) they are performed on apparently healthy individuals
(C) they are measured by sensitivity and specificity
(D) they are applicable to large numbers of individuals
(E) they are performed for diseases amenable to therapy prior to the onset of symptoms

9. All of the following are passive strategies for injury prevention and control EXCEPT

(A) child-resistant drug containers
(B) self-extinguishing cigarettes
(C) a home hot water setting at 120°F
(D) seat belts
(E) air bags

10. Efforts at primary prevention of mental disorder, which consists of the promotion of general mental health and protection against the occurrence of specific diseases, has been relatively successful with all of the following conditions EXCEPT

(A) Down's syndrome
(B) situational reaction formation
(C) organic brain syndrome
(D) schizophrenia
(E) none of the above

11. In a population of 5000 individuals, 20% have disease X. A screening test with a sensitivity of 95% and a specificity of 90% is used to screen for the disease. The probability that a person with a positive screening test will have disease X, that is, the positive predictive value, is

(A) 50/3650, or 1%
(B) 50/450, or 11%
(C) 950/1350, or 70%
(D) 3600/4000, or 90%
(E) 950/1000, or 95%

12. All of the following statements describe the advantages of a cohort study over a case-control study when assessing possible risk factors for disease EXCEPT

(A) prospective data collection is used
(B) there is less of a chance for bias in data collection or subject recall
(C) a cohort study is more likely to explain causation
(D) true incidence rates for disease can be determined
(E) none of the above

13. Which of the following factors distinguishes substance dependence from substance abuse?

(A) Intoxication during the day
(B) A pattern of pathologic use
(C) Symptoms of tolerance
(D) Impairment in occupational functioning
(E) Inability to stop

14. True statements concerning type I error include all of the following EXCEPT

(A) it is the rejection of a null hypothesis that is actually true
(B) it is often assigned a value of 0.05 in studies
(C) it is also called the alpha error
(D) it is used to determine sample size
(E) it is equal to 1 minus the beta error

15. All of the following statements describing the relationship between birth weight and neonatal mortality are true EXCEPT

(A) less than one-third of very low-birth-weight infants (i.e., infants weighing ≤ 1500 g) die in the neonatal period
(B) low-birth-weight infants (i.e., infants weighing ≤ 2500 g) account for more than 65% of neonatal deaths
(C) a birth weight of 2500 g or less is believed to increase the risk of neonatal mortality, regardless of gestational age
(D) as birth weight decreases, the neonatal mortality rate increases
(E) the major cause of neonatal mortality reflects inadequate intrauterine development

16. All of the following physical properties are important in determining the movement of chemicals between environmental mediums EXCEPT

(A) octanol water partition coefficient
(B) solubility
(C) viscosity
(D) bioconcentration factor
(E) vapor pressure

17. All of the following statements apply to both threshold and nonthreshold effects EXCEPT

(A) greater exposure increases response
(B) a chemical or metabolite causes the effect
(C) some exposure levels are safe
(D) the toxic effect is independent of the route of exposure
(E) none of the above

18. The Diagnosis Related Group payment system is best described by which of the following payment methodologies?

(A) Per diem
(B) Capitation
(C) Per admission
(D) Fee-for-service
(E) Risk corridor

Directions: Each question below contains four suggested answers of which **one or more** is correct. Choose the answer

A if **1, 2, and 3** are correct
B if **1 and 3** are correct
C if **2 and 4** are correct
D if **4** is correct
E if **1, 2, 3, and 4** are correct

19. Factors contributing to the dramatic growth in health care expenditures during the last 5 years include

(1) an increase in the number of hospitals
(2) an increase in private health insurance coverage
(3) a decrease in the physician to population ratio
(4) an increase in the percentage of the population over 65 years of age

20. Sociologic theories of addiction to alcohol have shown that

(1) there is a high degree of correlation between poverty and excessive drinking
(2) the degree of alcoholism is dependent on the cultural attitudes about drinking
(3) alcoholism is reduced if there are other means of satisfying inner tensions
(4) the prevalence of alcoholism is low if the religion of the culture prohibits its use

21. To calculate an indirect age-adjustment rate, you must

(1) know the age composition of the population being compared
(2) know the age-specific rates of the population being compared
(3) borrow age-specific rates from a standard population
(4) borrow the age composition of a standard population

22. The common sources of morality are

(1) social contract
(2) divine command
(3) natural law
(4) criminal law

SUMMARY OF DIRECTIONS

A	B	C	D	E
1, 2, 3 only	1, 3 only	2, 4 only	4 only	All are correct

23. A 2-year-old child is brought to the physician's office because of a broken arm. In taking a history, it is discovered that she had only two diphtheria-tetanus-pertussis immunizations (DTP) and one oral poliovirus (OPV) immunization during the first 6 months of life. The child has no other illnesses, and the mother is in her first trimester of pregnancy. The physician should

(1) administer DTP, OPV, and measles-mumps-rubella (MMR) vaccine to the child
(2) tell the mother that the immunization series has to be started all over again
(3) instruct the mother to bring the child back in 1 month for the *Hemophilus influenzae* vaccine and in 6 months for another DTP and OPV immunization
(4) instruct the mother that because of her pregnancy, she should avoid close contact with the child after immunization for 3 weeks

24. Individuals who have an increased risk of injuries include

(1) native Americans
(2) men
(3) those with osteoporosis
(4) the poor

25. Maternal exposure to which of the following substances or conditions is thought to harm the developing fetus?

(1) Alcohol
(2) Tetracycline
(3) Rubella
(4) Herpes

26. The Assistant Secretary of Health administers the Public Health Service together with the Surgeon General. Congress might seek the Assistant Secretary's testimony on which of the following topics?

(1) Vaccine liability legislation
(2) Funding for cancer research
(3) Prevention of drug abuse
(4) Smoking as a public health hazard

27. A chi-square test is used during an outbreak of gastroenteritis to test the association between eating chicken salad and becoming ill. The proportion of individuals who ate chicken salad who were ill is statistically significantly greater than the proportion of individuals who did not eat chicken salad and who were ill ($p = 0.02$). Correct interpretations of these data include which of the following?

(1) Two percent of those who ate the chicken salad became ill
(2) The null hypothesis is rejected
(3) The probability for becoming ill after eating the chicken salad was 98%
(4) There is a 2% probability that the difference noted is due to chance

28. An 18-month old child who attends a day-care center was diagnosed as having *Hemophilus influenzae* type b (Hib) meningitis. This day-care center has infants ranging from 6 months to 4 years of age. Every child over 18 months of age has already received Hib vaccine. Control recommendations should consist of

(1) rifampin (RMP) prophylaxis for those under 18 months of age
(2) RMP prophylaxis for all classroom staff except pregnant women
(3) booster Hib immunizations for all children over 18 months of age
(4) RMP prophylaxis for all classmates regardless of age

29. Expert testimony is required to establish a defendant's negligence in medical malpractice cases unless the

(1) case involves specialty care rendered by a board-certified specialist
(2) court is able to locate a recognized medical text from which the relevant information can be obtained
(3) plaintiff is unable to obtain an expert witness willing to testify against the defendant
(4) care rendered by a defendant was so obviously negligent that a lay jury can discern it without expert testimony

30. Crucial elements to taking an occupational medical history include

(1) a chronological list of all jobs
(2) a description of a temporal relationship between workplace exposure and illness
(3) a list of known hazards in the workplace
(4) a list of childhood immunizations

31. Community mental health centers have had which of the following effects on the care of the mentally ill?

(1) They have helped to reduce the patient population in state mental hospitals
(2) They have helped to reduce the number of readmissions to mental hospitals
(3) They were funded initially by the federal government to provide an impetus to local governments to provide for these services
(4) They have proven adequate to handle the large number of former state hospital patients

32. The standard error of the mean of a sample is

(1) an estimate of the standard deviation of the population
(2) based on a normal distribution
(3) used to determine confidence limits
(4) increased as the sample size increases

33. Asbestos may cause which of the following conditions?

(1) Bronchogenic carcinoma
(2) Interstitial lung disease
(3) Gastrointestinal cancer
(4) Mesothelioma

34. The International Classification of Diseases E codes classify causes of injuries and poisonings by

(1) body part affected
(2) apparent intent
(3) nature of injury
(4) cause of injury

35. Natural immunity, which eliminates the need for further immunizations against disease, is conferred by which of the following diseases?

(1) Influenza
(2) Polio
(3) Tetanus
(4) Measles

36. The starting point for the statute of limitations applicable to medical malpractice suits in United States jurisdictions is the date that the

(1) alleged malpractice took place
(2) alleged malpractice was discovered by the patient
(3) alleged malpractice was discovered, or should have been discovered, by the patient
(4) the physician-patient relationship was terminated

37. Which of the following statements describe the Occupational Safety and Health Administration (OSHA)?

(1) It is a branch of the United States Department of Labor
(2) It conducts scientific research and professional training
(3) It establishes environmental standards for toxic chemicals in the workplace
(4) It enforces standards for toxic chemicals released from industries into the environment

Directions: The groups of questions below consist of lettered choices followed by several numbered items. For each numbered item select the **one** lettered choice with which it is **most** closely associated. Each lettered choice may be used once, more than once, or not at all.

Questions 38–42

For each situation listed below, select the rate which most closely relates to it.

(A) Crude rate
(B) Direct age-adjusted rate
(C) Indirect age-adjusted rate
(D) Incidence rate
(E) Age-specific rate

38. Can be compared in different populations
39. Is used as an attack rate in epidemic investigations
40. Is a summary rate for the entire population
41. Is expressed as a standardized ratio
42. Borrows a standard population

Questions 43–47

Match each of the following phrases describing the origin or basis of medical philosophies with the school of medical thought it best describes.

(A) Naturopathy
(B) Allopathy
(C) Chiropractic
(D) Osteopathy
(E) Homeopathy

43. Founded by Andrew Taylor Still
44. Founded on the principle of the law of similars
45. Directly descended from the age of heroic medicine
46. Founded by Samuel Hahnemann
47. Employs therapeutic manipulation of the skeletal system to assist in treating disease

Questions 48–50

For each disease listed below, select the description of the screening program that is most likely to be associated with it.

(A) Screening programs are cost-effective for selected populations
(B) Screening programs do not exist for this condition
(C) Screening programs are not cost-effective for this condition
(D) Screening programs are only cost-effective for men over 40 years of age
(E) Screening programs are only cost-effective for women after the menopause

48. Cerebrovascular disease
49. Peptic ulcer disease
50. Colorectal cancer

Questions 51–55

Match the following control strategies with the appropriate communicable disease.

(A) Shigella
(B) Tuberculosis
(C) Rabies
(D) Acquired immune deficiency syndrome
(E) Measles

51. Administer a chemoprophylactic agent to kill the biologic agent inside the patient so that it cannot infect others.
52. Eliminate the reservoir so that the agent has no place to live, multiply, or die in its natural state.
53. Avoid contact with a potentially dangerous reservoir.
54. Use a barrier to prevent the transfer of bodily fluids containing organisms from one person to another.
55. Prevent spread of disease by good handwashing techniques and good personal hygiene.

Questions 56–60

For each of the legal principles listed below, select the case that is credited with establishing that principle.

(A) *Helling v. Carey*
(B) *Hawkins v. McGee*
(C) *Canterbury v. Spence*
(D) *Tarasoff v. Regents of University of California*
(E) *Claire Conroy*

56. When a physician makes an express promise of cure, he or she can be held liable on contract grounds (breach of warranty) for failure to deliver the promised result.

57. A court may insist upon a higher standard of care than is currently observed in practice in the medical community.

58. With proper safeguards to help assure that it would be the patient's own choice, a health care provider may legitimately discontinue the provision of nutrition and water through a nasogastric tube to a seriously ill and failing patient even though death is certain to result.

59. In obtaining a patient's consent to treatment, a physician must disclose all that a reasonably prudent patient would consider *material* to the decision of whether or not to accept treatment.

60. A psychotherapist whose patient states that he or she intends to harm a specific third party has the duty to warn that party of the danger.

ANSWERS AND EXPLANATIONS

1. The answer is B. [*Chapter 10 IV A 2 a (1)–(2)*] Cerebromacular degeneration involves a group of disorders in which there is progressive mental deterioration as a result of the accumulation of lipid substances called gangliosides in the nerves cells throughout the central nervous system. There are four different types, which differ as to age of onset. Tay-Sachs disease begins at 4 to 8 months of age. Infants appear normal at birth, but progressive mental and physical deterioration follow, resulting in death in 2 to 4 years. Jansky-Bielschowsky disease has its onset at 2 to 4 years of age. Spielmeyer-Stock-Vogt-Koyangi disease, the juvenile form, occurs in children 5 to 6 years of age. Kuf's disease, the late juvenile form, is rare, occurring after 15 years of age.

2. The answer is D. (*Chapter 14 III B 1 a–d*) An individual can sue for damages as a result of alleged failures in medical care. However, in order to recover damages the plaintiff must prove that duty of care (an obligation recognized by the law for the breach of which the law imposes sanctions) was breached, that dereliction (that the defendant performed significantly below the legally required standard of care) existed, that damage (that the plaintiff was harmed) resulted from a failure of medical care, and that the defendant's negligence was the proximate cause of the plaintiff's injuries.

3. The answer is C. (*Chapter 2 III B 1–3*) A case series report is an objective report of a clinical characteristic or outcome from a group of clinical subjects. A case series report can address almost any clinical problem, including the natural history of a specific disease, the clinical characteristics of a disease, screening test results, and treatment outcomes. It is particularly useful to describe the natural history of disease or treatment outcomes. The major limitation of case series reports is that no control group is included for comparison. Hence, the results or observations may not be valid or generalizable to other populations since the population studied may be highly selected as may be the treatment or other evaluations. It is not acceptable or logical to compare the results of one case series with those of other studies since there is no way to ensure that the subjects, interventions, or treatments were equal.

4. The answer is B. (*Chapter 3 III E 3*) The critical ratio or z score is the number of standard deviations that a value in a normally distributed population lies away from the mean. The critical ratio is used in testing the null hypothesis and in calculating confidence limits in large samples and populations.

5. The answer is E. (*Chapter 11 II A 1–5*) Although 100 million people in the United States drink alcohol, only 9 million Americans suffer from alcoholism. Population surveys indicate that between 3% and 5% of adult men and between 0.1% and 1% of adult women are alcoholics. American Indians have a particularly high rate of alcoholism. Heavy drinkers are most likely to be between 45 and 49 years of age and belong to the low socioeconomic groups. Alcoholic individuals are associated with 15,000 homicides and suicides annually.

6. The answer is C. (*Chapter 5 VIII A 1 b, 2, B 2–4*) In 1980, the death rate from homicide was 10.5 individuals per 100,000 population in the United States. Homicide comprised 10% of all deaths in the United States in 1983. Currently, homicide rates for most age groups of both sexes are as high or higher than any previously recorded in the United States. Homicide is the leading cause of death for black American men between the ages of 15 and 24. Men are 4 times more likely to be victims of homicide than women; nonwhites are 8 to 15 times more likely to be victims than whites; and Hispanic men are 2 to 3 times more likely than white men to be victims of homicide. The use of alcohol and other drugs has been documented in 45% of all homicides.

7. The answer is C. (*Chapter 10 I A, B 1–2*) According to the American Association on Mental Deficiency (AAMD), mental retardation refers to significantly below average intellectual functioning that coexists with nonadaptive behavior during the developmental period. In more than 90% of cases, mental retardation exists at birth or occurs within the first 2 years of life; in more than 95% of cases, mental retardation occurs before the fifth year. The AAMD definition excludes mental deficiency that is acquired as an adult as well as conditions in which intelligence may be masked by illness or disease.

8. The answer is A. (*Chapter 3 IV A*) Screening is the initial examination of an individual to detect disease not yet being treated. Screening tests are applicable to large numbers of individuals and are best if highly sensitive and specific. The ability of the screening test to identify correctly those individuals who truly have the disease is the sensitivity, and its ability to identify correctly those who truly do not have the disease is the specificity. Diagnosis testing is done to determine the cause of a patient's disease and treatment testing to monitor the effectiveness of and the patient's response to therapy. Individuals for whom a screening test is positive should be given follow-up evaluation.

9. The answer is D. (*Chapter 8 VI A 1, 2*) Passive strategies for injury prevention and control are automatic, require no individual or repetitive action to be protective, and are generally the most effective. Active strategies, on the other hand, are voluntary, require repetitive, individual action to be protective, and generally are less effective than passive strategies. Child-resistant drug containers, self-extinguishing cigarettes, a safe hot water setting, and air bags require no individual or repetitive action to be protective and thus are considered passive strategies. Seat belts, however, must be buckled by the occupant of the automobile each time the vehicle is used in order to be effective and thus is considered an active strategy.

10. The answer is D. (*Chapter 9 VI A 1–2*) Primary prevention of mental disorder focuses on the promotion of general mental health and protection against the occurrence of specific disease. However, not all of these efforts have been successful; for example, all evidence suggests that the rate of schizophrenic breakdown has remained stable for many years in spite of prevention efforts. Organic brain syndrome, resulting from diseases such as syphilis and vitamin deficiencies, is rare today, although it was the leading cause of mental hospital admissions 50 to 75 years ago. Caplan has worked successfully with prevention of situational reaction formation by developing a theory and techniques for preparing individuals in advance to deal with crises in order to avoid the distress that usually results. Amniocentesis can detect Down's syndrome in utero for those couples who are interested in prenatal screening for mental disorders.

11. The answer is C. (*Chapter 3 IV C 3*) The positive predictive value is the ability of a test to identify those individuals who truly have a disease from among all those whose screening tests were positive. A fourfold table based on the data provided (shown below) reveals that of 1350 persons with positive screening tests, 950 had disease X. The positive predictive value is equal to 950 divided by 1350, or 70%.

	Disease X		
Screening Test	**Yes**	**No**	**Total**
Positive	950	400	1350
Negative	50	3600	3650
Total	1000	4000	5000

12. The answer is C. (*Chapter 2 III D–E*) A case-control study is an observational or descriptive analytic study in which diseased and nondiseased subjects are identified after the fact and then compared regarding specific characteristics to determine possible risk for the disease in question. A cohort study is an observational or descriptive analytic study in which exposed and nonexposed populations are identified and followed prospectively over time to determine the rate of a specific disease or event. Although costly and time-consuming, a cohort study allows for determination of a population-based rate of the event under question. A case-control study, on the other hand, is relatively easy and inexpensive to conduct since prospective or long-term follow-up is not required. In a cohort study, potential bias is lessened because exposure can be determined prior to the onset of disease, while with a case-control study, there is a potential for bias in the selection of subjects since a case-control study is not population based. The incidence rate of an event or disease for exposed and nonexposed populations must be calculated for a cohort study but cannot be determined in a case-control study. Causality cannot be determined for either a case-control study or a cohort study. Causation is defined by various criteria in addition to risk assessment. These include biologic plausibility, appropriate temporal relationships between exposure and disease or event, consistent outcomes and observations across several studies, dose-response relationships, and finally an experimental or animal study confirmation of association.

13. The answer is C. (*Chapter 11 I B 1–2*) Nonpathologic substance use is distinguished from substance abuse by three criteria: a pattern of pathologic use characterized by intoxication throughout the day, inability to stop drinking even in the face of medical contraindications, and a need for daily use for adequate functioning; impairment in social or occupational functioning; and duration of at least 1 month. Substance dependence, on the other hand, is distinguished from substance abuse by the physical dependence on the substance being abused as evidenced by either tolerance or withdrawal.

14. The answer is E. (*Chapter 3 III B 4*) The type I error, or alpha error, is the rejection of a null hypothesis that is actually true. Type I error is used to determine sample size and to test the null hypothesis, which is often rejected at the arbitrary cutoff of 5% probability due to chance. The beta error is the acceptance as true of a false null hypothesis, and the formula 1 minus the beta error is used to calculate the power of a study.

15. The answer is A. (*Chapter 7 I C 1*) The major cause of neonatal mortality reflects failure of intrauterine growth, which can occur as prematurity or as weight gain inappropriate to gestational age.

Between one-third and one-half of very low-birth-weight infants (i.e., infants weighing $\leq$ 1500 g) die in the neonatal period. As birth weight decreases, the neonatal mortality rate increases sharply. In general, low-birth-weight infants (i.e., infants weighing $\leq$ 2500 g) account for more than 65% of neonatal deaths, regardless of the gestational age of the infant.

16. The answer is C. (*Chapter 13 IV A 1 b–c*) Viscosity is a measure of how readily a liquid flows, and movement between environmental mediums cannot be predicted from viscosity information. However, all of the other properties are measures that directly predict the tendency of chemicals to concentrate in a medium. The octanol water partition coefficient predicts partitioning between water and oil-like materials such as soil or sediment. The vapor pressure predicts partitioning between water and air. Solubility predicts the potential for concentration in water. Bioconcentration factor (BCF) predicts the affinity of a chemical for aquatic organisms; thus, high BCF values indicate an accumulation of the chemical in fish as compared to the water in which they swim.

17. The answer is C. (*Chapter 13 II A–B*) Some exposure is safe for toxic effects that show thresholds; however, for nonthreshold effects, there is some risk associated with any exposure. Increases in exposure or dose is expected to increase either the intensity of a toxic effect or the percent responding in a population regardless of whether the effect is a threshold or nonthreshold effect. For both classes of effect, the chemical or metabolite does cause the effect, although the exact mechanism of action may not be known. Both threshold and nonthreshold effects can be independent of route of exposure because a chemical can enter the systemic circulation from inhalation or ingestion. Both nonthreshold effects that require chemical interaction with genetic material and threshold effects that require that the chemical or metabolite reach the sensitive target organ depend on absorption of the chemical.

18. The answer is C. (*Chapter 18 III B 1–4, C*) Four payment methodologies are used by third-party payers to reimburse providers. Per diem is an all-inclusive flat rate for each day of hospital care provided. It usually includes all ancillary services, supplies, and other services billed by the hospital. Capitation is a fee that the provider agrees to accept per patient per month for each patient enrolled in the practice in exchange for providing all specified health services to enrollees. "Risk corridor" is a capitation adjustment whereby additional payments to or refunds from the provider would occur if the variance from the budget exceeded a certain threshold percentage. Per admission is an all inclusive flat rate for each hospital admission. This admission reimbursement consists of different rates according to the admitting service or diagnosis. The Diagnosis Related Group payment system is based on a fixed hospital per admission payment rate for each of 470 treatment classifications. Fee-for-service charges are billed on an itemized invoice.

19. The answer is C (2, 4). (*Chapter 18 I B*) Health care costs do not obey the usual economic laws of supply and demand whereby an increase in supply would result in a price decrease. The increase in health insurance coverage has reduced the patient's direct responsibility and concern for cost. Neither has the increase in the physician to population ratio (supply) resulted in lowered physician fees because the patient is often insulated from direct costs by insurance coverage. The number of hospitals has declined due to mergers and health planning regulations. Health costs have increased due to the "graying" population.

20. The answer is A (1, 2, 3). (*Chapter 11 IV C 1–2*) Horton showed a high degree of correlation between subsistence insecurity and excessive drinking. Bales reported that attitudes of a culture toward drinking are responsible for alcoholism. Bales related the amount of alcoholism in a culture to the degree to which the culture provides suitable substitute means of satisfaction for the relief of inner tensions. There is no evidence to support the statement that the prevalence of alcoholism is low if the religion or the culture prohibits its use.

21. The answer is B (1, 3). [*Chapter 1 IV C 2 b (2) (a), (b)*] An indirect age-adjustment rate is a summary rate for the entire population. It is used to compare two populations and is used when the age-specific rates are unknown (as in developing countries) or when the age-specific rates of a population are unstable because of small numbers. In order to calculate the indirect rate, the age composition of the populations being compared must be known, and age-specific rates from a standard population must be borrowed.

22. The answer is A (1, 2, 3). (*Chapter 15 I G 1–4*) Morality may rest on common consent of a social unit, on adherence to the will of a god, or on what is deemed consistent with normal human behavior. It may also be based on individual perception of what is right either through common sense or intuition. Criminal law is generally based on one or more of the moral sources; however, there may often be a major discrepancy between the (criminal) law and morality.

23. The answer is B (1, 3). [*Chapter 4 III B 2 b (1), c (1)–(2), e (3)*] Children who are behind in their immunizations should be given multiple vaccines at the same time to catch up on their immunization schedule. The simultaneous administration of multiple antigens has been shown to produce effective immunity without any increase in adverse side reactions. Since the immune system can remember previous immunizations, there is never any need to start an immunization series all over again. Since persons immunized with measles, mumps, and rubella virus vaccines do not transmit these viruses, these vaccines may be given to children of pregnant women. Although the live polio vaccine strain is shed by recently immunized children, this immunization should not be delayed because of a pregnancy in close adult contacts.

24. The answer is E (all). (*Chapter 8 II B 3 a–f, C 2 a–e; III A 1 b*) The host, or the individual affected, has been the principal focus of research related to injuries and preventive measures aimed at decreasing injury rates. Host factors that affect the risk of injuries differ according to the type of injury; for example, native Americans have a higher rate of all injuries than other racial groups, even when income is controlled. Men have an increased incidence of almost all injuries and mortality resulting from these injuries as compared to women. Osteoporosis increases the risk of fall-related injuries such as hip fractures. Social environmental factors that increase the risk of injuries include violent behavior; alcohol and drug use; and economic deprivation, racism, and sexism.

25. The answer is A (1, 2, 3). (*Chapter 6 IV F 1, 2, 6; V A 1*) Excessive alcohol intake during pregnancy can result in the fetal alcohol syndrome, consisting of excessive irritability, delayed mental and physical growth, and particular facial characteristics. Tetracycline exposure can cause discolored teeth in the child. Rubella exposure can result in mental retardation, deafness, and blindness. While a herpes infection in the mother during delivery can be fatal to a new infant, the harm is done during the birthing process not during gestation.

26. The answer is E (all). (*Chapter 17 I B 1 b; Figure 17-2*) The Assistant Secretary for Health is responsible for virtually all areas of personal and public health within the federal government. Thus, vaccine programs, cancer research at the National Cancer Institute, drug abuse issues through the Alcohol, Drug Abuse, and Mental Health Administration, and public health issues of smoking all are vital areas within the Public Health Service.

27. The answer is C (2, 4). (*Chapter 3 III B 2*) The probability is 2% that the distribution of illness in those who ate chicken salad compared with those who did not is due to chance. Because the report states that the difference is statistically significant, the null hypothesis (i.e., that the difference is due to chance) can be rejected, and alternative hypotheses (e.g., the chicken salad was contaminated) must be considered. The proportion of individuals who were ill cannot be deduced from the given probability value.

28. The answer is C (2, 4). (*Chapter 4 III C 4 a–d; VIII A 3 c*) Rifampin (RMP) prophylaxis should be offered to all staff (except pregnant women) and classmates regardless of prior immunization. Although previously immunized individuals are at decreased risk of disease, *Hemophilus influenzae* vaccine does not affect nasopharyngeal carriage of the organism, which may be passed to susceptible classmates. Also, immunologic response to either natural disease or immunization under 24 months is not considered sufficient to prevent future disease. In order to be effective, RMP should be given to at least 75% of the contacts during the same 4-day period. Because this is difficult to accomplish, some authorities would not implement these recommendations until a second case has occurred.

29. The answer is D (4). [*Chapter 14 III B 1 a (1), (2), 2 a (1), (2), b, 3 a (1), (2)*] In cases where the court can see that "the matter speaks for itself" (*res ipsa loquitur*), most jurisdictions will excuse the plaintiff from introducing expert testimony to establish the appropriate professional standard of care. Specialty care may have a bearing upon the standard of care to be applied—that is, a local versus a national standard—but does not address how the plaintiff goes about proving what that standard is. Some states allow the plaintiff to use medical texts in lieu of expert testimony to establish a point about the standard of care, but the burden of proof lies with the plaintiff. Under our adversary system, the court, with very rare exceptions, does not undertake independent research to answer questions upon which a subject piece of litigation turns. When the plaintiff is unable to secure an expert witness—perhaps because of the so-called conspiracy of silence—it generally means that the plaintiff's suit will fail as a result of the plaintiff's inability to provide the burden of proof. The doctrine of *res ipsa loquitur* provides the only major exception to this unfortunate fact of life.

30. The answer is A (1, 2, 3). (*Chapter 12 II A 1–3, B 1–5*) Because occupational diseases frequently present as common medical conditions, a key factor in a physician's ability to recognize an occupational disease is the occupational history. Screening questions related to work exposure should be asked of all patients and should include a chronological list of all jobs, a description of any temporal relationship between a work exposure and a presenting illness, and known hazards in the workplace.

Occupational information should also be sought from the employer, records of the Occupational Safety and Health Administration, the labor union, or by a visit to the workplace. Childhood immunizations, while important in pediatric histories, rarely have any relevance to diseases of workers and are therefore not crucial to an occupational history.

31. The answer is B (1, 3). (*Chapter 9 V C 1–2*) Although community mental health centers have helped to reduce the patient population in state mental hospitals, the number of readmissions has risen so sharply that psychiatrists have begun to reevaluate this system. These centers have also proved inadequate to handle the large number of former state hospital patients, resulting in an extraordinary number of homeless mentally ill people. Although community health centers were initially funded by the federal government to provide an impetus to local government to provide for these services, the results have been disappointing.

32. The answer is A (1, 2, 3). (*Chapter 3 III G 1 a*) The standard error of the mean is an estimate of the standard deviation of the population based on the standard deviation of a sample. The standard error of the mean is equal to the standard deviation of the sample divided by the square root of the sample size; therefore, the standard error of the mean decreases as the sample size increases. The standard error of the mean is based on the fact that the means of the samples follow a normal distribution, even if the samples do not. The standard error of the mean is used to determine confidence limits.

33. The answer is E (all). [*Chapter 12 IV C 1 a (3)*] Asbestos, an inorganic dust used as insulation, in fireproofing and roofing materials, and in automotive parts is toxic when inhaled or ingested. Asbestos exposure may cause asbestosis, an interstitial lung disease; mesothelioma, a cancer of the pleural covering of the lung; bronchogenic carcinoma, the most common lung cancer; and gastrointestinal cancer.

34. The answer is C (2, 4). (*Chapter 8 IV C 1–2, D 1–3*) The International Classification of Diseases (ICD) is the principal classification scheme that defines the nature of injuries (N codes) and the external cause of injuries (E codes). The N codes classify injuries by the part of the body that was injured, the type of damage that occurred, and the infectious or parasitic etiology (if applicable). The E codes classify injuries by apparent intent and by external environmental cause.

35. The answer is D (4). [*Chapter 4 III C 1 b (4), 2 a, 3 a (1); IV A 2 f (2), (3), B 2 a (2)–(3), f (2), 3 b (2)*] Since the H and N component of the influenza A virus can undergo minor and major antigenic shifts, natural disease does not confer immunity. In fact, the composition of the vaccine must be continually updated to provide protection against the current strains. Clinical tetanus does not confer immunity, and it is possible to have this disease many times. Apparently, the amount of toxin necessary to cause disease is not sufficient to stimulate the immune response. Since there are three distinct types of poliovirus, it is possible to get polio on three separate occasions. Polio vaccine provides protection against all three types. Although a case of measles confers lifelong immunity, it is important to document immunity since a measles-like illness can be caused by a number of other viral illnesses. A history of having had measles disease is not sufficient for a child to attend school; a child must have serologic evidence of immunity or a documented measles immunization to attend school.

36. The answer is E (all). (*Chapter 14 II F 3 a–d*) The statute of limitations is a procedural rule that establishes a maximum period of time during which a legal suit may be initiated. The beginning of the statutory period for medical malpractice suits in the United States is generally defined as the date: (1) the alleged malpractice took place, (2) the alleged malpractice was discovered by the patient, (3) the alleged malpractice was discovered or should have been discovered by the patient, and (4) the physician-patient relationship was terminated. Definition (1) is the simplest, but perhaps the most unfair to the plaintiff if the statutory period is running against him while he is unaware that there has been an act of malpractice. Definition (2) guards against the unfairness to the plaintiff but is arguably unfair to the potential defendant, since the plaintiff (patient) could be lax in investigating symptoms that would lead to the discovery of an error in treatment. Definition (3) is favored by most jurisdictions as the fairest, although it may be difficult to determine when a reasonably diligent patient should have discovered the malpractice. Definition (4), which is used in very few jurisdictions, assumes that while the patient is still under the care of the same physician, it is unfair for the statutory period to run because it is unlikely that the patient would discover that he has been the victim of malpractice.

37. The answer is B (1, 3). (*Chapter 12 I D 12*) The Occupational Safety and Health Administration (OSHA) was established in 1970 as part of the United States Department of Labor to assure safe and healthful working conditions for American workers. It is charged with establishing, enforcing, and educating the public concerning workplace health and safety standards. The National Institute for Occupational Safety and Health (NIOSH) was established to provide for scientific research and professional education in the field of occupational safety and health. The Environmental Protection Agency (EPA) was established to provide research, standard setting, and enforcement of guidelines for protection of human health in the environment.

38–42. The answers are: 38-E, 39-D, 40-A, 41-C, 42-B. (*Chapter 1 IV B 2 a, c, C 1, 2 b (1), (2), 3 b*) Rates are precise terms with precise definitions in terms of what constitutes the numerator and the denominator when they are expressed mathematically. They were developed to quantify or describe certain events in a population.

Age-specific rates are calculated for various segments of the population. Although they are difficult to calculate because more information about the demographic composition of the community must be known than with other rates, they can be used to compare events in similar age groups in different populations.

Attack rates are a form of incidence rates—that is, the number of new cases of a specified disease during a specific time interval divided by the total population at risk during the same time interval. They are used in epidemic investigations using a particular population, which is observed for a limited period of time.

Crude rates are summary rates for an entire population. They are easy to calculate because only the number of events and the total population are needed. They cannot, however, be used to compare events in different populations because the rate is dependent on the age-sex composition of the total population.

The indirect age-adjusted rate calculates the number of events that would have been observed if the two populations being compared had the same age-specific rates, which in this case are unknown. The age composition of the populations being compared and the total number of observed events in each population must be known but age-specific rates from a larger population with stable rates must be borrowed. The total observed events is divided by the total expected events in that population times 100 and is expressed as a standardized ratio.

The direct age-adjusted rate calculates the rate that would have been observed if the populations being compared had the same age distribution; the age-specific rates in the populations being compared must be known but the standard population from elsewhere must be borrowed.

43–47. The answers are: 43-D, 44-E, 45-B, 46-E, 47-D. (*Chapter 16 II A 1, B 1*) Andrew Taylor Still, a Missouri physician who learned primarily by apprenticeship, established the first schools of osteopathy. Still, who was wary of the poisonous compounds used in the therapies of the day, developed his theories of musculoskeletal manipulation to replace these medications. At present, manipulation is an adjunct to other modes of treatment.

Samuel Hahnemann's law of similars was the belief that a set of symptoms could be treated by minute doses of a chemical causing the same symptoms when given in larger doses. The concept of using increasingly rarer dilutions, which were assigned greater therapeutic strength, was called the law of infinitesimals.

Allopathy, a termed coined by Hahnemann to describe traditional therapies which were "other than the disease" (i.e., the treatments bore no particular relationship to the illness) was actually the term applied to heroic medicine in the 1800s. We continue to use the term to this day, though purging and bloodletting, the cornerstones of heroic medicine, have largely disappeared in the United States.

Homeopathy was established in Germany near the end of the eighteenth century and spread to the United States with the founding of the Hahnemann Medical School in Philadelphia.

Chiropractic, developed by Palmer in Davenport, Iowa, adheres to the belief that all illness stems from dislocations of the vertebrae. Chiropractors, therefore, concentrate on therapy of the spine.

48–50. The answers are: 48-C, 49-B, 50-A. (*Chapter 5 III D 1; IV D 3 a–b; XI D 2*) Measurement of blood pressure, which is recommended every 5 years for men and women 16 to 64 years of age and every 2 years after age 65, is the primary screening method for cerebrovascular disease; however, widespread screening of target populations is not considered cost-effective.

Risk factors such as cigarette smoking, regular use of aspirin and acetaminophen, and prolonged use of large doses of steroids are closely associated with peptic ulcer disease. Less conclusive associations have been reported for alcohol, caffeine, diet, and psychologic stress. In spite of the awareness of these risk factors, no tests for determining a preulcerous condition in asymptomatic individuals exist.

Screening for colorectal cancer is by testing the stool for occult blood in men and women over 46 years of age. Target populations include individuals with a history of colitis, familial polyposis or villous adenomas, or familial cancer of the colon. Screening is considered cost-effective for potential cases of colorectal cancer.

51–55. The answers are: 51-B, 52-E, 53-C, 54-D, 55-A. (*Chapter 4 II A 1 a, 3, B 2 a, D 1 a; VII C 2*) Chemotherapeutic or chemoprophylactic agents kill biologic agents inside patients so that they cannot infect others. Isoniazid prophylaxis, for example, is administered to patients with a positive skin test for tuberculosis to prevent reactivation of a latent infection and secondary spread to other individuals.

Certain diseases, such as measles and smallpox, die out when the agent has no natural place to multiply. Thus, immunization of a susceptible population with a live attenuated measles vaccine eliminates the reservoir so that the measles virus has no place to live in its natural state.

Humans should avoid contact with potentially rabid animals and should not keep certain wild animals (e.g., skunks and raccoons) as pets. They should also make certain that their pet is properly immunized against rabies.

The transfer of organisms directly from one person to another can be blocked by simple processes such as hand washing and using a condom. Hand washing is the most important procedure for preventing the spread of many enteric diseases, such as *Shigella*. Condoms can block the transmission of many sexually transmitted diseases, such as acquired immune deficiency syndrome.

56–60. The answers are: 56-B, 57-A, 58-E, 59-C, 60-D. [*Chapter 14 III B 2 d (1)–(3); IV D 2; V B 2; VI B 2 b; VIII D 2 d (1), (2)*] In general, courts do not like to entertain medical negligence cases under the rubric of contract suits. However, at least one court has held (*Hawkins v. McGee*) that where a very specific promise of improvement or cure is made, a health care provider may be liable if the promised result is not forthcoming. Some states insist that the promise not only be expressly stated but also that it be in writing if it is to be the basis of a breach of warranty suit.

Helling v. Carey, although not widely followed, held that customary professional practice is not absolutely determinative of reasonably prudent care. A court is normally reluctant to substitute its judgment as to what is reasonable care for that of the medical community but will do so in a clear-cut case. What made the *Helling* case clear-cut was the fact that the test involved was simple, inexpensive, painless, risk-free, and highly definitive, whereas the disease it might detect (glaucoma) was serious, degenerative, and irreversible. *Helling* stands as a limited, but significant, symbol that the medical profession cannot absolutely determine the standards by which its performance is to be judged.

The *Claire Conroy* case goes well beyond that of *Karen Quinlan* by allowing withdrawal of food and water, which some consider not to be an *extraordinary* means of life support. In the *Quinlan* case, the court authorized removal of a respirator, but intravenous feeding was continued until Karen's death in 1985. Moreover, in the *Quinlan* case, the patient was comatose and was thought to have no significant chance of ever returning to consciousness. In *Conroy*, the patient was partially responsive and had some degree of interaction with her environment. The court established elaborate criteria by which to determine what the patient would have wished regarding the continuation of care had she been able to do so, and thus, the doctrine of substituted judgment was established.

Canterbury v. Spence is the landmark case that moved the physician's obligation to disclose information to the patient from a physician-based to a patient-based standard. Under this new approach, the relevant inquiry focuses on what a patient would want to know in deciding on treatment, rather than, as previously, on what physicians normally disclose to patients in such situations. It is a question of fact for the court—and for a jury where one of the parties to the suit has requested one—to determine whether a particular item of information would have been material to an individual in the patient's situation.

The *Tarasoff v. Regents of University of California* case was very controversial in the mental health community since it unsettled the traditional belief that there was an absolute privilege protecting information a patient divulged to his or her psychotherapist in the course of treatment. The case recognized that the mental health professional has a duty to the public that can supersede that owed to his or her client. The *Tarasoff* ruling, which has been adopted in a number of other jurisdictions, is limited to cases in which the therapist has sound reason to believe that the patient threatens danger to an identifiable third party. The therapist's duty is to inform the authorities or warn the intended victim.

Index

Note: Page numbers in *italics* denote illustrations; those followed by (t) denote tables.

A

AAMD, *see* American Association on Mental Deficiency
Abandonment, definition of, 6, 12
legal implications of, 275, 281, 282
Abortion, mortality rate associated with, *140*, 141(t)
rate of, 139
trends in, 143–144, *145*, *146*
Absorption, examples of, 248–249
Accidents, *see* Injuries
Accreditation, definition of, 4, 10, 320
2-Acetylaminofluorene (2AAF) exposure, cancers and, 240, 240(t), *241*
ACGIH, *see* American Conference of Governmental Industrial Hygienists
ACIP, *see* Advisory Committee on Immunization Practices
Acquired immune deficiency syndrome (AIDS), casual contact and, 97
control strategies for, 98, 342, 350
disinfectants and, 79
epidemiology of, 95–97
human immunodeficiency virus (HIV) as the cause of, 97
infectious disease process of, 97–98
quarantine and, 277
screening blood for, 114, 116
Act deontology, definition of, 286, *287*
ethics and, 293, 294
Act utilitarianism, definition of, 287
Action levels of chemicals, Food and Drug Administration and, 259
Addiction, definition of, 345
Adjusted rates, 8
age-specific, 342, 346, 349
calculation of, 22, 23
Adler, A., addiction and, 7, 13, 203
Adolescence, alcohol use in, 159, 161, 163
health problems in, 158–159
injuries in, 159
mortality, causes of, 158
Adoption studies, alcoholism and, 203
Advisory Committee on Immunization Practices (ACIP), 83
Aflotoxin, peanut butter and, 251
Agar-agar, food and, 258
Agents, disease-causing, 16–17, 19, 31, 34
elimination of, 79
injury-causing, 166–167, 174, 175, 176, 177
substance abuse and, 204
Aid to Dependent Children, 160
AIDS, *see* Acquired immune deficiency syndrome
Air, Clean Air Act (CAA) and, 255
Airborne spread of disease, 18
Alcohol, abuse of, 201–202
epidemiology of, 337, 344
adolescent use of, 161, 163
cirrhosis and, 126–127
colorectal cancer and, 124
homocide and, 128
mortality and, 201
patterns of use, 204–205
toxicity and, 218
withdrawal from, 205
Alcohol addiction, family studies of, 203, 208, 209
theories related to, 203–204
Alcoholism, definition of, 345, 346
immunization and, 86
maternal, fetal mental retardation and, 195
Aldehydes, toxicity and, 219
Aliphatic hydrocarbons, toxicity and, 217
Allied health professionals, qualifications and training for, 302, 303(t)
Allopathic medicine, 296, 297(t)
Allopathy, definition of, 342, 349
Alpha error, 36, 39, 338, 345
AMA, *see* American Medical Association
Ambulatory care, 307
facilities for, 318–319, 319(t)
American Association on Mental Deficiency (AAMD), 191
mental retardation and, 338, 344
American Conference of Governmental Industrial Hygienists (ACGIH), description of, 211
American Medical Association (AMA), Code of Medical Ethics and, 2, 8
Ames test, mutagenesis and, 238–239, 265, 266
Amino acid metabolism, mental retardation and, 192
Amniocentesis, pregnancy and, 146
Amphetamines, abuse of, 202
Anatomic asplenia, *see* Asplenia
Anemia, epidemiology of, 131–132, 135, 137
incidence and prevalence of, 132
iron deficiency and, 132
mortality rates for, 131–132
screening for, 132, 136, 137
sickle-cell, 132
Antigenic drift, influenza virus and, 90
Antigenic shift, influenza virus and, 90
Antitoxin, definition of, 82
Aromatic hydrocarbons, toxicity and, 217–218
Arsenic, toxicity and, 215–216, 233, 234
Asbestos, in insulation, 249
regulations concerning, 259
toxicity and, 219, 341, 348
Asphyxiant gases, definition of, 223, 232, 234
Asplenia, immunization and, 86
Asthma, occupations and, 226
schoolchildren and, 156
Atomic Energy Act, radioactive substances and, 260
Attack rates, definition of, 21, 342, 349
Autonomy, definition of, 290

B

Bacterial diseases, occupations and, 225
Baden formula, addiction rates and, 202, 209
Bar chart, description of, 49, *49*
Barbiturates, abuse of, 202, 208, 209
Bard, M., research in crisis intervention and, 184
Barrier method of contraception, 99, 142, 150, 151
Battery, definition of, 6, 12
deliberate torts and, 270–271
Bayes theorem, screening tests and, 71
BCF, *see* Bioconcentration factor
Beneficence, definition of, 290
Benefit of the bargain, contract law and, 271, 272
Bennett Amendment, Social Security Act and, 321
Beryllium, toxicity and, 216, 233, 234
Beta error, cohort study and, 42
definition of, 5, 11, 36
Bias, clinical trial and, 40, 42
cohort study and, 41, 42
definition of, 36, 37
Binomial distribution, applications of, 56–57
definition of, 44
Bioassay tests, animal, definition of, 237
Bioconcentration factor (BCF), definition of, 346
edible fish and, 247, 247(t), 250
example of, 266
Birth canal, infectious diseases of, 147
Birth control pills, 143, 150, 151
see also Oral contraceptives
smoking and, *143*
Birth injury, neonatal mortality from, 154
Birthing centers, description of, 319
Blood pressure, heart disease and, 119
Blood, screening of, 81
Boards of health, responsibilities of, 308
Breach of confidentiality, deliberate torts and, 271
see also Confidentiality
Breach of contract, bad faith, 272
contract law and, 272
deliberate torts and, 271
Breach of warranty, contract law and, 272
Hawkins v. McGee and, 343, 350
Breast cancer, epidemiology of, 122, 122(t)
risk factors for, 7, 13, 123–124
screening for, 125
Bronchitis, occupations and, 226
Bronchogenic carcinoma, asbestos and, 341, 348
Burden of proof, malpractice suits and, 340, 347

C

Cadmium, toxicity and, 216

Cancer, *see also specific sites of*
adolescent mortality and, 158
asbestos-induced, 237(t), 240, *240*
epidemiology of, 122, 122(t)
occupations and, 229(t), 230(t), 232, 234
radiation-induced, dose-response curves and, 240–242
Canterbury v. Spence, consent and disclosure and, 343, 350
informed consent obligations and, 273, 279
Capitation, definition of, 312, 329, 330, 346
Carbon monoxide, toxicity and, 223, 232, 234
Carbon tetrachloride, toxicity and, 219
Carcinogenesis, nonthreshold effects and, 235–236
Carcinogens, animal, tumor sites of, 242–243, 242(t)
dose-response evaluation, 240
epidemiologic studies of, 236–239
food and, 259
human, latency periods for, 237(t)
tumor sites of, 242, 242(t)
weight of evidence classification system, 239, 239(t)
Cardiovascular diseases, *see also* Heart disease
occupations and, 227
Care, *see also* Health care and Long-term care
access to, 275–276
duty to render, 281, 282
emergencies and, 280, 282
free, 280, 282
Carriers, agents and, 17
Case-control study, description of, 38, 39, 338, 345
example of, 41, 42
Case fatality rate, 1, 8
Case report, description of, 37
example of, 41, 42
Case series report, description of, 37, 38, 337, 344
example of, 41, 42
Causation, informed consent obligations and, 273
Centers for Disease Control (CDC), immunization and, 83
injuries and, 171
responsibilities of, 307–308
Cerebromacular degeneration, mental retardation and, 193, 337, 344
Cerebrospinal fluid leaks, immunization and, 86–87
Cerebrovascular disease, epidemiology of, 121
prevention of, 122
risk factors for, 121
screening for, 342, 349
Certificate of need statutes, major health care expenditures and, 322–323, 324, 326
Cervical cancer, epidemiology of, 122, 122(t)
risk factors for, 7, 13, 124
screening for, 125, 136, 137
Chemicals, analysis of, all mediums and materials and, 252–253
physical properties of, 247, 247(t), 252
regulation of environmental, 255–261
safe doses for, 10
states of, 251
Chiropractic, definition of, 349
Chi-square tests, 62, 73, 74, 76, 77
definition of, 62–64, 63(t)
example of, 340, 347
Chlamydia, 2, 8
control strategies for, 99
epidemiology of, 98
infectious disease process and, 98–99
Chlordane, animal fat and, 259
Cholesterol, control of, 120, 135, 137
heart disease and, 119
Chorionic villus biopsy, pregnancy and, 146
Chronic illness, epidemiology of, 119
prevention of, 119
Chronic obstructive pulmonary disease (COPD), epidemiology of, 125–126
risk factors for, 126
screening for, 126
Cirrhosis, epidemiology of, 126
immunization and, 86
risk factors for, 126–127
Civil suits, definition of, 267
Claire Conroy, substituted judgment and, 275, 279, 283, 343, 350
Clinical decisions, medical ethics and, 288–289, *289*, 290
Clinical trial, definition of, 4, 5, 9, 11
examples of, 40, 41, 42
principles of, 35
subject selection in, 36
Coal dust, toxicity and, 219
Codes of conduct, professional, 288
Coefficient of variation, definition of, 47
Cohort study, bias in, 42
description of, 39, 40, 338, 345
examples of, 41, 42
Coitus interruptus, 142
Cold, toxicity and, 224
Colorectal cancer, epidemiology of, 122, 122(t)
risk factors for, 7, 13, 124
screening for, 125, 342, 349
Community mental health centers, progress of, 182–183, 341, 348
Competency, definition of, 274
Comprehensive Health Planning and Public Service Amendment, 321
Condoms, prevention of disease by, 80
Confidence limits, calculation of 3, 9
definition of, 61–62
disregard of, 278
guidelines for, 293, 294
information and, 278
medical ethics and, 290
Confidentiality, *Tarasoff v. Regent of University of California* and, 343, 350
Congenital anomalies, infant mortality and, 154
Consent, *see also* Informed consent
adult, 273
disclosure and, 343, 350
emergency, 6, 12, 274
minors and, 274
next of kin and, 274
Conspiracy of silence, malpractice cases and, 270, 347
Consumer Product Safety Commission, 174, 176
products and, 259
Contamination levels, maximum (MCL), 256
Contingency tables, 55–56, 55(t), 56(t), 73, 76
Contraception, methods of, 140, 142–145, 149, 150, 151
Contract law, definition of, 271
Contractual allowance, 329
Cook v. Ochsner Foundation Hospital, hospital financing laws and, 276, 279
Copay, definition of, 312, 329
COPD, *see* Chronic obstructive pulmonary disease
Correlation coefficient, application of, 66–67, 67(t), 67, 74, 76–77
Cosmetics, chemical exposure and, 260–261
Cost(s), assessment of, Peer Review Organizations (PROs) and, 321
Professional Standards Review Organizations (PSROs) and, 321
cancer treatment, 123
cerebrovascular disease, 121
chronic obstructive pulmonary disease, 126
diabetes, 129
health care, moral problems concerning 291
heart disease, 119
increases in, 339, 347
injuries and, 168
renal disease, 130
sexually transmitted diseases, 92
Cotton dust, toxicity and, 220
Court cases, 279
Criminal suits, definition of, 267
Crisis intervention, mental illness and, 184
research and, 188, 189
Crisis reaction, prevention of, 183
Critical ratio, definition of, 57, 57(t), *58*
normal distribution and, 337, 344
Crude rates, calculation of, 22, 342, 349
Cumulative frequency graph, 50, *52*
Cyclamate, food and, 259
Cyclic hydrocarbons, toxicity and, 218
Cytomegalovirus, screening blood for, 114, 116

D

Damages, compensatory, 268
contract action and, 271
negligence and, 280, 282
nominal, 269
punitive, 269
tort law and, 269
Data, collection, in clinical studies, 36
definition of, 43–44
graphic presentations of, 47–51
Deductible, definition of, 312, 329
Defamation, deliberate torts and, 271
Degrees of freedom, definition of, 55–56, 56(t), 73, 76
Deliberate wrongdoing, 280, 282
Delivery, obstetric concerns at the time of, 147–148
types of, 147
Dental caries, prevention of, 158
Dentists, educational requirements for, 301
specialization of, 301
Deontological theories, definition of, 286
Department of Health and Human Services (DHHS), organization of, 307, *308*
Dependence, drug and alcohol, 201–202, 208, 209
Dereliction, negligence and, 280, 282
proof of, 270
tort law and, 269
Descriptive ethics, definition of, 285, *285*
Deviation *see* Standard deviation
DHHS, *see* Department of Health and Human Services
Diabetes, epidemiology of, 128–129
pregnancy and, 147
renal disease and, 130
screening for, 129
Diagnosis Related Groups (DRG), 329, 330
Diagnostic and Statistical Manual for the Classification of Mental Disorders (DSM), description of, 183, 188, 189, 201
Diarrheal disease, postneonatal mortality and, 154
Dioxins, regulations for, 260
Diphtheria, immunization and, 84, 87(t)
Diphtheria and tetanus toxoids (DT) vaccine, 84, 157(t)
Diphtheria, tetanus, and pertussis (DTP) vaccine, 84
immunization schedules for, 87(t), 157(t)
Disability, epidemiology of, 174, 176
Disclosure, informed consent and, 273
Disease, control of, 79–82
eradication of, 20
index of, 8
limiting risk of, 292

natural history of, 35
prevention of, 79, 82–83
rates of, 20–21
reporting of, 278
surveillance of, 7, 13, 20
Dispersion, measures of, 46
Distributions, definition of, 44, 45
Dix, Dorothea Lynde, 181
Doses, high, definition of, 237
Down's syndrome, characteristics of, 6, 12
mental retardation and, 191, 194
test for, in pregnancy, 345
Drift hypothesis, schizophrenia and the, 180
DRG, *see* Diagnosis Related Groups
Drugs, abuse of, 202, 261
adolescent mortality and, 158
adolescent use of, 159
homicide and, 128
risks of, 261
toxicity and, 251
withdrawal from, 205–206
DSM, *see Diagnostic and Statistical Manual for the Classification of Mental Disorders*
DTP, *see* Diphtheria, tetanus, and pertussis
Dusts, toxicity and, 219–220
Duty, negligence and, 280, 282
statutory imposition of, 275
tort law and, 269

E

E codes, *see also* International Classification of Disease (ICD)
poisonings and the, 170, 170(t), 341, 348
Ectopic pregnancy, definition of, 139, *142*
Egoism, ethics and, 287, 293, 294
Elderly, care of, 317
Emissions, controls for, 256
hazards of, 255–256
Emotional problems, adolescent, 156, 158
Encephalitis, measles and, 82
viral, 25
Endrin, asparagus and fish and, 259
Energy, as injury-causing agent, 166–167 175, 176
Environment, diseases and, 19
injuries and, 166, 175, 177
Environmental exposures, mental retardation and, 195
Environmental fate, definition of, 246
Environmental mediums, movement of chemicals between, 339, 347
Environmental monitoring, analysis and, 253
Environmental Protection Agency (EPA), definition of, 211
Environmental releases, duties of, 348–349
examples of, 254–255
EPA, *see* Environmental Protection Agency
Epidemic, investigation of, 27–28, 30, 33
Epidemic curve, definition of, 49, *51*
uses of, 26
Epidemiologic triangle, 7, 13, 18–19
Epidemiologic variables, definition of, 23, 28
Epidemiology, definition of, 15, 16, 31, 33
EPOs, *see* Exclusive Provider Organizations
Equity, issues of, 268
Esters, toxicity and, 218
Ethambutol (EMB), 108–109
Ethanol, toxicity and, 251
Ethers, toxicity and, 218
Ethical decision, definition of, 5, 12
Ethics, consequence-based, 287
definition of, 285, *285*
Exclusive Provider Organizations (EPOs), definition of, 311, 312
Exposure, definitions of, 235
evaluation of, 251–255
food, 251
land disposal and, 250
monitoring individuals for, 253
occupational recommendations and, 245
routes of, 245, 246–251
water, 249–250

F

Family history, alcoholism and, 203
breast cancer and, 123
diabetes and, 129
heart disease and, 120
lung cancer and, 123
peptic ulcer disease and, 131
prostate cancer and, 124
Family studies, alcohol addiction and, 208, 209
Fat metabolism, mental retardation and, 193
Febrile illness, immunization and, 116
Federal agencies, injury surveillance and, 171, 171(t)
Fee-for-service, definition of, 346
Fellowship, definition of, 298
Fetal alcohol syndrome, mental retardation and, 195
Fidelity, medical ethics and, 289
Fifth pathway, American foreign medical graduates and, 2, 8, 297
Fisher's exact test, 65–66, 66(t), 74, 76
Food additives, examples of, 258
Food and Drug Administration and, 258, 259
Generally Recognized as Safe (GRAS) and, 258–259
toxicity and, 251
Formaldehyde, offgassing of, 249, 259
toxicity and, 219
Foundry workers, occupational hazards and, 232, 234
Fraud, deliberate torts and, 271
Freestanding outpatient surgery centers, description of, 319–320, 320(t)
Frequency polygon, description of, 2, 8, 49–50, *51, 52*
Freud, S., addiction and, 203
Fungal diseases, occupations and, 226
Fungicides, toxicity and, 221

G

Gases, toxicity and, 222
Gastrointestinal cancer, asbestos and, 341, 348
Gates v. Jensen, court-imposed standard of care and, 270, 279
Gaucher's disease, mental retardation and, 194
Gaussian distribution, *see* Normal distribution
Genetic marker studies, alcoholism and, 203
Genotoxic tests, discussion of, 238–239
Glass, A.J., research in crisis intervention and, 184, 188–190
Glycols, toxicity and, 218
GMENAC, *see* Graduate Medical Education National Advisory Committee
Gonorrhea, 6, 13
control strategies for, 95, 115, 116–117
epidemiology of, 93–94
infectious disease process and, 94
rates for, 96
screening women for, 95
"Good samaritan," definition of, 6, 12
statutes, 275
Graduate medical education, osteopathic physicians and, 298–299
postgraduate year-I (PGY-I), PGY-II, and PGY-III, 297–298
Graduate Medical Education National Advisory Committee (GMENAC), physician manpower and, 295, 304, 306
Guerro v. Copper Queen Hospital, hospital licensure and, 276

H

Haddon Matrix, definition of, 174, 176
prevention of injuries and the, 172–173, 172(t)
Hahnemann, S., homeopathy and, 342, 349
Halogenated hydrocarbons, toxicity and, 219
Hand washing, disease prevention by, 80
HAV, *see* Hepatitis A virus
Hawkins v. McGee, breach of warranty and, 272, 279, 343, 350
Hazardous substances, alcohols as, 218
aldehydes as, 219
aliphatic hydrocarbons as, 217
aromatic hydrocarbons as, 217–218
arsenic as, 215
asbestos dust as, 219
beryllium as, 216
cadmium as, 216
carbon monoxide as, 223
coal dust as, 219
cotton dust as, 220
cyclic hydrocarbons as, 218
dusts as, 219–220
esters as, 218
ethers as, 218
fungicides as, 221
glycols as, 218
halogenated hydrocarbons as, 219
herbicides as, 221
hydrogen cyanide as, 223
hydrogen sulfide as, 223
insecticides as, 220–221
iron oxide dust as, 219
ketones as, 218–219
lead as, 216–217
mercury as, 217
metal as, 215–216
mold as, 220
nematocides as, 222
nickel as, 217
nitrohydrocarbons as, 218
rodenticides as, 221–222
silica as, 219–220
solvents as, 217–219
talc as, 220
tungsten carbide as, 219
zinc as, 217
Hazardous wastes, treatment of, 257–258
HBV, *see* Hepatitis B virus
HDV, *see* Hepatitis D virus
Health care, Department of Health and Human Services (DHHS) and, 307, *308*
employer contributions to, 327
expenditures for, 327, *327*, 335, 336
financing administration and, 324, 326
funding sources for, 327–328, *328*
government funding for, 327, 328
injuries and, 168
labor costs for, 296
methods of payment for, 329
private insurance for, 328
quality of, 320–321
services, annual cost of, 307
Health Care Financing Administration (HCFA), Medicaid and, 330
Health care workers, acquired immune deficiency syndrome and, 96–97
occupational hazards and, 232, 234
Health Insurance Organizations (HIOs), definition of, 332
Health Maintenance Organizations (HMOs), description of, 311, 325, 326
models of, 3, 9, 330–331, 332(t)
operations of, 313

prepaid health care and, 312, *313*
regulation of, 267
Health Professions Education Assistance Act, physician shortage and, 1, 8
Health services for children, 159–160
Heart diseases, epidemiology of, 119
prevention of, 120–121
risk factors for, 119–120, 135, 137
screening for, 136, 137
Heat, toxicity and, 224
Helling v. Carey, standard of care and, 270, 279, 283, 343, 350
Hemophilus influenzae, see Meningitis, *Hemophilus influenzae* type b
Hemophilus influenzae type b (Hib) polysaccharide vaccine, use of, 86
Henry's law constant (H), definition of, 247
Hepatic diseases, occupations and, 227
Hepatitis, infectious, natural history of, 25
non-A, non-B, epidemiology of, 106, 115, 117
reported cases of, 26
viral, reported cases of, *25, 27*
Hepatitis A virus (HAV), control strategies for, 4, 10, 101
epidemiology of, 100, 115, 117
infectious disease process, 100–101, 115, 116
isolation and, 79
Hepatitis B virus (HBV), control strategies for, 103–104, 115, 117
disinfectants and, 79
epidemiology of, 101–104, 103(t)
immunization and, 5, 11, 79
infectious disease process and, 102–103, 114, 116
prophylaxis for, 104–105, 105(t)
screening blood for, 114, 116
screening pregnant women for, 104(t)
Hepatitis D virus (HDV), epidemiology of, 115, 117
infectious disease process and, 106
Herbicides, toxicity and, 221
Herd immunity, 7, 13, 19
Heroin, abuse of, 202, 208, 209
methadone and, 208, 209
Herpes simplex virus (HSV), long-term effects of, 6, 13
Hib, *see* Meningitis, *Hemophilus influenzae* type b
Hill-Burton free care obligation, 276, 281, 282
HIOs, *see* Health Insurance Organizations
Histogram, description of, 8, 49, *50*
HIV, *see* Human immunodeficiency virus
HMOs, *see* Health Maintenance Organizations
Hodgkin's disease, immunization and, 86
Home health care services, 300, 317, 318
Homeopathy, 342, 349
Homicide, epidemiology of, 127–128, 338, 344
prevention of, 128
risk factors for, 128
Hospitals, accreditation of, 316
admissions to, 276
ancillary services of, 315, 315(t)
cost of care in, 316
free care and, 276, 282
licensure, statutes for, 276
operations of, 315
payments to, 339, 347
tax-exempt status of, 276
types of, 314–315, 315(t)
Host, characteristics of, 26–27, 30, 31, 33, 34
disease and, 17, 19, 81, 82
immunity to disease and, 18
injuries and, 166, 175, 177
substance abuse and, 204
Human exposure data, occupational recommendations and, 245
Human immunodeficiency virus (HIV), 97
disinfectants and, 79
Hydrocarbons, toxicity and, 217–218, 219
Hydrogen cyanide, toxicity and, 223
Hydrogen sulfide, toxicity and, 223
Hypersensitivity pneumonitis, occupations and, 226
Hypertension, cerebrovascular disease and, 121, 135, 137
coronary heart disease and, 135, 137
diabetics and, 137
mortality and, 120
pregnancy and, 147
renal disease and, 130, 135, 137
screening for, 120
Hypothesis, application of statistical test to, 28

I

ICD, *see* International Classification of Diseases
Illness, *see* Chronic illness
Immune serum globulin (IG), administration of, 4, 10, 83, 106
definition of, 82
hepatitis A virus and, 101, 116
hepatitis B virus and, 103–104, 105(t)
live vaccines and, 116
Immunity, types of, 82
Immunization, childhood, 340, 347
prevention of disease by, 79, 111, 156
schedules for, 157(t), 162, 163
vaccines available for, 84–87
Immunobiologic agents, 82–87
see also specific agents
Implants, contraception and, 143
Incidence, *see also specific diseases*
definition of, 1, 8, 21
examples of, 342, 349
injury morbidity and, 174, 176
Incidence study, description of, 38
Independent Practice Associations (IPAs), description of, 311, 325, 326, 331
Health Maintenance Organizations and, 313
Index, definition of, 21, 22
Infant, management of health problems in, 153–155, 162, 163
Infant mortality, causes of, 154
definition of, 139, 153
rates of, *154*, 161, 163
risk factors for, 155
Infectious disease, occupations and, 227
process of, 16, 18
sources of, 27
spectrum of, 7, 13, 19
Influenza, antigenic variation of, 90, 90(t)
control strategies for, 90–91
epidemiology of, 89
infectious disease process and, 90
Influenza A virus, immunity and, 341, 348
Informed consent, basic concepts of, 272–274
ethics and, 291–292, 293, 294
examples of, 280, 281, 282, 283
Injectables, contraception and, 143
Injuries, adolescence and, 158, 159
countermeasure strategies, 173(t)
epidemiology of, 165–167
individuals prone to, 340, 347
intentional and unintentional, 168–169
morbidity related to, 167, 169, 175, 177
mortality related to, 167–168, 169, 175, 176, 177
occupational, 211
places of occurrence of, 169
postneonatal mortality and, 155
prevention of, 158, 172–173, 172(t), 173(t)
screening strategies for, 338, 344, 345
surveillance of, 170–172, 171(t), 174, 176
years of potential life lost due to, 168
Insecticides, toxicity and, 220–221
Insurance coverage, mental illness and, 182, 187, 189
Intelligence quotient (IQ), definition of, 191–192, 199, 200
International Classification of Diseases (ICD), 183
N and E codes and, 169–170, 341, 348
Internship, *see* Postgraduate year-I
Intrauterine device (IUD), pros and cons of, 142–143, 150, 151
Intrauterine growth retardation, neonatal mortality and, 154
Intrauterine infections, prevention of infant health problems from, 155
Invasion of privacy, deliberate torts and, 271
Iodine deficiency, mental retardation and, 195
IPA, *see* Independent Practice Associations
Iron oxide, toxicity and, 219
Isoniazid (INH), 108–109

J

Jansky-Bielschowsky disease, mental retardation and, 193
onset of, 344
Joint Commission on Accreditation of Hospitals, 276
composition of, 316
national standards set by, 270, 276
June, acknowledgment of, xiii
Justice, definition of, 290

K

Karen Quinlan, substituted judgment and, 275, 279
Ketones, toxicity and, 218–219
Khantzian, drug addiction and, 7, 13
onset of, 344
Kufs' disease, mental retardation and, 193

L

Labor force, composition of, 211
distribution of, 211(t)
hospital care and, 316
women in, 3, 9
Lactation, contraception and, 142
Land, cleanup provisions for, 258
Comprehensive Environmental Response, Compensation, and Liability Act (CERCLA or Superfund) and, 257, 258
disposal issues and, 258
Resource Conservation and Recovery Act (RCRA) and, 257, 258
Latency periods, human carcinogens and, 237, 237(t)
Lead, mental retardation and, 195
toxicity and, 4, 10, 11, 216–217, 233, 234
Learning disorders, 156
Legal age, 273–274
Liability, definition of, 267
negligence, 269
Licensed practical nurses (LPNs), duties of, 304, 306
educational requirements for, 300
Licensure, definition of, 321
of dentists, 301
of licensed practical nurses, 300
of physicians, 298, 299, 304, 306
of registered nurses, 300

Lifecare centers, needs of the elderly and, 318, 318(t)
Life-support treatment, moral problems concerning, 291
terminally ill patients and, 274–275, 281, 282–283
Lindemann, E., research in crisis intervention and, 184, 188, 189
Living will, definition of, 275
Locality rule, definition of, 270
Log-normal distribution, 45
Long-term care, 307
costs of, 317
definition of, 316
facilities for, 317–318
nursing and, 317, 317(t)
Loss of chance theory, 269
Low-birth-weight, mental retardation and, 195
Low density lipoprotein (LDL), heart disease and, 119–120
Low-doses, cancer risks at, 243, 243(t)
Low octanol water partition coefficients (K_{ow}), example of, 266
Lung cancer, epidemiology of, 122, 122(t), 135, 137
occupations and, 226–227
risk factors for, 7, 13, 123
screening for, 125, 136, 137

M

Macroallocation, ethical questions and, 291
Malpractice, *see* Medical malpractice litigation
Mammalian cell transformations, definition of, 239
Manic-depressive illness, epidemiology of, 180, 187, 189
Mantoux skin test, 109
schedules for, 157
Maple syrup urine disease, mental retardation and, 193
Marijuana, abuse of, 202
Maternal mortality, 139, *140*, 141(t), *142*, 149, 151
McNemar test, 64, 64(t), 65(t), 74, 77
Mean, arithmetic, definition of, 45, 77
geometric, definition of, 46
normal distribution and, 1, 8
Measles, consequences of, 82
control strategies for, 88–89, 342, 350
immunity and, 341, 348
immunization schedules for, 85, 87(t)
infectious disease process and, 88
reported cases of, *89*
Measles, mumps, and rubella (MMR) vaccine, 85
history of, 88, *89*
schedules for, 157
Measures of central tendency, definition of, 5, 12
Measures of dispersion, 12, 73, 76
Median, definition of, 5, 11, 45, 77
Medicaid, benefit payments, 334
disadvantaged children and, 160
hospital admissions and, 276
overview, 333–334, 335, 336
Medical education, characteristics of, 297
costs of, 295, 304, 306
enrollment, 295, 296(t)
Medical ethics, definition of, *285*, 287–288
morality and, 293, 294
principles of, 289–290
Medical malpractice litigation, 267
burden of proof and, 337, 344
statute of limitations and, 341, 348
Medical practice, characteristics of, 308–314
Medicare, benefit limitations of, 333, 335, 336
description of, 4, 10
hospital admissions and, 287
overview of, 332–333
Mediums, examples of, 248–251
Meningitis, *Hemophilus influenzae* type b, 86
control strategies for, 111–112, 114, 116
epidemiology of, 11,
infectious disease process of, 111
immunization schedules for, 87(t)
prophylaxis for, 79, 340, 347
meningococcal, 31, 34
control strategies for, 112–113
epidemiology of, 112
Meningococcal polysaccharide vaccine, 112–113
Menninger, K.A., addiction and, 7, 13, 203
Mental disorder, definition of, 179, 188, 189
Mental health, definition of, 179
Mental health centers, *see* Community mental health centers
Mental illness, care for, 180, 181–182, 187, 189
case definitions in, 179–180
cost of, 181
educating the public about, 184
epidemiology of, 179–180
extent of, 180
hospitals for, 181–182
insurance coverage of, 182, 187, 189
patients in hospitals with, 3, 9
prevention of, 183–185, 338, 345
rehabilitation for, 187, 189
screening for, 184
Mental retardation, classification of, 198, 200
definition of, 191, 338, 344
epidemiology of, 191
etiology of, 192
future research and, 197, 198, 200
genetic diseases and, 3, 9
treatment of, 196–197, 198, 200
Mercury, mental retardation and, 195
toxicity and, 217, 233, 234
Mesothelioma, asbestos and, 341, 348
Metabolism, routes of exposure and, 248
Metaethics, definition of, 285, *285*
Metals, toxicity and, 215–217
Methadone maintenance, heroin addiction and, 206
Microallocation, ethical questions and, 291
Midlevel practitioners, definition of, 301–302
duties and salaries of, 310
Midwife, definition of, 5, 12
educational requirements for, 301–302, 305–306
MMR, *see* Measles, mumps, and rubella vaccine
Mode, definition of, 5, 11, 45, 77
Modeling, chemical concentrations and, 265, 266
chemicals in mediums and, 254–255
Models, air exposure and, 253
description of, 253–254
fish ingestion and, 254, 255(t)
Mold, toxicity and, 220
Monitoring, chemical concentrations and, 265, 266
Monosodium glutamate (MSG), food and, 258
toxicity and, 251
Moral codes, medical ethics and, 288
Morality, medical ethics and, 290–292
sources of, 286, 339, 346
Morbidity, *see also specific diseases*
children and, 156
definition of, 21
Mortality, *see also specific diseases*
adolescent, 156, 162, 163
age-adjusted, 24(t), 25(t)
childhood, 156
crude, 23(t)
infant, 153, 154
leading causes of, 1, 8, 174, 176
maternal, 139
motor vehicle related, 3, 5, 9, 11
preschoolers, 155
rates of, 21, *120*, *121*
schoolchildren, 155–156
Mumps, immunization against, 86
Musculoskeletal disease, occupations and, 227–228
Mutagenesis, threshold effects and, 236

N

Narcotic antagonists, addiction and, 206
Natality rates, 21
Natanson v. Kline, informed consent and, 272, 279
National Association for Mental Health, 181
National Health Planning and Development Act, 322
National Institute for Occupational Safety and Health (NIOSH), definition of, 212, 348
safe doses and, 245
National Safety Council, injuries and, 171
Natural family planning, 140
N codes, *see also* International Classification of Disease (ICD)
nature of injuries and, 341, 348
Negligence, tort law and, 269
Neisseria gonorrhoeae, 94, 116
Neisseria meningitidis, rifampin and, 79
Nematocides, toxicity and, 222
Neonatal mortality, *see also* Infant mortality
definition of, 139
major causes of, 154, 339, 345–346
rate of, 153, 154, *154*
Nickel, toxicity and, 217
Niemann-Pick disease, mental retardation and, 193–194
NIOSH, *see* National Institute for Occupational Safety and Health
Nitrohydrocarbons, toxicity and, 218
Noise, toxicity and, 223–224
Noncarcinogens, thresholds and, 243–246
Nonmaleficence, definition of, 290
Nonparametric tests, applications of, 68, 68(t)
definition of, 4, 10, 74, 77
types of, 67–68
Nonthreshold effects, definition of, 4, 10, 235–236
exposures and, 339, 347
Normal distribution, applications of, 57–58, *58*
definition of, 44
examples of, 73, 76
Normative ethics, definition of, 285, *285*, 286, *287*
Null hypothesis, definition of, 53–55, 54(t)
example of, 74, 77, 340, 347
Nurse midwife, *see* Midwife
Nurse practitioners, educational requirements for, 301
Nurses, *see* Registered nurses and Licensed practical nurses
Nursing, long-term care facilities and, 317, 317(t)
specialization in, 299
Nursing homes, *see* Long-term care facilities

O

Obesity, diabetes and, 129
heart disease and, 120
Obstetric attendants, 148
Occupational diseases, 211, 226–228
medical history for, 341, 347–348
screening for, 212

Occupational hazards, artists and, 214
bacterial diseases and, 225
cancer and, 229(t), 232, 234
chronic obstructive pulmonary disease and, 126
foundry workers and, 213, 232, 234
fungal diseases and, 226
health care workers and, 215, 232, 234
lung cancer and, 123
machinists and, 215
office workers and, 214
painters and, 213
pregnancy and, 147
prostate cancer and, 124
renal disease and, 130
rickettsial disease and, 225
screening the workplace for, 212–213
trauma disorders and, 224
viral diseases and, 225
welders and, 214
workplace and, 341, 347–348
Occupational injuries, rates of, 3, 9, 211
mortality and, 174, 176
Occupational medical services, 228, 230–231
Occupational Safety and Health Act, 260
Occupational Safety and Health Administration (OSHA), definition of, 212
workplace and, 341, 348
Octanol water partition coefficient, chemicals and, 247
definition of, 346
O'Neill v. Montefiore Hospital, abandonment, 276, 279
One-tailed tests, 54
Opioids, abuse of, 202
Optometrists, 303
Oral attenuated poliovirus vaccine (OPV), immunization and, 85
immunization schedules for, 87(t), 157(t)
Oral contraceptives, cerebrovascular disease and, 121
cervical cancer and, 124
diseases and, 4, 10
heart disease and, 120
Organic brain syndrome, prevention of, 183
Origin hypothesis, schizophrenia and, 180
OSHA, *see* Occupational Safety and Health Administration
Osteopathic medicine, 297(t), 298
founding of, 342, 349
physicians, primary care and, 305, 306

P

Pain and suffering, compensation for, 269
Parens patriae, 276, 281, 282–283
Patient's rights, 274–275
PCBs, *see* Polychlorinated biphenyls
PDR, *see Physician's Desk Reference*
Peer Review Organizations (PROs), federal performance requirements for, *322*
organization of, 321
Pelvic inflammatory disease (PID), ectopic pregnancies and, 6, 13, 92
gonorrhea and, 95
human casualties of, 92
Peptic ulcer disease, epidemiology of, 130–131
risk factors for, 131, 135, 137
screening for, 131, 342, 349
Per admission, definition of, 346
Per diem, definition of, 346
Perinatal mortality, definition of, 139, 149, 151
Periodicity, definition of, 25
Personal health care, definition of, 307
Personality disorders, prevention of, 184
Pesticides, definition of, 220, 232, 234
Pertussis, immunization and, 85
Pharmacists, 303
Phenylketonuria (PKU), characteristics of, 198, 200
mental retardation and, 192–193
Philosophical ethics, definition of, 285, *285*
PHS, *see* Public Health Service
Physician's assistants (PAs), qualifications and training for, 302
Physician's Desk Reference (PDR), 83
Physicians, annual net income of, 310–311, 311(t)
geographic distribution of, 295, 297(t)
numbers of, 1, 8, 304, 305, 306, 310
office visits by children to, 161, 163
regional differences in income of, 311(t)
salaried versus self-employed, 310
specialty differences in income of, 311(t)
PID, *see* Pelvic inflammatory disease
PIE chart, description of, 48, 73, 76
PKU, *see* Phenylketonuria
Podiatrists, 303
Point mutations, chemicals and, 138
Poisson distribution, 45
Police power, protection of the public and, 1, 8
public health and, 276, 277, 280, 282
Poliomyelitis, immunization for, 31, 34, 85, 341, 348
paralysis and, 83
Pollutants, *see also* priority pollutants
conventional water, 257, 257(t)
criteria, 255, 256
hazardous air, 256, 256(t)
limits for discharge of, 256–257
Polychlorinated biphenyls (PCBs), epidemiologic study of, 265, 266
regulation of, 260
Portals of entry, *see also infectious disease process of specific diseases*
disease and, 17, 31, 34, 81
Portals of exit, *see also infectious disease process of specific diseases*
diseases and, 17, 80
Postgraduate year-I (PGY-I), 6, 12, 297–298
Postneonatal mortality, 153, 154, 155, 161, 163
Postpartum medicine, 148
Potency, cancer-causing, 242
Power of attorney, 273
Pneumoconioses, occupations and, 226
Pneumococcal pneumonia, penicillins and, 83
Pneumococcal polysaccharide vaccine, 86–87
Practice, solo and group, description of, 309–310, 324, 326
Precedent, definition of, 267
Predictive values, screening tests and, 70–71, 75, 77, 338, 345
Preferred Provider Arrangements (PPAs), definition of, 331–332, 332(t)
Preferred Provider Organizations (PPOs), description of, 311, 325, 326
Pregnancy, adolescent, 3, 9, 159
alcohol and, 340, 347
bacteriuria screening for, 130
care during, 145–147
high-risk, 155
prenatal care and, 5, 12
prevention of, 140, 142–145
rubella and, 86, 340, 347
sexually transmitted diseases and, 92
tests for Down's sydrome in, 345
tetracycline and, 340, 347
vaccination and, 84
Prematurity, neonatal mortality and, 154
Preschoolers, health of, 155–158
Prevalence, *see also specific diseases* 8, 21, 31, 33, 75, 77
Prevalence study, description of, 38
Primary care physician, gatekeeper role of, 309, 325, 326
keystone role of, 309, 325, 326
role of, 308–309, 324, 326
Primary care specialties, definition of, 309
Priority pollutants 252–253, 252(t)
PROs, *see* Peer Review Organizations
Probability, definition of, 52
Professional Standards Review Organizations (PSROs), 321
Proof, burden of, 268
Proportion, definition of, 20
Prostate cancer, epidemiology of, 122(t), 123
risk factors for, 124
screening for, 125
Protective apparel, disease prevention by, 80
Proximate cause, negligence and, 280, 282
tort law and, 269
PSROs, *see* Professional Standards Review Organizations
Psychosocial problems, high-risk groups for, 158
Psychotropic drugs, mental illness and, 182
Public health, definition of, 307
government power and, 276–278
nursing care and, 300
Public Health Service (PHS), description of, 307, *309*, 324, 326
measles and, 88–89, *89*
vital areas of, 340, 347
Punitive damages, definition of, 5, 11, 269
Pyelonephritis, definition of, 130

Q

Quarantine, public health and, 277
Querido, A., research in crisis intervention and, 184, 188, 190
Quid pro quo, 271

R

Rabies, control strategies for, 342, 350
Radiation, controls of, 260
ionizing, sources of, 260
toxicity and, 224–225
Radioactivity, food and, 258
Radon, insulated homes and, 249
Range, definition of, 5, 11, 46, 73, 76, 77
Rates, adjusted, 30, 33
calculation of, 22–23
definition of, 21
types of, 22–23
Ratio, definition of, 20
r × c chi-square test, 62
Registered nurses (RNs), availability of, 9, 305, 306
educational requirements for, 299, 299(t), 305–306
training for, 304, 305, 306
Rehabilitation, hospitals for, 316, 317–318
mental disorders and, 187, 189
objectives of, 184–185
substance abuse and, 205–206
Reliability, clinical studies and, 36
Renal disease, epidemiology of, 129–130
risk factors for, 130
screening for, 130
Renal failure, immunization and, 86
Reproductive disorders, occupations and, 228
Research, moral limits on, 291–292
Reservoirs, *see also specific diseases*
control of, 79–80
definition of, 17, 31, 34
Res ipsa loquitur, negligence and, 270, 280, 281, 282, 283, 347
Respiratory tract infection, postneonatal mortality and, 154
Reversibility of effects, definition of, 236
Rh testing, pregnancy and, 146

Rickettsial diseases, occupations and, 225
Rifampin (RMP), 108–109
 exposure to *Hemophilus influenzae* type b (Hib) meningitis and, 340, 347
Right of bodily inviolability, deliberate torts and, 271
Right of privacy, 274
Risk corridor, definition of, 346
Risks, environmental, 261–264
 assessment of, 235
 chemical exposure and, 263(t)
 management of, 262, 263
 voluntary and involuntary, 261, 261(t)
Rochin v. California, due process and, 277, 279
Rodenticides, toxicity and, 221–222
Root premise, informed consent and, 272
Rubella, *see also* Measles
 congenital birth defects and, 83, 155
 immunization against, 86
 mental retardation and, 195
Rule deontology, definition of, 287, *287*
 ethics and, 293, 294
Rule utilitarianism, definition of, 287, *287*
 ethics and 293, 294

S

Saccharin, Food Additive Amendment and, 259
Safe dose, toluene as an example of, 246, 246(t)
Salgo v. Stanford University Hospital, informed consent and, 272, 279
Salmonella, isolation and, 79
Sampling errors, the null hypothesis and, 54–55, 54(t)
Schizophrenia, epidemiology of, 5, 11, 180
 progress with, 184–185
 screening for, 183
Schloendorff v. Society of New York Hospital, informed consent and, 272, 279
Schmerber v. California, judicial warrants and, 277, 279
Schneidman, E.B., research in crisis intervention and, 184, 188, 189
Schoolchildren, health of, 155–158
 mortality in, 161, 163
Screening, blood, for infectious diseases, 114, 116
 conditions for, 69
 cost-effectiveness of, 156, 161, 163, 342, 349
 criteria for, 156, 158, 161, 163
 definition of, 68–69
 for hypertension, 120
 for mental illness, 184
 parameters of tests for, 69–71, 69(t), 70(t), 75, 76, 338, 344
 prenatal, 145–147
 for tuberculosis, 108
Senility, prevention of, 183–184
Sensitive population, occupational exposure to chemicals and, 245
Sensitivity, clinical study and, 37
 screening tests and, 5, 11, 70, 75, 77
Sex problems in adolescents, management of, 159
Sexual assault, deliberate torts and, 271
Sexually transmitted diseases (STDs), 31, 34
 see also specific diseases
 in adolescents, 159
 cancer and, 92
 discussion of, 91–100
 high-risk groups for, 91
 incidence of, 91
 primary prevention of, 99–100
 tests for, 91
Shigella, control strategies for, 342, 350
 isolation and, 79
Shilkret v. Annapolis Emergency Hospital, standards of care and, 270, 279
Sickle-cell anemia, definition of, 132
SIDS, *see* Sudden infant death syndrome
Silica, toxicity and, 219–220
Skewd distribution, 44
Smoking, cerebrovascular disease and, 121
 cervical cancer and, 124
 chronic obstructive pulmonary disease and, 126
 heart disease and, 120
 peptic ulcer disease and, 131
Social Security Act, 160
Sodium benzoate, food and, 258
Solubility, definition of, 247
Solvents, hobbies and, 249
 toxicity and, 217–219
Sonography, pregnancy and, 146
Specificity, clinical study and, 37
 screening tests and, 70, 75, 77
Spermicides, contraception and, 142
Spielmeyer-Stock-Vogt-Koyanagi disease, mental retardation and, 193, 337, 344
Spina bifida, mental retardation and, 195
Splenic dysfunction, immunization and, 86
Spot map, description of, 50, *53*
Standard of causation, subjective, 281, 283
Standard deviation, definition of, 47, 73, 76, 341, 348
 normal distribution curve and, 1, 8
Standard error, definition of, 61, 74, 76
Standard error of the mean, definition of, 341, 348
Standards of care, 269–270, 273, 281, 283
 court-imposed, 270
 Helling v. Carey and, 343, 350
 local and national, 270
 malpractice suits and, 340, 347
 professional, 272
Stare decisis, 267, 280, 282
Statistical analysis, clinical studies and, 36
Statistical significance, 53
Statistics, analytic, 52–68
 definition of, 43
 history of, 43
 uses of, 43
Statute of limitation, contract law and, 272
 definition of, 268
 medical malpractice and, 341, 348
STDs, *see* Sexually transmitted diseases
Sterilization, contraception and, 144–145
Still, A.T., osteopathy and, 342, 349
Stillbirth, definition of, 139
Streptococcus pneumoniae, immunization against, 86, 113
Student's t tests, description of, 58–61 60(t), 73, 76
Substance abuse, in adolescents, management of, 159
 definition of, 201, 338, 345
 epidemiology of, 201–202
 pregnancy and, 147
 prevention of, 204–205
 treatment for, 205–206, 208, 209
Substituted judgment, *Claire Conroy* and, 275, 281, 283, 343, 350
 Karen Quinlan and, 275
Sudden infant death syndrome (SIDS), postneonatal mortality and, 155
Suicide, epidemiology of, 127
 prevention of, 127
 risk factors for, 127
Sulfite, toxicity and, 251
Sullivan v. O'Connor, breach of warranty and, 272, 279
Surgery centers, procedures of, 320, 320(t)
Synanon, addiction and, 205, 208, 209
Syphilis, control strategies for, 93
 epidemiology of, 92
 infectious disease process of, 92–93
 long-term effects of, 6, 13
 mental retardation and, 195
 screening blood for, 81, 114, 116

T

t distribution, definition of, 58, 59(t)
Talc, toxicity and, 220
Tarasoff v. Regents of University of California, confidential patient information and, 343, 350
Target organ dose, chemical concentration and, 248
Tax Equity and Fiscal Responsibility Act, 321
Tay-Sachs disease, characteristics of, 198, 200, 337, 344
 mental retardation and, 193
Td, *see* Tetanus and diphtheria toxoids
Technology, moral problems concerning, 291
Ten Countermeasure Strategies, 174, 176
Teratogenesis, threshold effects and, 236
Terminal illness, patient's rights and, 274–275
Testimony, expert, 269, 270
Tetanus and diphtheria toxoids (Td), immunization schedules for, 84, 87(t), 157(t)
Thalassemia, definition of, 132
Theological ethics, definition of, 285, *285*
Therapeutic privilege, 273, 281, 283
Threshold effects, 235–236
 definition of, 4, 10, 339, 346, 347
Thresholds, determination of, 243
Third-party payers, 328
Tolerance, definition of, 201
Torts, definition of, 269
 deliberate, 270
Toxic effects of chemicals, environment and, 235–239
Toxic end points, carcinogenesis and, 264
 description of, 236
 teratogenesis and, 264
Toxic Substances Control Act (TSCA), industrial chemicals and, 259–260
Toxicity, definition of, 235
 special tests for, 215, 217, 218, 219, 220, 221, 222, 223, 224, 225
Toxoid, definition of, 82
Transmission of disease, direct, 80–81
 indirect, 81
 modes of, 17–18, 30, 31, 33, 34
Trauma disorders, occupational health problems and, 224, 227–228
Treatment, individual rights to, 291
 outcome assessment of, 35
Treponema pallidum, 92
Trials, jury versus nonjury, 268
Trichloroethylene (TCE), epidemiologic study and, 265, 266
Tris, Flammable Fabrics Act and, 259
Trisomy 21, *see* Down's syndrome
Truman v. Thomas, informed consent, 274, 279
Truthfulness, medical ethics and, 290
Tubercle bacilli, 106, 114, 116
Tuberculin test, schedules for, 157(t)
Tuberculosis, 31, 34
 chemotherapy and chemoprophylaxis for, 108–109, 110
 control strategies for, 107–110, 342, 350
 epidemiology of, 106–107, 114, 116
 infectious disease process of, 107
 screening for, 108
Tularemia, 26
Tungsten carbide, toxicity and, 219
Twin studies, alcoholism and, 203
Two-tailed tests, 54
Tyhurst, J.S., research in crisis intervention and, 184
Type I error, *see also* alpha error
 definition of, 54
Type II error, definition of, 55

U

Uncertainty factors, description of, 244–245

Uncompensated care, *see* Hospitals, free care and
Urgent care centers, description of, 3, 9

V

Vaccine, definition of, 82
reaction to, 83–84
recommendations for use of, 83, 114, 116
schedules for, 87(t), 157(t)
Validity, clinical studies, 36, 41, 42
Values, moral and nonmoral, 286
Vapor pressure (P_V), definition of, 247
Variance, definition of, 46, 47(t)
Vasectomy, 144
Vectors, injuries and, 167, 174, 175, 176, 177
transmission of disease and, 18
Vehicles, transmission of disease and, 18
Venn diagram, description of, 48, *48*, 73, 76
Veterans Administration, services of, 313–314
Viral diseases, occupations and, 225
Virtues, definition of, 286
Viscosity, definition of, 346
Visiting Nurse Association (VNA), 317
Vital statistics, definition of, 43
Volatile organic chemicals (VOCs), location of, in mediums, 265, 266
water and, 249

W

Warranty, *see* Breach of warranty
Wastes, hazardous, *see* Hazardous wastes
Water, Clean Water Act (CWA) and, 257
Safe Drinking Water Act (SDWA) and, 257
Weight of evidence classification system, carcinogens and, 239, 239(t)
Wilcoxon tests, definition of, 67, 68(t)
Wilmington General Hospital v. Manlove, emergency care and, 276, 279
Withdrawal, definition of, 201
World Health Organization (WHO), disease control and, 90–91

Y

Yates correction factor, chi-square tests and, 62
Years of potential life lost, causes of, 168, 174, 176

Z

Z score, *see* Critical ratio
Zinc, toxicity and, 217